RESOURCE GROUPS

Crohn's and Colitis Foundation of America (CCFA)
444 Park Avenue South
New York, New York 10016-7374
212-685-3440
800-343-3637

United Ostomy Association (UOA)
36 Executive Park, Suite 120
Irvine, CA 92714-6744
714-660-8624
800-826-0826

Wound Ostomy and Continence Nurses Society
2755 Bristol St. Ste. #110
Costa Mesa, CA 92626
712-476-0268

American Cancer Society (ACS)
1599 Clifton Road NE
Atlanta, GA 30329
404-320-3333

Help for Incontinent People (HIP)
P.O. Box 544
Union, SC 29379
803-579-7900

Alcoholics Anonymous World Services
P.O. Box 459
Grand Central Station
New York, New York 10163
212-870-3400

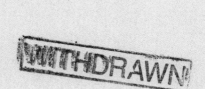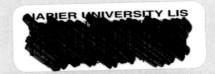

GASTROINTESTINAL DISORDERS

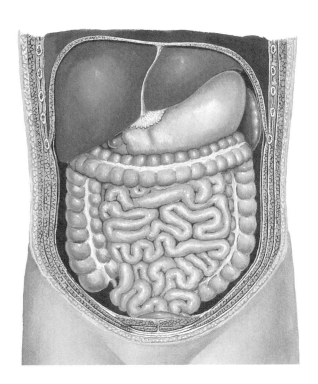

Mosby's Clinical Nursing Series

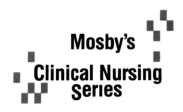

**Mosby's
Clinical Nursing
Series**

Cardiovascular Disorders
by Mary Canobbio

Respiratory Disorders
by Susan Wilson and June Thompson

Infectious Diseases
by Deanna Grimes

Orthopedic Disorders
by Leona Mourad

Renal Disorders
by Dorothy Brundage

Neurologic Disorders
by Esther Chipps, Norma Clanin, and
Victor Campbell

Cancer Nursing
by Anne Belcher

Genitourinary Disorders
by Mikel Gray

Immunologic Disorders
by Christine Mudge-Grout

Gastrointestinal Disorders
by Dorothy Doughty and Debra Broadwell Jackson

Blood Disorders
by Anne Belcher

Ear, Nose, and Throat Disorders
by Barbara Sigler and Linda Schuring

AIDS and HIV Infection
by Deanna Grimes and Richard Grimes

Skin Disorders
by Marcia Hill

Female Disorders
by Valerie Edge and Mirdi Miller

GASTROINTESTINAL DISORDERS

DOROTHY B. DOUGHTY, M.N., R.N., C.E.T.N.

Program Director
ET Nursing Education Program
Emory University
Atlanta, Georgia

DEBRA BROADWELL JACKSON, Ph.D., R.N.

Associate Professor and Department Head
Department of Health Science
College of Nursing
Clemson University
Clemson, South Carolina

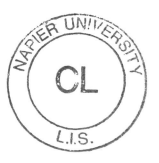

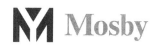 Mosby

St. Louis Baltimore Boston Chicago London Philadelphia Sydney Toronto

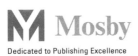

M Mosby

Dedicated to Publishing Excellence

Publisher: Alison Miller
Editor: Sally Schrefer
Developmental Editor: Penny Rudolph
Project Manager: Mark Spann
Production Editors: Julie Zipfel, Christine O'Neil
Designer: Liz Fett
Layout: Doris Hallas

Acknowledgments

The author gratefully acknowledges the following people; without their help this book would not have been possible: My parents, Warren and Vicky Beckley, for teaching me to set my goals high and then work hard to achieve them; my husband, Mac, and my sons, Matt and Michael, for months of unfailing computer assistance, moral support, and understanding of my non-availability; my editors, Sally Schrefer, for her expert guidance and much-needed perspective, and Penny Rudolph, for her constant encouragement and never-failing sense of humor that made "just one more thing" both possible and even (sometimes) enjoyable; and the staff of Emory University Hospital and the Emory Clinic (and especially Dr. William McGarity) for their support and assistance with illustrations.

Printed in the United States of America

Mosby–Year Book, Inc.
11830 Westline Industrial Drive
St. Louis, Missouri 63146

Library of Congress Cataloging in Publication Data

Doughty, Dorothy Beckley.
 Gastrointestinal disorders / Dorothy B. Doughty, Debra Broadwell
Jackson ; original illustrations by George J. Wassilchenko and
Donald P. O'Connor ; original photography by Patrick Watson.
  p. cm.
 Includes bibliographical references and index.
 ISBN 0-8016-2096-1
  1. Gastrointestinal system—Diseases—Nursing. I. Jackson, Debra
Broadwell, 1949- . II. Title.
  [DNLM: 1. Gastrointestinal Diseases—nursing. 2. Nursing Care-
-nursing. WY 156.5 D732g]
RC802.D7 1993
616.3′3′0024613—dc20
DNLM/DLC
for Library of Congress   92-49975
                                                           CIP

93 94 95 96 97 CL/VH 9 8 7 6 5 4 3 2 1

Consultants

REBECCA WILLS BUTLER, R.N., M.N.
Liver Transplant Nurse
Emory University Hospital
Atlanta, GA

THERESE WRIGHT, R.N., B.S.N.
Nutritional Support Nurse
Emory University Hospital
Atlanta, GA

Original illustrations by
GEORGE J. WASSILCHENKO
Tulsa, Oklahoma
and

DONALD P. O'CONNOR
St. Peters, Missouri

Original photography by
PATRICK WATSON
Poughkeepsie, New York

Preface

Gastrointestinal Disorders is the tenth volume in *Mosby's Clinical Nursing Series*, a new kind of resource for practicing nurses.

The *Series* is the result of the most elaborate market research ever undertaken by Mosby–Year Book, Inc. We first surveyed hundreds of working nurses to determine what kinds of resources practicing nurses require to meet their advanced information needs. We then approached hundreds of clinical specialists—proven authors and experts—and asked them to develop a consistent format that would meet the needs of nurses in practice. This format was presented to nine focus groups composed of working nurses and refined between each group. In the later stages we published a 32-page full-color sample so that detailed changes could be made to improve physical layout and appearance, page by page.

Gastrointestinal Disorders is a comprehensive nursing resource for the nurse caring for patients with gastrointestinal disorders. Chapter 1 is a focused review of relevant anatomy and physiology. Multiple illustrations serve to clarify anatomic relationships, and physiologic functions are discussed in terms of clinical applications. Chapter 2 provides guidelines for nursing assessment of patients with gastrointestinal disorders; a detailed interview guide is boxed for easy reference, and a pictorial guide depicts step-by-step physical assessment. In Chapter 3, current diagnostic procedures are presented according to a structured format that focuses on nursing concerns; each procedure is briefly described and is discussed in terms of indications, contraindications, preprocedural and postprocedural nursing care, and guidelines for patient teaching.

Chapters 4 through 7 focus on the nursing care of patients with commonly occurring pathologic states: inflammatory disorders, obstructive disorders, interferences with nutrient intake and absorption, and interferences with fecal elimination. A consistent format makes these chapters "user-friendly". Each disorder is discussed in terms of epidemiology and pathophysiology; boxed material outlines and highlights potential complications, diagnostic studies and results, and medical-surgical management. Nursing management is the focus of this book, and these pages have a color border to enhance quick access. Each nursing care plan is presented in the nursing process sequence, utilizing nursing diagnoses that are accepted by the North American Nursing Diagnosis Association (NANDA). This material can be used to develop individual care plans quickly and accurately. Each nursing care plan is further enhanced by an additional section that outlines key content to be included in patient teaching.

Chapter 8 focuses on the management of patients requiring gastrointestinal intubation or nutritional support, and Chapter 9 presents common surgical procedures. All therapies are discussed according to a structured format that emphasizes nursing management; the therapy or procedure is described, and boxed material outlines indications, contraindications, and potential complications. Nursing management is then detailed, using nursing diagnoses and the nursing process sequence.

In response to requests from scores of nurses participating in our research, a distinctive feature of this book is its usefulness for patient teaching. Background material increases the nurse's ability to answer common patient questions with authority. The illustrations in the book, particularly those in the anatomy and physiology, assessment, and diagnostic procedures chapters, are specifically designed to support patient teaching. The book concludes with chapter 10, which is a compilation of patient teaching guides that supplement the patient teaching sections of each care plan. The patient teaching guides are ideal for reproduction and distribution to patients.

This book is intended for medical-surgical nurses who are frequently involved in the care of individuals with gastrointestinal disorders. The book will provide valuable information for nurses in acute care settings, gastrointestinal diagnostic units, surgical units, outpatient settings, extended care settings, and home health settings. The book also serves as a comprehensive resource for students and nurses returning to practice.

We hope this book contributes to the advancement of professional nursing by providing a comprehensive resource that supports a scientific and holistic approach to professional nursing practice.

Contents

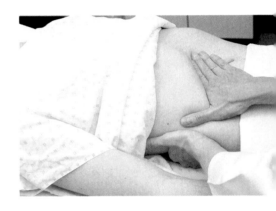

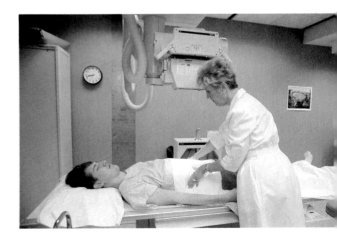

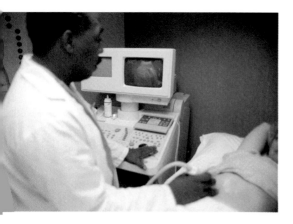

4 Inflammatory Disorders of the Gastrointestinal System, 71

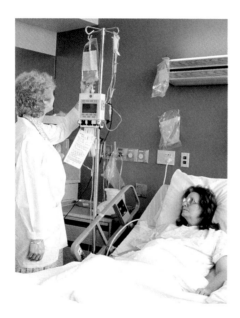

5 Obstructive Disorders of the Gastrointestinal System, 173

6 Disorders of Nutrient Intake and Absorption, 228

7 Interference with Fecal Elimination, 254

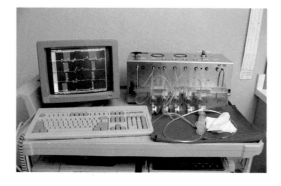

8 Gastrointestinal Intubation and Nutritional Support, 284

9 Surgical Procedures, 303

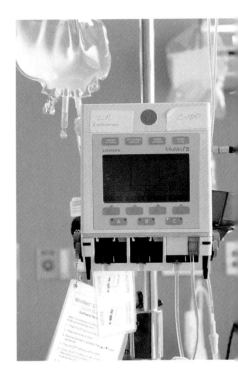

10 Patient Teaching Guides, 344

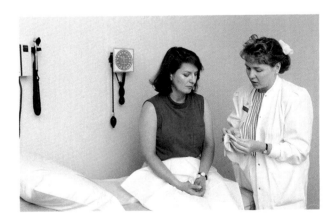

Color Plates

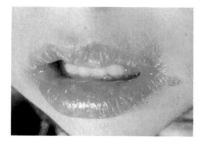

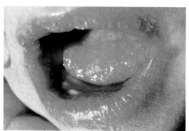

PLATE 1
Primary gingivostomatitis showing lesions on the lips, tongue, and gums.

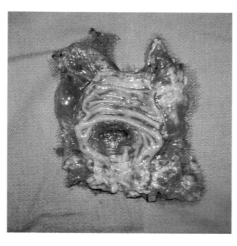

PLATE 2
Adenocarcinoma of distal rectum.

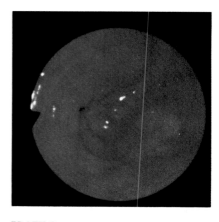

PLATE 3
Erosive gastritis (as seen through endoscope).

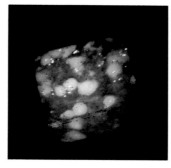

PLATE 4
Pseudomembranous colitis (as seen through endoscope).

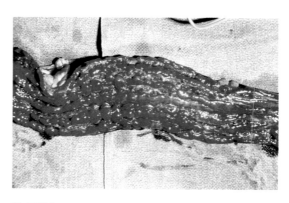

PLATE 5
Crohn's disease showing deep ulcers and fissures creating "cobblestone" effect.

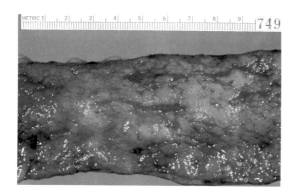

PLATE 6
Ulcerative colitis showing severe mucosal edema and inflammation with ulcerations and bleeding.

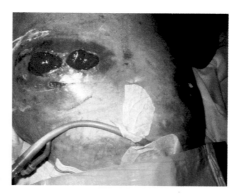

PLATE 7
Caput medusae around abdominal stoma in patient with portal hypertension.

CHAPTER 1

Color Atlas of Gastrointestinal Structure and Function

The gastrointestinal (GI) tract is critical to life and health, because it regulates the ingestion, digestion, and absorption of nutrients. It also is responsible for storing and eliminating waste products. Normal function of the gastrointestinal tract depends on a number of interrelated physiologic processes such as hormone production, enzyme secretion, carrier-mediated absorption, peristalsis, and voluntary control of defecation.

The organs within the GI tract are commonly divided into the alimentary canal and the accessory organs. The alimentary canal is the long tube that extends from the mouth to the anus; it includes the mouth, esophagus, stomach, small intestine, colon, rectum, anal canal, and anus (Figure 1-1). Accessory organs are structures outside the alimentary canal that contribute to the processes of nutrient digestion and absorption; the liver, pancreas, and gallbladder are important accessory organs (Figure 1-1).

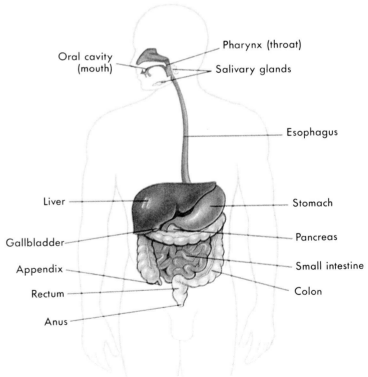

FIGURE 1-1
Digestive system depicted in place in the body. (From Seeley.[53])

A LIMENTARY CANAL

MOUTH

The mouth, also referred to as the buccal cavity or oral cavity, is the beginning of the alimentary canal. Structures in the oral cavity assist with speech, nutrient ingestion, initiation of mechanical and chemical digestion, and swallowing. Important structures in the mouth are the teeth, the tongue, the hard and soft palates, and the salivary glands (Figure 1-2).

Teeth begin mechanical digestion through the process of chewing; they tear and cut food into smaller pieces. Chewing increases the surface area of food particles, and since digestive enzymes work only on exposed surfaces, this promotes chemical breakdown. Mechanically breaking down food into smaller pieces also makes swallowing easier. Thus chewing contributes significantly to the digestive process.

The **teeth** also contribute to the ability to clearly articulate words.

The **tongue** is a muscular organ covered with moist, squamous epithelium. It contains both mucous and serous glands.

The anterior surface of the tongue is covered with papillae, where the taste buds are located. Adults have approximately 10,000 taste buds; however, with age the taste buds begin to degenerate, and the sensation of taste becomes less acute. This can contribute to reduced appetite and nutrient intake in older adults.

In addition to taste, the tongue contributes significantly to speech, chewing, and swallowing.

The **palates** form the "roof" of the mouth, with the "hard" (or bony) palate located anteriorly and the "soft" (or muscular) palate located posteriorly (see Figure 1-2). The soft palate is attached to the posterior portion of the hard palate; it forms the partition between the mouth and the nasopharynx. During swallowing, the soft palate moves upward to close off the nasopharynx and prevent food and fluids from entering.

There are many **glands** in the mouth that contribute to the production of saliva; the three largest pairs are the parotid, the submandibular and the sublingual glands (see Figure 1-2). The parotid glands produce ptyalin (salivary amylase), which begins the chemical breakdown of starches. The submandibular glands produce a mixture of mucus and serous secretions. The sublingual glands produce a lubricating fluid composed primarily of mucus. Daily production of saliva ranges from 1,000 to 1,500 ml, with a pH of 6 to 7. The amount of saliva produced is determined by salivatory nuclei in the brainstem. These nuclei are stimulated by taste and tactile stimuli, with pleasant taste and

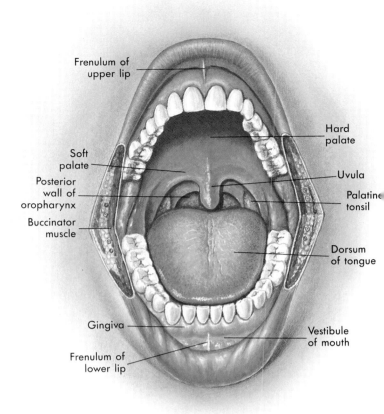

FIGURE 1-2
Anatomic structures of the oral cavity. (From Seidel.[52])

smooth texture providing a greater stimulus than unpleasant tastes and rough-textured foods. Salivation after ingestion of irritants helps dilute or neutralize the irritant.

Saliva also helps prevent infections of the oral cavity, because it constantly "bathes" the mouth, and it has some degree of antibacterial activity.

Initiation of Digestion

Mechanical digestion of nutrients begins in the mouth with the process of chewing, or mastication. Chewing breaks large food particles into smaller bits and increases the surface available for enzymatic action.

Enzymatic digestion of carbohydrates is also initiated in the mouth by the action of salivary amylase (ptyalin), which reduces polysaccharides to maltose and isomaltose. Only a small percentage (5% to 10%) of ingested starches are digested in the mouth, because most starches are covered with cellulose and thus are protected from enzymatic action. The activity of ptyalin continues in the stomach until the gastric pH drops low enough to inactivate the enzyme.

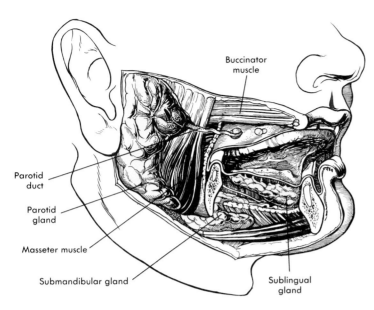

FIGURE 1-3
Salivary glands. The large salivary glands are the parotid glands, the submandibular glands, and the sublingual glands. The minor salivary glands include the buccal and labial glands. The parotid duct extends anteriorly from the parotid gland. (From Seeley.[53])

Swallowing

A very important function of the mouth and related structures is swallowing, which begins transport of the nutrients along the digestive pathway. Any condition that interferes with the ability to swallow places an individual at risk for nutritional compromise as a result of inadequate intake.

Swallowing is a complex act involving the tongue, the soft palate, the muscles of the oropharynx, the upper esophageal sphincter, the epiglottis, the muscles of the esophagus, and gravity (Figure 1-3).

Swallowing is mediated by the swallowing center, which is located in the pons and medulla. Swallowing is begun as a voluntary act and completed by reflex activity. Swallowing is facilitated by the presence of saliva, which acts as a lubricant for food particles.

GENERAL HISTOLOGY OF ALIMENTARY CANAL STRUCTURES

The histology of the alimentary canal is essentially the same from the esophagus to the anal canal, with minor variations; it consists of four tissue layers: the mucosa, the submucosa, the muscularis, and the serosa, or adventitia (Figure 1-4).

Mucosa

The mucosa is the innermost layer of the gut wall, and it has three distinct layers: the mucous epithelium, or surface layer; the lamina propria, a connective tissue layer; and the muscularis mucosa, a thin layer of circular muscle that separates the mucosa from the submucosa. Because the mucosal layer has many mucus-secreting glands, it is always moist.

Submucosa

The submucosa is the second layer of the gut wall; major structures within this layer include connective tissue, blood and lymph vessels, nerve fibers, and reticuloendothelial cells. The nerve fibers in the submucosal layer are known as Meissner's plexus; this plexus is a component of the enteric nervous system.

Muscularis

The muscularis is the third layer of the gut wall; it actually consists of two layers of smooth muscle, an inner layer of circular muscle and an outer layer of longitudinal muscle. The myenteric plexus, also known as Auerbach's plexus, is located between these two muscle layers. Auerbach's plexus and Meissner's plexus jointly form the intramural plexus, also known as the enteric nervous system. The nerve fibers of the intramural plexus originate in receptors located on the mucosal surface and in the bowel wall. These receptors respond to stretch and may respond to chemical stimuli. The intramural plexus is important, because it is the primary mediator for intestinal secretion and motility.

Serosa

The outermost layer of alimentary canal structures is known either as the serosa or as the adventitia. For structures within the peritoneal cavity, the outer layer is the serosa; it is a connective tissue layer that in turn is covered by the visceral peritoneum. This continuity with the visceral peritoneum helps explain the severe abdominal pain frequently felt by patients with transmural inflammatory bowel disease (Crohn's disease); inflammation involving the serosa may spread to the peritoneum, causing a generalized peritonitis.

Because the serosa has no mucus-secreting glands, exposure to air results in inflammation with edema and eventual necrosis and sloughing of the serosal layer. This is why nurses are taught to cover exposed loops of bowel with sterile, saline-soaked towels in the event of evisceration.

Structures outside the peritoneal cavity, such as the esophagus, are covered with a connective tissue layer known as adventitia.

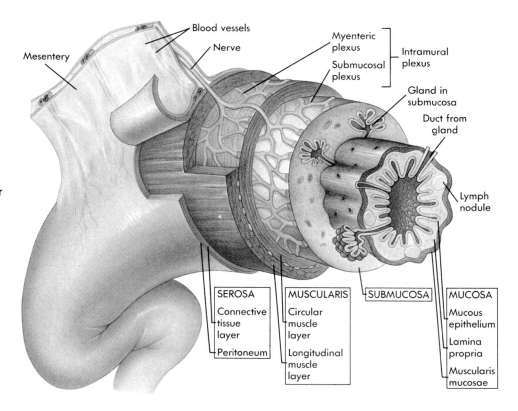

FIGURE 1-4
Digestive tract histology. The four layers are the mucosa, submucosa, muscularis, and serosa or adventitia. (From Seeley.[53])

SEROSA
Connective tissue layer
Peritoneum

MUSCULARIS
Circular muscle layer
Longitudinal muscle layer

SUBMUCOSA

MUCOSA
Mucous epithelium
Lamina propria
Muscularis mucosae

ESOPHAGUS

The esophagus is the muscular tube that connects the oropharynx to the stomach; it is about 25 cm long. The esophagus passes through the diaphragm and into the abdominal cavity at the tenth thoracic vertebra.

The walls of the esophagus are composed of the four layers discussed in the preceding section, with the following variations. The mucosal layer is made up of moist, stratified squamous epithelium, which changes to a simple columnar epithelium at the distal end of the esophagus. The submucosal layer contains mucus-secreting cells in addition to blood vessels, nerves, and connective tissue. These cells secrete an amphoteric mucus that can neutralize both acids and bases; this mucus helps protect the wall of the esophagus. The muscle layer is unique in that the esophagus contains both striated and smooth muscle. The upper third is striated and is innervated by the vagus nerve, whereas the lower two thirds is primarily smooth muscle and is innervated by both the vagus nerve and the intramural plexus. This is significant, because loss of vagal stimulation causes loss of voluntary swallowing; however, because the intramural plexus can still cause peristalsis in the distal esophagus, any food delivered to the lower esophagus by gravity will still be transported to the stomach. The outer layer of the esophagus is adventitia.

The esophagus is bounded proximally and distally by the upper esophageal (pharyngoesophageal) sphincter and the lower esophageal (esophagogastric) sphincter. These sphincters prevent reflux from the esophagus into the oropharynx and from the stomach into the esophagus.

The major function of the esophagus is to transport food from the mouth and oropharynx into the stomach. The esophageal sphincters normally are closed but open in response to a food bolus. The lower esophageal sphincter is actually an area of hypertrophied circular muscle that creates a high-pressure zone. It relaxes in response to peristalsis but remains tonically contracted at all other times, protecting the esophageal mucosa from gastric contents. Certain factors are known to increase or decrease the resting pressure in the lower esophageal sphincter. Factors that increase the resting pressure include cholinergic agents, antacids, adrenergic agonists, protein meals, and small amounts of alcohol. Factors that reduce the resting pressure include anticholinergics, adrenergic antagonists, glucagon, fat meals, and large amounts of alcohol.

ABDOMINAL CAVITY AND PERITONEUM

Most of the organs in the gastrointestinal tract are contained in the abdominal cavity, which actually is continuous with the pelvic cavity and is separated from the thoracic cavity by the diaphragm (Figure 1-5).

The peritoneum is a serous membrane that lines much of the abdominal cavity and covers most of the abdominal organs (Figure 1-6). Organs outside the peritoneum are said to be retroperitoneal. The peritoneum lining the abdominal cavity is known as the parietal peritoneum, and the peritoneum covering the abdominal organs is referred to as the visceral peritoneum. The *mesentery* is a double layer of peritoneum with a central layer of loose connective tissue; the mesentery encircles most of the small intestine (the jejunum and ileum) and attaches it to the posterior abdominal wall. The mesentery is a vital support structure for the bowel, because it contains the blood vessels and nerves that nourish and innervate the intestine. The mesentery that attaches the lesser curvature of the stomach to the liver and diaphragm is known as the *lesser omentum;* the mesentery that attaches the greater curvature of the stomach to the transverse colon and posterior abdominal wall is called the *greater omentum.* The greater omentum frequently is referred to as the "fatty apron," because it hangs down loosely over the bowel, and large amounts of fat tend to accumulate in and between its double folds.

STOMACH

The stomach is a distensible organ located in the left upper quadrant of the abdomen; its major function is to liquify ingested food and to provide controlled emptying into the duodenum. The stomach's size depends on its state of fullness; at capacity (about 1 to 2 L) the stomach is approximately 10 inches long and about 4½ inches wide.

The gastric wall is made up of the four layers common to GI tract histology, with the following variations: (1) The gastric wall has an inner oblique muscle layer in addition to the middle circular layer and the outer longitudinal layer, which increases the stomach's ability to "churn" the gastric contents; (2) the submucosal and mucosal layers are arranged in deep folds known as rugae, which permit the gastric lining to "stretch" as the stomach fills with ingested nutrients; (3) the mucosal layer invaginates to form openings known as gastric "pits," which communicate with the gastric glands and provide drainage for their secretions (Figure 1-7). The gastric mucosa is covered with simple columnar epithelium.

The stomach can be divided into four anatomic regions (Figure 1-7): the *cardiac region*, the *fundus*, the *body*, and the *antrum*, or pyloric region.

Cells

Five types of cells are found within the stomach. The gastric glands contain mucous neck cells, parietal (ox-

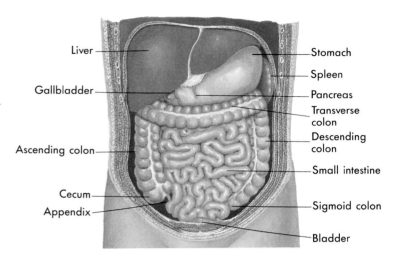

FIGURE 1-5
Anatomic structures of the abdominal cavity. (From Seidel.[52])

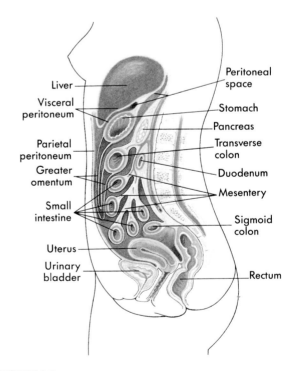

FIGURE 1-6
Sagittal section through the trunk showing the peritoneum and mesenteries associated with some abdominal organs.

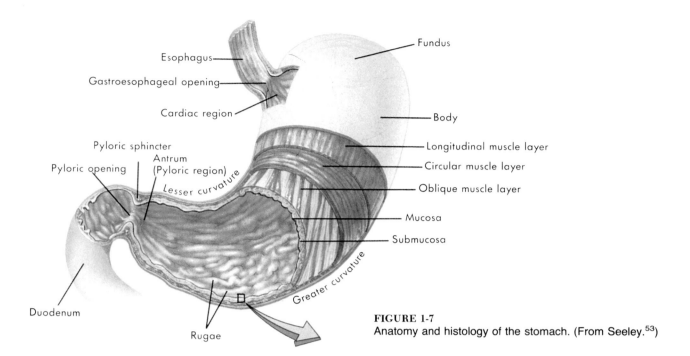

FIGURE 1-7
Anatomy and histology of the stomach. (From Seeley.[53])

yntic) cells, zymogenic (chief) cells, and endocrine cells (G cells). The fifth cell type is the surface mucous cell; these cells line the gastric pits and cover the gastric surface. The surface mucous cells and the mucous neck cells are responsible for secreting a viscous, alkaline mucus that coats the surface epithelial cells of the stomach. This mucous blanket, which normally is about 1 to 1.5 mm thick, provides a barrier against the proteolytic and highly acidic gastric contents. Any gastric irritation causes a tremendous increase in the production of mucus. The surface membranes of the mucosal cells and the tight junctions between these cells serve as an additional barrier to gastric contents. This barrier helps prevent diffusion of hydrogen ions from the gastric lumen into the mucosal cells. If the barrier is damaged, ulcers may result. Substances known to be "barrier breakers" include aspirin, alcohol, and bile salts (which come into contact with the gastric mucosa when duodenal reflux into the stomach occurs).

The parietal (oxyntic) cells produce hydrochloric acid (HCl) and intrinsic factor (IF). The low pH created by secretion of hydrochloric acid inactivates the salivary amylase, thus inhibiting carbohydrate digestion; however, it also serves to convert pepsinogen to the active enzyme pepsin, which initiates protein digestion. Conversion of pepsinogen to pepsin requires a pH below 6, and the optimum pH for pepsin activity is between 1.8 and 3.5. Vagal stimulation, gastrin, and histamine increase the secretion of hydrochloric acid; basal secretion of HCl is lowest in the morning and

highest in the afternoon and evening. Intrinsic factor is also produced by the parietal cells; it is a mucoprotein that binds with vitamin B_{12} and facilitates its absorption at specific receptor sites in the terminal ileum.

The chief cells (zymogenic cells) secrete pepsinogen, which is the precursor of the proteolytic enzyme pepsin. As noted, pepsinogen is converted to pepsin in the acidic environment created by secretion of hydrochloric acid. Production of pepsinogen is stimulated by gastrin, calcium, histamine, and secretin.

The endocrine cells, or G cells, are located in antral glands. These cells secrete gastrin, which stimulates the parietal cells to increase secretion of hydrochloric acid. Gastrin production is increased by gastric distention, vagal stimulation, calcium ions, and the presence of protein breakdown products; it is inhibited by a gastric pH below 1.5.

Gastric Secretion

The total volume of gastric secretions normally is about 2 to 3 L a day. Gastric secretion is regulated by neural phenomena and by hormonal secretion.

A number of factors are known to increase or decrease gastric secretion. Stimulating factors include pleasant thoughts, the taste and smell of food, tactile stimulation from chewing and swallowing, gastric distention, partially digested proteins in the stomach, and moderate amounts of caffeine and alcohol (which explains why caffeinated and alcoholic beverages increase appetite). Factors that inhibit gastric secretion include

FACTORS THAT AFFECT RATE OF GASTRIC EMPTYING

Factors that reduce gastric motility	Factors that increase gastric motility
Chyme	Vagal stimulation (e.g., by cholinergic drugs such as metoclopramide)
Narcotics	Surgical procedures that bypass or alter the pylorus
Pathologic conditions (e.g., hypokalemia, peritonitis, uremia)	
Emotions	
Surgical vagotomy	
High-fat foods	
Consistency of ingested nutrients (solids empty more slowly than liquids)	
Temperature extremes of ingested nutrients	

FUNCTIONS OF THE STOMACH

Reservoir for ingested nutrients
Provides controlled emptying into the duodenum
Continues digestive process begun in the mouth
Produces intrinsic factor
Provides for limited absorption
Inhibits bacterial proliferation by low gastric pH

The rate of gastric emptying is primarily determined by the pH, fat content, and osmolality of the chyme. The duodenum is equipped with osmoreceptors, acid-sensitive receptors, and fat-sensitive receptors; when stimulated, these receptors produce substances that increase the pressure within the pylorus and inhibit gastric emptying.

Digestion

The stomach contributes to mechanical digestion by mixing the ingested nutrients with gastric secretions to form the semifluid chyme. In addition, the stomach begins enzymatic digestion of proteins. The hydrochloric acid produced by the parietal cells converts pepsinogen to pepsin, a proteolytic enzyme that splits intact protein into peptide chains.

Secretion of Intrinsic Factor

The most essential function of the stomach is to produce intrinsic factor, which is required for effective absorption of vitamin B_{12} (cyanocobalamin) in the terminal ileum. If the stomach has been surgically removed or if the parietal cells fail to secrete intrinsic factor (as may occur with chronic gastritis and achlorhydria), lifelong parenteral administration of vitamin B_{12} is required to prevent pernicious anemia.

Absorption

The stomach provides only limited absorption; substances that can be partially absorbed in the stomach include carbohydrates that were chemically digested in the mouth, alcohol, and some medications, such as aspirin.

Antibacterial Effect

The stomach's antibacterial action is produced by the low gastric pH; this acidity eliminates most ingested bacteria.

distention or irritation of the duodenum, and duodenal contents that are very acid, hypertonic, or hypotonic. Emotions are also believed to affect gastric secretion; anger and hostility have been associated with increased gastric secretion, whereas fear and depression are thought to be inhibiting factors.

Reservoir for Nutrients

The stomach provides a reservoir for ingested nutrients, with gradual and controlled emptying into the duodenum; this allows a healthy individual to eat at intervals. (When the stomach has been removed or bypassed, enteral feedings must be provided on a more continuous basis.)

Ingested nutrients remain in the stomach until they have been thoroughly mixed with the gastric contents and converted to the semifluid material known as chyme. This process involves both mixing waves and peristaltic waves. Both types of waves proceed from the proximal end of the stomach to the distal (pyloric) end; the difference is that the weaker mixing waves primarily act to combine the ingested nutrients with the gastric secretions, whereas the stronger peristaltic waves actively sweep the liquid chyme toward the pylorus. This process of mixing and movement continues until the gastric contents have all been converted to a semifluid state and emptied into the duodenum.

SMALL INTESTINE

In adults, the small intestine is approximately 660 cm long and has about 7,000 cm of absorptive surface. The small intestine is divided into three anatomic and functional sections: the duodenum, the jejunum, and the ileum.

Histology

The wall of the small intestine is made up of the four layers common to the GI tract. However, the small intestine has several unique characteristics that tremendously increase its absorptive ability (Figure 1-8): (1) The submucosal and mucosal layers are arranged in folds, known as the plicae circulares. (2) The mucosal surface is covered with villi, fingerlike projections 0.5 to 1 mm long. Each villus contains a capillary network, a lymphatic vessel, and smooth muscle fibers. (3) The villi are covered with absorptive cells that have cytoplasmic extensions known as microvilli. The total increase in absorptive surface provided by the plicae circulares, villi, and microvilli is about 600%.

The microvilli form what is known as the *brush border*. The cells that make up the brush border and the mucopolysaccharide that covers it contain many digestive enzymes and carrier substances, which facilitate the digestion and absorption of nutrients.

The villi actually have the ability to elongate, or hypertrophy, which partly explains the phenomenon of bowel "adaptation" following segmental small bowel resection. The converse is also true; patients maintained on nothing by mouth (NPO) status for more than a few days may experience temporary atrophy of the villi, resulting in loss of absorptive surface and diarrhea.

The mucosal layer of the small intestine contains solitary lymphoid cells, and the submucosal layer contains aggregated lymphatic nodules known as Peyer's patches; these are particularly common in the ileum. It is now recognized that a number of immunoglobulins are produced in the small bowel, and that the small bowel plays a significant part in the functioning of the immune system. Loss of bowel wall integrity is thought to play a role in the overwhelming sepsis that occurs in some critically ill patients maintained on NPO status for prolonged periods.

The small intestine is the primary organ responsible for the digestion and absorption of nutrients, vitamins, minerals, fluids and electrolytes, and miscellaneous substances such as drugs. Specific functions that contribute to the digestive process include intestinal motility, intestinal secretion, digestion, and absorption.

Intestinal Motility

Two types of contractions occur regularly in the small intestine, segmentation and peristalsis. Segmental contractions are mixing waves that produce a back-and-forth motion, which churns the intestinal contents and increases exposure of the chyme to the absorptive mucosal surface. Peristaltic waves propel the chyme distally through the bowel. Peristalsis occurs in response to intestinal distention; a strong contraction begins just behind the point of stimulus and sweeps along the intestine toward the ileocecal valve. Normally peristalsis occurs almost continuously, propelling the chyme distally at a rate of 2 to 25 cm per minute.

Small bowel motility is affected by both extrinsic and intrinsic innervation, but the intrinsic system is far more important. Extrinsic innervation includes sympathetic stimulation, which inhibits intestinal motility, and parasympathetic (vagal) stimulation, which increases intestinal motility. However, motility is most affected by local factors such as bowel wall distention, hypertonic or hypotonic intestinal contents, very acid chyme, and some products of digestion. Response to these stimuli is mediated primarily by the intramural plexus; extrinsic innervation plays only a minor, "modulating" role. In fact, both segmentation and peristalsis can be mediated by an intact myenteric plexus, even in the absence of extrinsic innervation.

Transit time from the mouth to the colon averages 4 to 9 hours.

Intestinal Secretion

There are two types of small bowel secretions, mucus and intestinal fluid. Mucus is produced in large amounts by goblet cells located throughout the mucosal layer. Mucus protects the mucosal epithelium, and irritating stimuli increase mucus production. In addition to mucus, a large volume of watery intestinal fluid is produced by intestinal glands known as the crypts of Lieberkühn. These glands secrete as much as 2 to 3 L of fluid a day, with a pH of about 6.5 to 7.5. This intestinal fluid does not contain digestive enzymes; the enzymes needed to complete the digestive process are found in the cells of the brush border and in the mucopolysaccharide covering of the brush border, as explained above. The watery intestinal fluid functions primarily to facilitate absorption.

Digestion

Most nutrient digestion takes place in the small intestine as a result of enzymatic action. Enzymes produced by the mouth, stomach, pancreas, and small intestine break the complex molecules of ingested foods into simple substances that can be absorbed into the bloodstream. Breakdown of these complex mole-

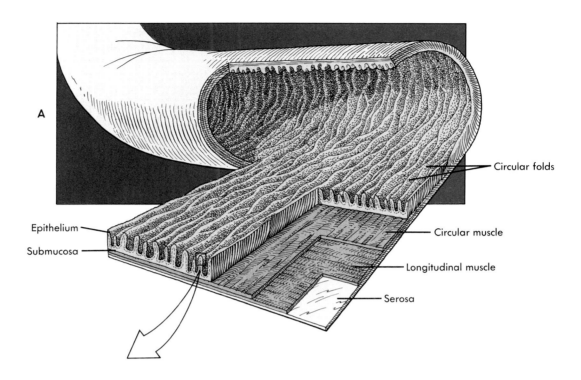

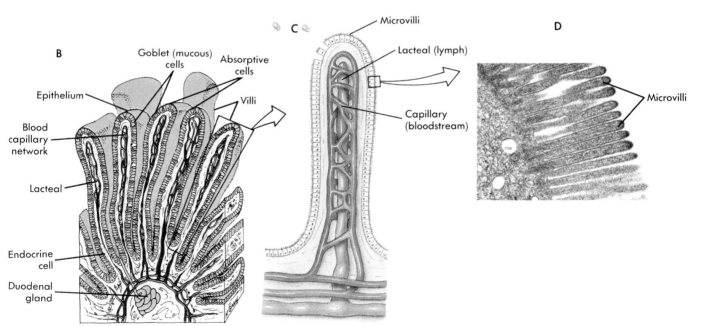

FIGURE 1-8
Anatomy and histology of the duodenum and pancreas. **A,** Wall of the duodenum showing the circular folds. **B,** The villi, and **C,** a single villus showing the lacteal and capillary network. **D,** Electron micrograph of the microvilli. (From Seeley.[53])

cules involves enzymatically mediated reactions that replace hydrogen and hydroxyl ions (hydrolysis), which causes separation of the bound molecules.

Absorption

The end products of carbohydrate, protein, and fat digestion are absorbed into the epithelial cells of the brush border and from there into the bloodstream through the processes of facilitated diffusion and active transport. Nutrient absorption is a complex process involving several carrier substances; absorption of specific nutrients is influenced by factors such as the nutrient mix and concurrent electrolyte absorption.

Carbohydrate absorption illustrates the complexity of the absorptive process. Galactose and glucose are more rapidly absorbed than other carbohydrate breakdown products, suggesting that the various monosaccharides must "compete" for carrier substances and that the carrier substances preferentially select galactose and glucose. Carbohydrate absorption is also significantly affected by sodium absorption; this is because the carrier substance for glucose and galactose does not transport the monosaccharide unless sodium is also being transported, and does not transport sodium without a monosaccharide. This explains why many oral rehydration solutions contain a mix of glucose and sodium.

Protein absorption parallels carbohydrate absorption; certain amino acids are absorbed more readily than others, carrier systems are required, and amino acid transport occurs simultaneously with sodium transport. One of the carrier systems for amino acid transport is a derivative of the vitamin pyridoxine.

Fat absorption occurs as a result of diffusion; bile salts transport the monoglycerides to the brush border, where they dissolve in the lipid membranes of the epithelial cells and thus are transported to the interior of the cell. Inside the cell the monoglycerides are reconstituted into triglycerides, which combine with cholesterol and phospholipids to form globules. These globules are extruded from the epithelial cell of the brush border into the intercellular space and then into the central lacteal of the villi, which empties into the thoracic duct and then into the venous system.

Electrolyte and water absorption: In addition to providing for absorption of the end products of nutrient digestion, the small intestine plays a vital role in maintaining fluid and electrolyte balance through its reabsorption of intraluminal fluids. The volume of fluid secreted into the small intestine may be as much as 7 to 9 L per day; with the average oral intake being 2 L daily, the volume of secreted and ingested fluids may reach 11 L a day. Most of this fluid is reabsorbed into the bloodstream, with less than 2 L passing through the ileocecal valve daily. These absorptive processes involve complex mechanisms of active transport as well as simple diffusion along the concentration gradient.

Chloride absorption is achieved by passive diffusion in the proximal small bowel; however, in the distal small bowel and colon, chloride ions are actively absorbed and bicarbonate ions are actively secreted. The purpose of bicarbonate ion secretion is to neutralize the acidic products formed by colonic bacteria; chloride ions are reabsorbed to maintain electrical balance. Certain bacterial toxins, such as those produced by cholera and staphylococci, stimulate this exchange mechanism; this results in secretion of a large volume of bicarbonate, which carries with it both sodium and water. The secretory diarrhea that results can rapidly cause death.

Water is absorbed readily by the process of osmosis; the flow of water occurs in response to the concentration of the chyme in the intestinal lumen. When the chyme is dilute, large volumes of water are absorbed into the brush border and thus into the bloodstream; concentrated chyme causes water to pass out of the bloodstream and into the intestinal lumen.

Because the small bowel plays such an important role in the reabsorption of electrolytes and water, any abnormal intestinal losses may result in fluid and electrolyte imbalance; hypokalemia, hyponatremia, and metabolic acidosis commonly occur along with fluid volume deficit.

Digestion and absorption of specific nutrients are summarized in Table 1-1.

Blood Supply

The superior mesenteric artery supplies blood flow for most of the small intestine (i.e., the jejunum, ileum, and distal duodenum). The proximal duodenum (the portion above the ampulla of Vater) derives its blood supply from the celiac vessels. Venous drainage for the small bowel is provided by the superior mesenteric vein; the superior mesenteric vein empties into the portal vein, which drains into the liver. This vascular arrangement provides the necessary "detoxification" of the blood draining the intestinal tract before it reenters the systemic circulation. It also explains the frequency of metastatic disease in the liver in an individual with a malignancy of the GI tract.

DUODENUM

The first section of the small bowel is the duodenum, an immobile, C-shaped segment 20 to 30 cm long. The duodenum lies just distal to the pylorus and is secured to the pyloric region of the stomach by the ligament of Treitz, which divides the duodenum from the jejunum (Figure 1-9). The proximal portion of the duodenum is

Table 1-1

NUTRIENT DIGESTION AND ABSORPTION

	Digestive enzymes	Site of action/absorption
Carbohydrates	Amylase	Produced in mouth/(salivary glands)
		Absorbed in stomach (limited)
		Produced in small intestine (pancreas)
		Absorbed in small intestine
	Disaccharidases (sucrase, maltase isomaltase, lactase)	Produced in small intestine (brush border)
		Absorbed in small intestine
Proteins	Pepsin	Produced in stomach (chief cells)
		Absorbed in small intestine
	Trypsin, chymotrypsin	Produced in small intestine (pancreas)
		Absorbed in small intestine
	Carboxypeptidase / Peptidases	Produced in small intestine (brush border)
		Absorbed in small intestine
Lipids	Bile (not enzyme)	Produced in liver and delivered to duodenum
		Absorbed in small intestine
	Lipase	Produced in small intestine (pancreas, brush border)
		Absorbed in small intestine
	Esterase	Produced in small intestine (pancreas)
		Absorbed in small intestine

located within the peritoneal cavity, and the distal portion is located retroperitoneally. The common bile duct and the pancreatic duct both empty into the duodenum at the ampulla of Vater, which is about 7 to 10 cm distal to the pyloric sphincter.

The duodenum's major function is to neutralize the very acidic gastric contents. This is accomplished partly by secretion of alkaline mucus by the duodenal (Brunner's) glands, which are located in the submucosal layer of the duodenum. In addition, the presence of acid chyme in the duodenum stimulates the release of secretin, which in turn stimulates the pancreas to secrete fluid with a high concentration of bicarbonate ions. This very alkaline fluid drains through the pancreatic duct into the duodenum and plays a major role in neutralizing the acidic chyme. If the ingested nutrients include fats, cholecystokinin is secreted; this stimulates contraction of the gallbladder, and the alkaline bile contributes to neutralization of the acidic chyme.

A second function of the duodenum is to continue the digestive process begun in the proximal alimentary canal. The presence of fats and proteins in the duodenum stimulates the release of cholecystokinin, which results in contraction of the gallbladder and secretion of enzymatic fluid by the pancreas. Bile emulsifies fats, and the pancreatic juice contains the primary digestive enzymes for each of the nutrient categories.

The duodenum also plays a role in absorption; carbohydrates and minerals such as iron, calcium, and magnesium are absorbed in the duodenum.

JEJUNUM

The midportion of the small intestine is the jejunum, which is about 270 cm long and about 2.5 to 3.8 cm wide. The jejunum is the major organ for absorption of nutrients; most of the fats, proteins, and vitamins are absorbed in this area, as well as carbohydrates not absorbed in the stomach and duodenum. The jejunum has very prominent villi, consistent with its role in nutrient absorption.

ILEUM

The ileum is the third segment of the small intestine. It is about 360 cm long and about 2.5 cm wide. There is no clear demarcation between the jejunum and the ileum; however, the ileum is narrower than the jejunum, and the villi are less prominent in the ileum. The ileum provides for absorption of any nutrients not absorbed by the duodenum and jejunum; if the jejunum is diseased, removed, or bypassed, the ileum can take over many of the absorptive functions.

The ileum also contains the only receptor sites for absorption of the intrinsic factor–vitamin B_{12} complex and for bile salts; these sites are found in the terminal ileum. Patients who undergo resection of significant lengths of the terminal ileum may require lifelong parenteral replacement of vitamin B_{12} to prevent pernicious anemia and may also experience fat intolerance and weight loss. This fat intolerance is based on the fact that failure to reabsorb bile salts in the terminal ileum retards bile production in the liver. Normally the bile emulsifies the fats, and bile salts then transport the monoglycerides and fatty acids to the cells of the brush border for absorption. The bile salts are then released back into the intestinal lumen. When the bile salts reach the terminal ileum, they are reabsorbed into the bloodstream by active transport and are delivered back to the liver, where they are again used to produce bile. This recycling of bile salts is known as the enterohepatic circulation; it promotes bile production and therefore fat absorption.

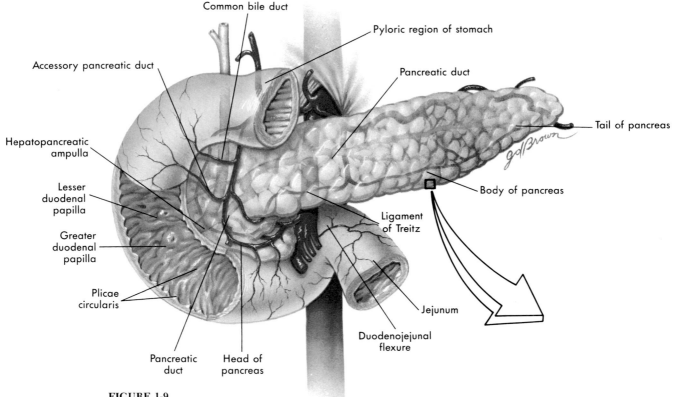

FIGURE 1-9
Anatomy and histology of the duodenum and pancreas. The head of the pancreas lies within the duodenal curvature, with the pancreatic duct emptying into the duodenum. The greater pancreatic duct joins the common bile duct to form the hepatopancreatic duct, which opens into the duodenum at the greater duodenal papilla. (From Seeley.[53])

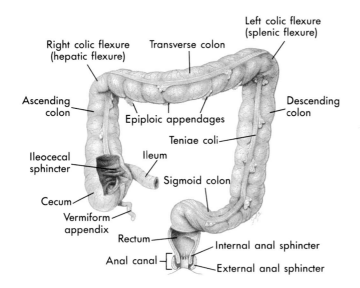

FIGURE 1-10
Large intestine (i.e., cecum, colon, and rectum) and anal canal. The teniae coli and epiploic appendages are along the length of the colon. (From Seeley.[53])

ILEOCECAL VALVE

The ileocecal valve is a one-way valve located at the junction between the ileum and the colon (Figure 1-10). The ileocecal valve functions in conjunction with the ileocecal sphincter, a ring of smooth muscle, to regulate emptying into the colon and to prevent reflux of contents into the small intestine. Normally the ileocecal sphincter is partially contracted; peristaltic waves in the distal ileum cause the sphincter to relax, allowing chyme to pass into the colon. In contrast, distention of the cecum increases sphincter tone, preventing reflux of large bowel contents into the small intestine.

The ileocecal valve and sphincter provide some delay in the passage of chyme from the small bowel into the colon; this delay may be important for the patient who has undergone significant small bowel resection or who has compromised absorptive capacity, because it increases the exposure of nutrients to the absorptive surface of the small bowel.

LARGE INTESTINE (COLON)

The colon is the organ responsible for storing and eliminating waste products produced by nutrient di-

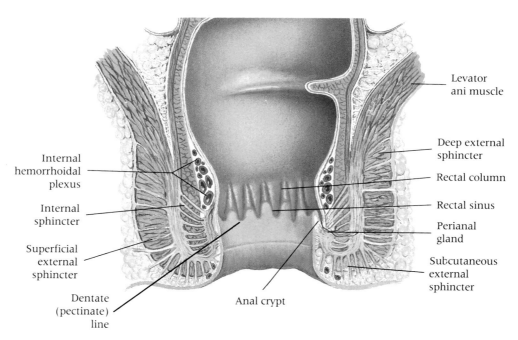

FIGURE 1-11
Anatomy of the anus and rectum. (From Seidel.[52])

gestion and absorption. The colon is approximately 150 cm long and 3.8 to 5 cm in diameter.

The cecum, which is the first segment of the large intestine, connects the ileum to the colon. The colon itself is divided into four anatomic sections: ascending colon, transverse colon, descending colon, and sigmoid colon. The colon is continuous with the rectum, which connects to the anal canal. The anal canal terminates at the anus, the most distal structure of the alimentary canal (Figure 1-10).

The **cecum,** which contains the ileocecal valve, is the junction between the small and large intestines. The cecum extends inferiorly past the ileocecal valve to form a blind pouch; attached to the cecum is the appendix, a small, blind tube about 9 cm long that contains many lymph nodes.

The **ascending colon** extends from the cecum to the hepatic flexure, where the colon curves to the left and becomes the transverse colon. The **transverse colon** extends across the abdominal cavity and curves slightly upward to form the splenic flexure, and then turns downward to become the **descending colon.** The descending colon continues down the left side of the abdominal cavity to the opening of the pelvic cavity, where it curves to the right to form the **sigmoid colon.** The sigmoid colon is an S-shaped tube that ends at the rectum.

The **rectum** begins at the midsacral level; the proximal portion of the rectum is within the peritoneal cavity but the distal portion has no peritoneal covering.

The rectum is about 12.7 cm long. In men, the distal portion of the rectum is adjacent to the prostate gland; in women, this portion of the rectum is attached to the posterior vaginal wall. The rectum joins the anal canal, which is the last 2 to 3 cm of the alimentary canal.

The junction of the rectum and the **anal canal** is known as the dentate, or pectinate, line (Figure 1-11). Above this line the rectum is lined with mucus-secreting epithelium that is relatively insensitive, whereas distal to this line the anal canal is lined with squamous epithelium rich in sensory receptors. Two sphincters encompass the anal canal and support fecal continence (Figure 1-11). The internal sphincter is a continuation of the circular muscle layer of the rectum; it encircles the anorectal junction and the anal canal, except for the most distal centimeter of the anal canal, and is under autonomic control. The external sphincter is a skeletal muscle that surrounds the internal sphincter and the distal centimeter of the anal canal; it is under voluntary control. The external sphincter is actually continuous with the puborectalis muscle, which forms a sling that encircles the anorectal junction and attaches to the pubic symphysis (Figure 1-12); this means that contraction of the external sphincter causes contraction of the puborectalis, which renders the anorectal angle more acute and thus supports continence.

The **anus** is the superficial portion of the striated external sphincter. The anal verge marks the boundary between the anal canal epithelium and perianal skin.

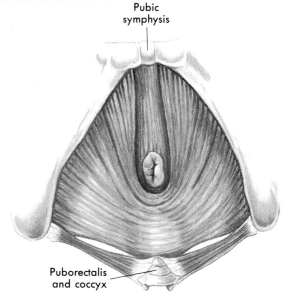

Pubic
symphysis

Puborectalis
and coccyx

FIGURE 1-12
Puborectalis and levator ani muscles, which form pelvic floor.

Histology

The wall of the large intestine is composed of the same four layers that make up the rest of the alimentary canal. However, there are marked variations in the mucosal and muscular layers compared to those of the small intestine (Figure 1-13).

The mucosal layer of the large intestine is made up of simple columnar epithelium; it has no plicae circulares, no villi, and no microvilli. Instead this layer has straight tubular glands called crypts, which produce epithelial cells and mucus-producing goblet cells.

The muscle layer differs in two ways: (1) The muscle layer in the rectum is thicker than in the proximal alimentary canal; and (2) the longitudinal muscle layer does not completely encase the colon wall, but instead forms three muscle bands, known as the teniae coli, that run the length of the colon (see Figure 1-10). One of these muscle bands attaches to the anterior surface of the colon, one to the posteroinferior surface, and one to the posterosuperior surface. Contraction of the teniae causes the sacculations in the colon known as haustrations. This feature of the colon wall is advantageous for the patient who requires a loop colostomy; if the colostomy is opened parallel to the teniae, the natural haustrations create separate openings into the proximal and distal bowel, thus providing complete fecal diversion.

Another feature of the colon wall not seen in the small intestine is the presence of epiploic appendages; these are small, fat-filled, connective tissue pouches attached to the outer surface of the colon (Figure 1-13).

The transverse colon and the sigmoid colon each have a mesentery, which contributes to the mobility of these two colonic segments. This increased mobility renders these segments more prone to volvulus and intussusception. The ascending and descending colons, on the other hand, are located retroperitoneally against the abdominal wall and have no mesenteric attachments; this is also true of the distal rectum.

Lymphatic drainage of the colon is provided by the epicolic nodes, located on the surface of the colon; the paracolic nodes, located along the mesenteric border; the intermediate nodes, located along the superior and inferior mesenteric arteries; and the paraaortic nodes, which are adjacent to the abdominal aorta.

Colonic Secretion

There are two types of colonic secretions, mucus and an electrolyte solution. The mucosal layer normally produces large amounts of mucus that protect the colonic wall from the intraluminal contents and also provide adherence for the fecal mass. Mucus production is regulated by local reflexes and direct tactile stimuli affecting the mucus-producing cells and by parasympathetic stimulation, which can markedly increase both mucus production and colonic motility. Extreme parasympathetic stimulation, which may result from emotional disturbances, can increase the rate of mucus production so much that the individual has a bowel movement of mucus every 30 minutes.

The colonic mucosa can actively secrete bicarbonate ions while absorbing chloride ions in an exchange process described previously. The purpose of this alkaline fluid secretion is to neutralize the acidic end products formed by the colonic bacteria.

Colonic Motility

Like the small intestine, the colon has two types of movements, mixing movements and propulsive movements. However, movements in the colon are more sluggish and less frequent than those in the small intestine, and this type of motility is uniquely suited to the colon's functions of fluid absorption and fecal storage.

Mixing movements are provided by simultaneous contraction of a section of circular muscle and the three longitudinal muscle bands known as the teniae coli. These combined contractions are called haustral contractions, because they cause the colon to bulge outward, intensifying the natural haustrations. These haustral contractions increase exposure of the colon contents to the absorptive surface; haustral contractions in the cecum and ascending colon also move the contents very slowly toward the anus. It can take as long as 8 to 15 hours to move the colonic contents from the ileocecal valve to the transverse colon by

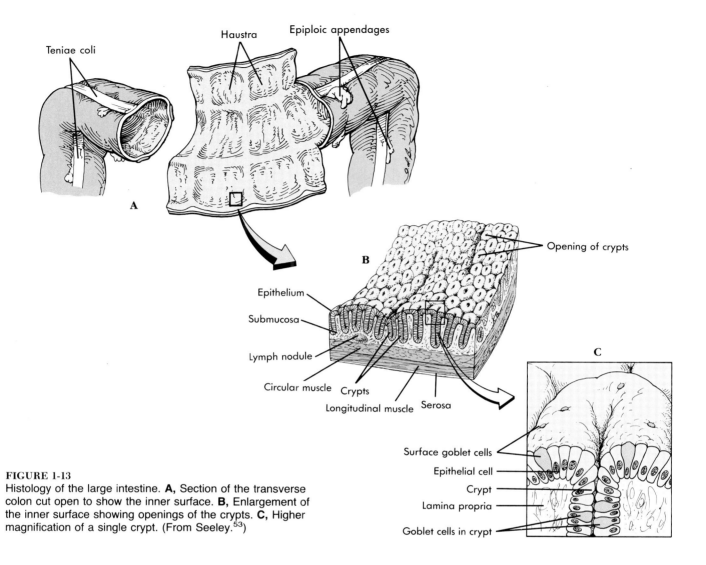

FIGURE 1-13
Histology of the large intestine. **A,** Section of the transverse colon cut open to show the inner surface. **B,** Enlargement of the inner surface showing openings of the crypts. **C,** Higher magnification of a single crypt. (From Seeley.[53])

means of these haustral contractions; during this process the semifluid chyme is converted to a semisolid slush.

Propulsive movements in the colon occur as mass movements, which are a series of peristaltic waves that sweep stool rapidly through the colon. Mass movements occur most commonly in the transverse and descending colons; peristalsis begins at a point of distention or irritation and initiates a peristaltic wave that continues 20 cm or farther distally, forcing stool toward the rectum. These peristaltic waves occur at intervals for about 10 to 15 minutes two to three times daily; mass movements are particularly common in the first hour after breakfast. This increased colonic motility after meals is triggered by the gastrocolic and duodenocolic reflexes, which are caused by distention of the stomach and duodenum. These reflexes are thought to be mediated primarily by local enteric reflexes, although parasympathetic stimulation further

stimulates colonic motility. These local and autonomic stimuli explain why bowel movements occur more commonly after meals, a principle of considerable importance in the establishment of a bowel training program.

The infrequency of mass movements contributes to the slow transit of fecal material through the colon. Total transit time from the ileocecal valve to the rectum usually is 24 hours or longer.

Storage and Elimination of Stool

The gradual passage of stool through the colon provides for absorption of water and conversion of the stool from a liquid to a solid state; it also reduces the frequency of rectal filling and stimulation of the defecation reflex. The defecation reflex can be explained as follows: rectal distention results in reflex inhibition of the internal sphincter and also stimulates peristaltic activity in the distal colon via activation of local myen-

MAJOR FUNCTIONS OF THE COLON AND RECTUM

Storage and elimination of stool
Absorption of water and electrolytes
Limited secretion
Synthesis of selected vitamins

FACTORS AFFECTING VOLUNTARY DEFECATION

Normal functioning of intestinal tract
Normal anorectal sensation
Normal sphincter function
Normal rectal compliance

teric reflexes and parasympathetic stimuli. Defecation can then be inhibited or promoted. In the precontinent child and in individuals with impaired cognition, defecation is promoted by the Valsalva maneuver, which is triggered by afferent stimuli and which tremendously augments the effectiveness of rectal emptying. In the continent individual, contraction of the external sphincter inhibits defecation.

GI Tract Function

Normal functioning of the intestinal tract results in delivery of soft, formed stool to the rectum at regular intervals, usually once or twice daily. Any changes in this pattern may affect fecal continence.

Sensory Status

Voluntary control of defecation also depends on normal sensory function, which provides awareness of rectal distention and the nature of rectal contents (i.e., solid, liquid, or gas). This awareness alerts the individual to seek an appropriate place for defecation or to inhibit the defecation reflex until a more convenient time. The sensation of rectal distention is mediated by stretch receptors in the muscles surrounding the rectum; normal sensation depends on intact sensory pathways and the cognitive ability to recognize the sensation of rectal distention. Accurate identification of rectal contents (i.e., discrimination between solid, liquid, and gas) is mediated by the epithelial cells of the proximal anal canal, at the junction of the rectal mucosa and the anal epithelium. This junction is known as the dentate or pectinate line. The relatively insensitive rectal mucosa lies proximal to this line, and the exquisitely sensitive anal epithelium is located distally.

Sphincter Function

Normal sphincter function is another critical factor in voluntary control of defecation. The normal response of the internal sphincter to rectal distention is receptive relaxation, which permits the rectal contents to come into contact with the sensitive epithelium of the

anal canal and provides for accurate identification of rectal contents; this is known as the sampling reflex. The external sphincter, which is under voluntary control, usually is contracted in response to rectal distention; this maintains fecal continence until a suitable time and place for defecation is found, at which point the external sphincter is voluntarily relaxed.

Rectal Capacity and Compliance

Rectal capacity and compliance also have a significant effect on bowel function and fecal continence. Capacity refers to the volume of stool that can be accumulated in the rectum before rectal distention overwhelms the sphincter mechanism and causes involuntary defecation; in a normal adult, capacity approaches 400 ml.

Compliance refers to the rectum's distensibility, its ability to accommodate increased fecal volume without marked increases in rectal pressure. Compliance is determined by measuring the changes in pressure that occur with specific changes in volume. Normally, intrarectal pressure rises to less than 20 cm H_2O even with volumes approaching 400 ml. The importance of rectal capacity and compliance is underscored by the fact that fecal continence depends on maintenance of rectal pressures that are lower than anal canal pressures. When a significant amount of stool is delivered to the rectum, rectal pressure increases suddenly and sharply; however, this is offset by a corresponding increase in anal canal pressure produced by contraction of the external sphincter. Maximum contraction of the external sphincter can be maintained for less than 60 seconds; continence beyond this point depends on a reduction in rectal pressure. In the normal rectum, the initial rise in pressure subsides as the rectum relaxes to accommodate the increased stool volume. This relaxation and corresponding drop in intrarectal pressure is known as the accommodation response. If the rectum is very inflamed or fibrotic, any stool volume tends to cause a significant and sustained increase in intrarectal pressure; these individuals experience fecal urgency and may experience fecal incontinence.

Defecation Process

In a normal individual, all of the above factors help to maintain a pattern of regular voluntary defecation. The defecation process can be summarized as follows: (1) Peristaltic waves transport soft, formed stool to the rectum; sometimes a small amount of stool is delivered, and sometimes a large amount. (2) When enough stool has been delivered to cause rectal distention and increased intrarectal pressure, sensory receptors signal rectal fullness and the urge to defecate. (3) Rectal distention causes the internal sphincter to relax (the rectoanal inhibitory reflex). This allows the rectal contents to come into contact with the sensitive epithelium of the anal canal, which provides for differentiation between solid, liquid, and gas. (4) The external sphincter is voluntarily contracted in response to the sensation of rectal fullness; temporary contraction of the external sphincter increases the anal canal pressure, which balances the increase in rectal pressure and thus maintains continence. (5) The rectum relaxes to accommodate the increased stool volume, which reduces the intrarectal pressure and maintains continence. (6) At an appropriate time and place, the individual voluntarily relaxes the external sphincter and initiates defecation by contracting the abdominal muscles, which increases intraabdominal and intrarectal pressures and forces the stool through the anal canal.

Composition of Feces

Feces normally is about three fourths water and one fourth solid material such as bacteria, fat, protein, inorganic matter, and undigested roughage. Additional components include epithelial cells and components of digestive juices. Stool normally is brown, due to derivatives of bilirubin; fecal odor is caused by bacterial action on the waste products and varies with diet and bacterial mix.

Absorption of Water and Electrolytes

Most of the fluid delivered to the large intestine each day is reabsorbed. Although about 1 L or more of fluid passes through the ileocecal valve, usually less than 100 ml is lost in the feces. Most of this fluid reabsorption occurs in the proximal colon. The colonic mucosa also has significant capacity for active absorption of sodium; this produces an electrical gradient that results in chloride reabsorption. The large bowel cannot absorb nutrients, because it lacks the enzymes and carrier systems that provide for nutrient absorption.

Secretion

As noted previously, the colonic mucosa actively secretes bicarbonate ions to help neutralize the acidic by-products of bacterial action. This secretion is balanced by active reabsorption of chloride ions.

Vitamin Synthesis

The colonic bacteria can synthesize folic acid, riboflavin, thiamine, vitamin B_{12}, and vitamin K. Synthesis of vitamin K is particularly important, because vitamin K plays an important role in coagulation, and usually only small amounts are obtained through the diet. Elimination of colonic bacteria prevents synthesis of vitamin K; parenteral administration may be required.

Flatus

The action of colonic bacteria on undigested food (usually complex carbohydrates) produces flatus. The volume and mix of flatus vary and depend largely on the foods eaten and colonic transit time. The foods known to increase flatus production are those that contain undigestible carbohydrates (e.g., beans, cabbage, and cauliflower) and those that act as irritants (e.g., vinegar). Transit time also affects the volume of flatus expelled; increased motility results in higher volumes of expelled flatus, because there is less time for the gas to be reabsorbed into the bloodstream. The amount of flatus produced daily averages 7 to 10 L, whereas the average volume of expelled flatus is only 600 ml.

Blood Supply and Innervation

The blood supply for the cecum, ascending colon, and proximal transverse colon is derived from branches of the superior mesenteric artery, which also supplies the small intestine. The inferior mesenteric artery supplies the distal transverse colon, descending colon, sigmoid colon, and rectum (Figure 1-14). A branch of the inferior mesenteric artery supplies the proximal anal canal; the middle and inferior rectal arteries, which are branches of the internal iliac artery, supply the remainder of the anal canal and the perianal area. Venous drainage parallels arterial supply, with the superior mesenteric vein draining the proximal colon and the inferior mesenteric vein draining the distal colon and rectum. The mesenteric veins drain into the portal system. The superior hemorrhoidal (rectal) vein empties into the inferior mesenteric vein and then into the portal system; the inferior hemorrhoidal veins drain into the pudendal vein and then directly into the systemic venous system.

With the exception of the inferior hemorrhoidal veins, all of the venous blood from the colon is drained into the portal system and then through the sinusoids of the liver before being returned to the systemic circulation; this pattern of blood flow provides

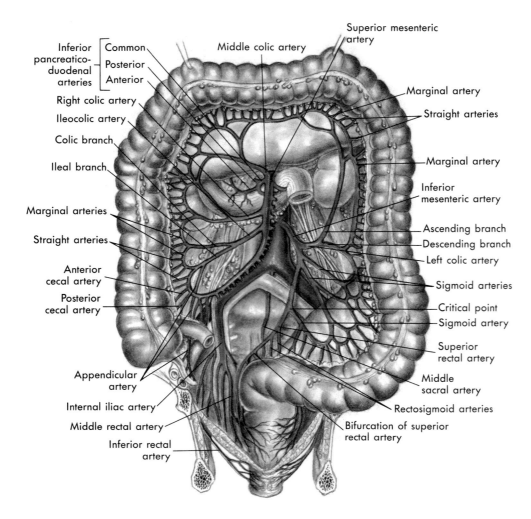

FIGURE 1-14
Arterial and venous blood supply to primary and accessory organs of alimentary canal. (From Thompson.[57])

for removal of bacteria and toxins from colonic blood.

Colonic secretion and motility are mediated by the enteric nervous system and by autonomic stimuli. The vagus nerves provide parasympathetic innervation of the right colon, whereas the pelvic nerves carry parasympathetic stimuli to the left colon. The pelvic nerves exit the cord at the S_2-S_4 level. Sympathetic stimuli are provided by the mesenteric hypogastric nerves, which exit the cord at the T_{12}-L_4 level. The anal canal and external sphincter are innervated by sensory and motor fibers. Somatic sensory pathways travel to the cord and enter at the S_2-S_4 level; they then travel to the cortex, where sensory stimuli are interpreted. Sensory innervation of the rectum is carried through parasympathetic pathways that enter the cord at the same level as the somatic pathways. Motor pathways providing voluntary control of the external sphincter exit the cord at the S_2-S_4 level; motor stimuli are provided through the pudendal nerve. These pathways explain why patients with spinal cord injuries experience loss of sensory awareness and sphincter control.

ACCESSORY ORGANS

Three organs outside the alimentary canal play important roles in nutrient digestion and absorption; they are the liver, gallbladder, and pancreas.

LIVER

The liver is one of the most important organs in the body; it plays a critical role in many functions that are essential to life and health.

The liver is located in the right upper quadrant of the abdominal cavity just under the diaphragm and normally extends from the fifth intercostal space to just below the right costal margin.

The liver is divided into two main lobes, the left and the right (Figure 1-15). The right lobe is further divided into three parts: the right lobe proper, the caudate lobe, and the quadrate lobe.

Major vessels, ducts, and nerves enter and exit the liver at the porta hepatis, located on the inferior surface of the liver (Figure 1-15). At this point the portal vein, the hepatic artery, and the hepatic nerve plexus enter the liver; this area is also the point of exit for lymphatic vessels and for the right and left hepatic bile ducts, which join to form the common hepatic duct.

The liver is covered by visceral peritoneum and by a connective tissue capsule (Glisson's capsule), which branches at the porta hepatis into a network of septa that extends throughout the liver tissue to provide support. The septa divide the liver tissue into approximately 1 million hepatic lobules, which are the anatomic and functional units of the liver. Key structures in each lobule are the portal triads, central veins, hepatic cords, bile canaliculi, and hepatic sinusoids (see Figure 1-15). The portal triads are located at the corners of each lobule. Each triad consists of a portal vein branch, a hepatic artery branch, and a bile duct, as well as nerves and lymphatics. The portal vein and hepatic artery branches supply blood flow to the liver, and the bile duct collects bile for transport out of the liver. The central vein is located in the center of each lobule and provides venous drainage; the central veins empty into the hepatic veins, which drain into the inferior vena cava. Hepatic cords are columns of hepatocytes, the functional cells of the liver; each lobule has numerous columns, or cords, of liver cells. The bile canaliculi are tiny bile capillaries located between the columns of hepatocytes; they collect the bile and transport it to the bile ducts in the portal triads. The sinusoids are blood channels that lie between the columns of hepatocytes. The sinusoids are lined with a thin squamous endothelium composed primarily of phago-cytic cells (Kupffer cells), which can engulf bacteria. Blood entering the lobule through branches of the portal vein and the hepatic artery drains into the sinusoids; blood from the sinusoids then drains into the central vein. Bile flows in the opposite direction, from the canaliculi in the lobule to the bile ducts in the portal triads and toward the hepatic duct at the porta hepatis.

Function

The liver plays a role in metabolic functions, bile production, storage of vitamins and minerals, coagulation, and detoxification.

Metabolic Functions

The liver is involved in the metabolism of all three major nutrients (carbohydrates, fats, and proteins). Its most important contribution to carbohydrate metabolism is its function as a glucose buffer; through the processes of glycogen storage, glycogenolysis, and gluconeogenesis, the liver helps maintain normal blood glucose levels. When the blood glucose level is low, the liver releases stored glucose (glycogenolysis); the liver also can convert amino acids into glucose (gluconeogenesis) if necessary to restore normal blood glucose levels. When blood glucose levels rise, the liver can convert glucose, fructose, and galactose to glycogen, thus restoring blood glucose levels to normal.

Fat metabolism occurs in cells throughout the body, but some components of fat metabolism occur much more rapidly in the liver than anywhere else. The liver can rapidly oxidize fatty acids to produce substances that can enter the citric acid cycle, where they are further oxidized to produce tremendous amounts of energy. The liver is also responsible for synthesis of cholesterol and phospholipids; phospholipids are essential components of cell membranes and are formed by combining fats with choline and phosphorus. An additional role of the liver is to convert carbohydrates and proteins to fat for storage in the adipose tissue.

The liver's role in protein metabolism is so important that serious morbidity or even mortality can occur within a few days after loss of these functions. One important function is deamination of amino acids, which must occur before the amino acids can be used for energy or converted into carbohydrates or fats. Another critical function is formation of urea, which removes ammonia from the bloodstream. Ammonia is continually produced by the colonic bacteria and is then absorbed into the bloodstream; ammonia is not

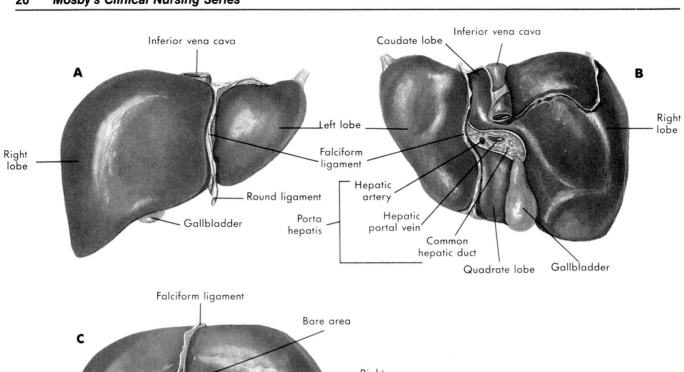

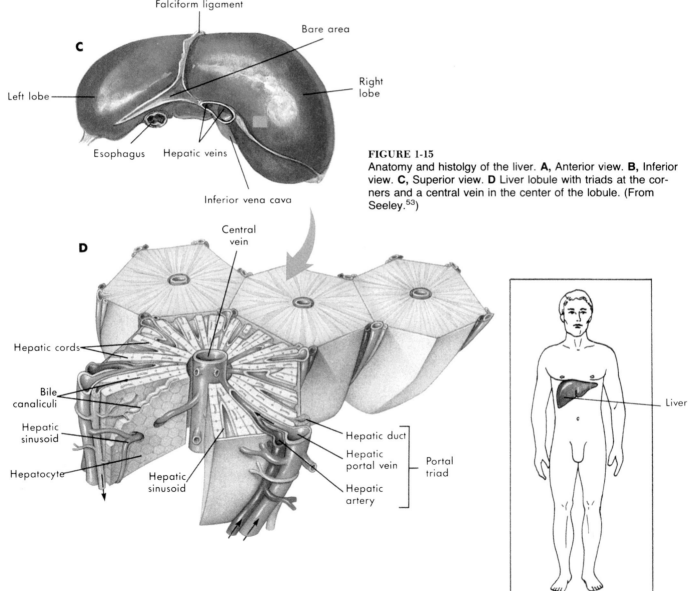

FIGURE 1-15
Anatomy and histolgy of the liver. **A,** Anterior view. **B,** Inferior view. **C,** Superior view. **D** Liver lobule with triads at the corners and a central vein in the center of the lobule. (From Seeley.[53])

readily eliminated by the kidneys, and high plasma ammonia levels are toxic and can result in hepatic coma or even death. Normally, however, all venous drainage from the colon empties into the portal system for delivery to the liver, where the hepatocytes remove the ammonia and convert it to urea, which is readily excreted by the kidneys. A third critical function performed by the liver is synthesis of plasma proteins; about 90% of the plasma proteins are produced by the liver. The plasma proteins play a major role in maintaining intravascular osmotic pressure, which in turn maintains intravascular volume and prevents abnormal shifts of intravascular fluid into the interstitial spaces. Patients with low levels of serum albumin usually have significant dependent edema, caused by a shift of fluid from the bloodstream into the tissues. Finally, the liver can synthesize needed amino acids and can convert amino acids into lipids or glucose.

Bile Production

One of the liver's most important functions is bile production. Bile is composed of bile salts, bilirubin, cholesterol, lecithin, electrolytes, and water. The usual daily volume of bile production is 600 to 1,000 ml.

Bile production is important in promoting digestion of fats and fat-soluble vitamins; bile production also provides for the excretion of bilirubin and the secretion of cholesterol. (The role of bile in the digestion and absorption of fats was described earlier in this chapter.) Absorption of the fat-soluble vitamins A, D, E, and K depends on absorption of fats; thus bile production is important in maintaining normal levels of these vitamins. This is particularly significant for maintaining adequate levels of vitamin K, a critical component of the clotting mechanism, because vitamin K is not stored in the body, unlike vitamins A, D, and E. An individual can develop a vitamin K deficiency within a few days after bile production stops.

Production of bile also provides a mechanism for excretion of bilirubin, one of the end products of hemoglobin breakdown. As red blood cells reach the end of their life cycle and rupture, they release hemoglobin, which is phagocytized to produce heme and globin. The heme ring breaks down and produces the pigment bilirubin, which combines with plasma albumin for transport in plasma and body fluids. The bilirubin is absorbed into the hepatocytes, where it is bound (conjugated) to other substances. This conjugated bilirubin is secreted by active transport into the bile canaliculi and is then transported through the bile ducts to the intestine, where bacterial action converts it to urobilinogen; small amounts of conjugated bilirubin are also absorbed into the bloodstream. Thus the bilirubin in the bloodstream is primarily of the unconjugated type, although small amounts of conjugated bilirubin are also present. Differentiation between free (unconjugated) bilirubin and conjugated bilirubin is an important diagnostic clue in cases of elevated bilirubin levels. Hemolytic disorders result in increased levels of *unconjugated* bilirubin, whereas obstructive syndromes cause increased levels of *conjugated* bilirubin.

Production of bile salts requires cholesterol, and some cholesterol is secreted into the bile. Cholesterol is almost insoluble in water, but in bile it is combined with bile salts and lecithin, which renders it soluble. Gallstones may develop when conditions cause precipitation of the cholesterol.

Storage of Vitamins and Minerals

The liver can store large amounts of vitamins A, D, and B_{12}; these liver "stores" prevent deficiency states for months or even 1 to 2 years. Iron is also stored in large amounts in the liver, in the form of ferritin, and is released when the body's iron is low.

Coagulation

The liver synthesizes a number of the clotting factors and is also responsible for bile production, which is required for absorption of vitamin K. The liver requires vitamin K to produce the clotting factors. In the absence of vitamin K, production of clotting factors is very limited and coagulation is severely compromised.

Detoxification

The liver is responsible for detoxifying or excreting a number of drugs and hormones; this explains why individuals with compromised liver function frequently require changes in medication to prevent toxicity.

Blood Flow and Innervation

The liver receives its blood supply from both the portal vein and the hepatic artery; blood flow averages 1,500 ml per minute, with 30% being delivered by the hepatic artery and 70% by the portal vein.

Venous drainage from the liver is provided by the hepatic vein, which drains into the vena cava. The pressure in the hepatic vein usually averages 0 mm Hg, which illustrates the low resistance to flow normally offered by the sinusoids. Any rise in hepatic vein pressure causes increased resistance to venous drainage; blood pools in the sinusoids, and the liver swells. This is common in right-sided heart failure, where elevated central venous pressure causes marked hepatomegaly stemming from vascular congestion.

Lymphatic Drainage

The endothelial lining of the sinusoids has very large pores, which permit large molecular substances such as proteins to pass through the endothelium into narrow spaces called Disse's spaces; these spaces connect directly with terminal lymphatic vessels, which absorb any proteins or fluid draining into Disse's spaces. One third to one half of all lymph formed in the body is formed in the liver.

GALLBLADDER

The gallbladder is the organ responsible for storing and concentrating bile and for delivering it to the small intestine.

The gallbladder is a pear-shaped sac 7.6 to 10 cm long that is attached to the inferior surface of the liver (Figure 1-16). The gallbladder empties into the cystic duct, which joins the hepatic duct to form the common bile duct. The common bile duct joins the pancreatic duct to empty into the duodenum at Vater's ampulla.

The liver constantly produces bile, which is delivered to the gallbladder through the cystic duct from the hepatic duct. Average daily production of bile far exceeds the gallbladder's storage capacity, which is about 40 to 70 ml; however, the gallbladder reabsorbs water and electrolytes from the bile, concentrating the bile salts and bile pigments fivefold to tenfold. Contraction of the gallbladder forces the concentrated bile through the cystic duct and common bile duct into the duodenum.

Blood Supply and Innervation

The gallbladder and biliary tree are innervated by the autonomic nervous system. Parasympathetic innervation causes the gallbladder to contract; sympathetic stimulation inhibits gallbladder contraction. Afferent fibers from the gallbladder follow the same course as the splanchnic nerves and the right phrenic nerve; the referred pain in the right shoulder associated with pathologic conditions of the gallbladder is explained by this shared course with the right phrenic nerve.

PANCREAS

The pancreas contributes significantly to the digestive process and performs essential endocrine functions.

The pancreas is approximately 25 cm long and lies in a transverse position in the posterior aspect of the upper abdominal cavity. It can be divided into three major areas: the head, which lies within the curve of the duodenum (see Figure 1-9); the body, posterior to the stomach; and the tail, which extends to the spleen.

The pancreas is composed of both endocrine and exocrine tissues. The bulk of the gland is made up of exocrine units and the ductal system, with endocrine units scattered among the exocrine units. The exocrine units are the acini, which are groups of cells that produce digestive enzymes. Clusters of acini form lobules, which are separated from each other by thin walls known as septa. Secretions drain into intercalated ducts located between the acini; these ducts are lined with secretory columnar epithelium. The intercalated ducts connect to intralobular ducts, which drain into interlobular ducts between the lobules (Figure 1-17). The interlobular ducts empty into the pancreatic duct running the length of the pancreas; the pancreatic duct joins the common bile duct to empty into the duodenum through the sphincter of Oddi at Vater's ampulla.

The endocrine units of the pancreas are the islets of Langerhans, which are clusters of endocrine cells; normally there are 500,000 to 1 million islets. These pancreatic islets contain both alpha and beta cells; alpha cells produce glucagon, and beta cells produce insulin. There is a third cell type, which may represent immature cells or may be delta cells, which secrete somatostatin. The endocrine secretions of the pancreas empty directly into the bloodstream.

Exocrine functions of the pancreas include production of an aqueous alkaline solution to neutralize duodenal contents, and production of an enzymatic solution capable of digesting fats, carbohydrates, and proteins. The total volume of pancreatic juice produced daily averages about 1,500 ml. Endocrine functions include production of glucagon, which raises blood sugar levels, and insulin, which lowers blood sugar levels.

Exocrine Functions

The delivery of acidic chyme to the duodenum stimulates the release of secretin from the mucosa of the proximal small intestine. Secretin stimulates the pancreas to produce large volumes of a watery, bicarbonate-rich solution; the key components of this solution, bicarbonate ions and water, are secreted by the epithelial cells lining the small pancreatic ductules. This very alkaline solution combines with the acidic chyme to neutralize it, which is a very important function because (1) the elevated pH inactivates the gastric enzyme pepsin, thus protecting the duodenal mucosa from ulceration, and (2) the elevated pH provides the optimum environment for the digestive activity of pancreatic enzymes.

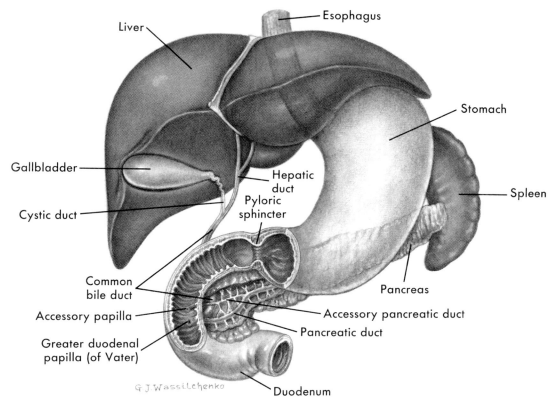

FIGURE 1-16
Liver, gallbladder, and pancreas. (From Thompson.[57])

The pancreas produces the key enzymes required for digestion of proteins, fats, and carbohydrates. These enzymes are secreted by the acini in response to neural and hormonal stimuli. Vagal stimuli cause moderate enzyme production; however, the major stimulus for secretion of enzymes is the hormone cholecystokinin, which is released from the duodenal mucosa in response to the presence of chyme in the duodenum. Cholecystokinin is produced in the greatest quantities when the chyme contains products of protein digestion.

The proteolytic enzymes have the potential to cause autodigestion of the pancreas, but two mechanisms prevent this: (1) The proteolytic enzymes are produced in precursor forms (i.e., trypsinogen, chymotrypsinogen, and procarboxypolypeptidase) that are enzymatically inactive; trypsinogen normally is activated in the duodenum and activated trypsin then activates the other precursor enzymes. (2) The acinar cells secrete a substance known as trypsin inhibitor, which prevents activation of trypsin within the pancreatic cells and ducts. These two mechanisms ensure that

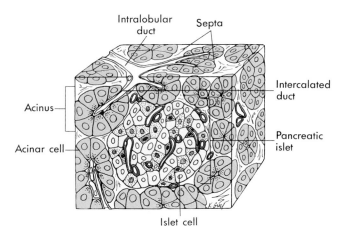

FIGURE 1-17
Histology of the pancreas, showing both the acini and the pancreatic ducts. (From Seeley.[53])

under normal conditions, the powerful pancreatic enzymes will not damage the pancreas.

The importance of pancreatic enzymes to nutrient digestion is underscored by the fact that loss of pancreatic function usually necessitates exogenous administration of pancreatic enzymes.

Endocrine Functions

The pancreas produces the hormones glucagon and insulin and may produce somatostatin. Glucagon is produced by the alpha cells in response to low blood glucose levels and sympathetic stimulation; glucagon stimulates glycogenolysis, the breakdown of glycogen to release glucose, and also increases glucose synthesis in the liver. Thus glucagon raises the blood glucose

levels. Insulin is produced by the beta cells in response to hyperglycemia, certain amino acids, parasympathetic stimulation, and gastrointestinal hormones. Insulin promotes uptake of glucose and amino acids by skeletal muscle, the liver, and adipose tissue; it also increases glucose uptake by the satiety center, which regulates appetite. Somatostatin has an inhibiting effect on gastrointestinal secretion, although factors regulating its production have not been clearly identified. Somatostatin has been used to reduce intestinal secretions for patients with small bowel fistulas.

Pancreatic endocrine function is essential to life; its loss requires exogenous administration of insulin and careful regulation of glucose intake.

CHAPTER 2

Assessment

HISTORY

The first step in assessment is the patient interview, which provides information about the patient's past and present health status from the patient's perspective. This subjective information is as important to effective care as is the most objective diagnostic data, and it can be obtained only through the interview process.

Historical data to be gathered specific to the gastrointestinal system are outlined in the box on the next page.

PRESENT PROBLEM

The patient's present problem must be thoroughly investigated. General data on any dysfunction or patient concern should include onset, duration, severity, associated factors, associated symptomatology, and exacerbating and relieving factors. Factors to be assessed for common presenting problems are briefly outlined.

Weight Loss

What is your usual weight? How much weight have you lost? In what time period? Was the weight loss deliberate or spontaneous? For deliberate weight loss: Describe your weight loss program (diet plan used, exercise program, use of support groups, weight goal). For

spontaneous weight loss: What other symptoms have you experienced (e.g., excessive thirst and urination, anorexia, nausea, vomiting, diarrhea)? What are the time frame and severity of the associated symptoms? Is your weight loss associated with a change in life-style, activity, or stress? Can you prepare your own meals, or do you have someone who does it for you? Does your income limit the kinds and amount of food you buy?

In assessing the patient with deliberate weight loss, the nurse must also evaluate the patient's concerns and perceptions about his or her weight and body dimensions. The nurse should explore the patient's use of excessive weight control behavior such as fasting, binge and purge cycles, excessive exercise, and excessive caloric restrictions.

Weight Gain

What is your usual weight? How much weight have you gained? Over what time period? Was the weight gain spontaneous or planned? Is the weight gain associated with a change in meal preparation patterns, eating patterns, exercise patterns, or stress? For premenopausal women: Is pregnancy a possibility? What concerns do you have about this weight gain?

HEALTH HISTORY

Demographic data

(Name, address, phone number, birthdate, sex, race, marital status, occupation, education, religious preference)

Chief complaint/reason for visit

(In patient's own words)

Present problem/current health status

Description to include onset, duration, severity, associated factors, associated symptoms, exacerbating or relieving factors, patient's concerns

Medical history

Chronic illnesses
Previous weight gain or loss
Tooth extractions or orthodontic work
Gastrointestinal disorders (e.g., peptic ulcer, inflammatory bowel disease, polyps, cholelithiasis, diverticular disease, pancreatitis, intestinal obstruction)
Hepatitis or cirrhosis
Abdominal surgery
Abdominal trauma
Cancer affecting gastrointestinal system
Spinal cord injury
Women: Episiotomy or fourth-degree laceration during delivery

Family history

(Investigate for history of following disorders, and document [+] or [−] responses)
Hirschsprung's disease
Obesity
Metabolic disorders
Inflammatory disorders
Malabsorption syndromes
Familial Mediterranean fever
Rectal polyps
Polyposis syndromes
Cancer of the GI tract

Personal and social history

Dietary habits
    Usual number of meals or snacks per day
    Usual fluid intake per day
Exercise patterns
Oral care patterns
    Frequency of toothbrushing/denture care
    Frequency of flossing
Alcohol intake (frequency and usual amounts)

Review of gastrointestinal system
General data

Usual height and weight
Nutrient intake
    Types of food usually eaten at each meal or snack
    Food likes and dislikes
    Religious or medical food restrictions
    Food intolerances
    Patient's perceptions and concerns about adequacy of diet and appropriateness of weight
    Effects of life-style on food intake, weight gain or loss
    Vitamins or nutritional supplements (type, amount, frequency)
Oral hygiene
    Last visit to dentist
    Presence of braces, dentures, bridges, or crowns
Bowel elimination
    Usual frequency of bowel movements
    Usual consistency and color of stool
    Ability to control elimination of gas and stool
    Any changes in bowel elimination patterns
    Use of enemas or laxatives (reason for use, frequency, type, response)
Medications (e.g., laxatives, stool softeners, antiemetics, antidiarrheals, antacids, frequent or high doses of aspirin, acetaminophen, corticosteroids)

Specific data

Oral lesions
Appetite
Digestion or indigestion (heartburn)
Dysphagia
Nausea
Vomiting
Hematemesis
Change in stool color or contents (clay colored, tarry, fresh blood, mucus, undigested food)
Constipation
Diarrhea
Flatulence
Hemorrhoids
Abdominal pain
Hepatitis
Jaundice
Ulcers
Gallstones
Polyps
Tumors
Anal discomfort
Fecal incontinence
Exposure to infectious agents (e.g., foreign travel, water source, other exposure)

Table 2-1

COMMON CONDITIONS PRODUCING ABDOMINAL PAIN*

Condition	Usual pain characteristics	Possible associated findings
Appendicitis	Initially periumbilical or epigastric pain; colicky; later becomes localized to RLQ, often at McBurney's point	Guarding, tenderness; + iliopsoas and + obturator signs, RLQ skin hyperesthesia; anorexia, nausea, or vomiting after onset of pain; low-grade fever
Cholecystitis	Severe, unrelenting RUQ or epigastric pain; may be referred to right subscapular area	RUQ tenderness and rigidity, + Murphy's sign, palpable gallbladder, anorexia, vomiting, fever, possible jaundice
Pancreatitis	Dramatic, sudden, excruciating LUQ, epigastric, or umbilical pain; may be present in one or both flanks; may be referred to left shoulder	Epigastric tenderness, vomiting, fever, shock; + Grey Turner's sign (blue/green discoloration on flank); + Cullen's sign (bluish discoloration around umbilicus): both signs occur 2-3 days after onset
Perforated gastric or duodenal ulcer	Abrupt RUQ pain; may be referred to shoulders	Abdominal free air and distention with increased resonance over liver; tenderness in epigastrium or RUQ; rigid abdominal wall, rebound tenderness
Diverticulitis	Epigastric pain, radiating down left side of abdomen especially after eating; may be referred to back	Flatulence, borborygmi, diarrhea, dysuria, tenderness on palpation
Intestinal obstruction	Abrupt, severe, spasmodic pain; referred to epigastrium, umbilicus	Distention, minimal rebound tenderness, vomiting, localized tenderness, visible peristalsis; bowel sounds absent (with paralytic obstruction) or hyperactive and high pitched (with mechanical obstruction)
Volvulus	Pain referred to hypogastrium and umbilicus	Distention, nausea, vomiting, guarding; sigmoid loop volvulus may be palpable
Leaking abdominal aneurysm	Steady, throbbing, midline pain over aneurysm; may radiate to back, flank	Nausea, vomiting, abdominal mass, bruit
Biliary stones, colic	Episodic, severe, RUQ or epigastric pain lasting 15 min to several hours; may be referred to subscapular area, especially right	RUQ tenderness, soft abdominal wall, anorexia, vomiting, jaundice, subnormal temperature
Splenic rupture	Intense LUQ pain, radiating to left shoulder (+ Kehr's sign); may worsen with foot of bed elevated	Shock, pallor, lowered temperature

*+, Positive; *RLQ*, right lower quadrant; *RUQ*, right upper quadrant; *LUQ*, left upper quadrant.
(From Seidel.)

Abdominal Pain

When did the pain start? Did it begin gradually or suddenly? Is it constant or does it come and go? How frequently does it occur? Have you had this kind of pain before? Is it related to anything else you are aware of (e.g., menstrual cycle, bowel movements, urinating, breathing, food or alcohol intake, change in position, stress, medications, time of day)? Describe the pain (i.e., dull, sharp, burning, gnawing, stabbing, cramping, aching, colicky). Point to the area where the pain is most intense. Does it spread to any other areas? If so, point to those areas. Has the location changed since the pain started? Do you have any other symptoms associated with the pain (e.g., nausea, vomiting, diarrhea, constipation, flatulence, belching, jaundice, fainting, increase in size of abdomen, fever)? Does anything relieve the pain? Have you been exposed to anyone with the same type of symptoms?

In assessing the patient with pain, it is very important to obtain complete data and to have the patient identify the location as accurately as possible. The location of the pain is a major diagnostic clue. Table 2-1 correlates the location of pain with the possible pathologic conditions.

Indigestion

Describe what you mean by indigestion (e.g., feeling of fullness, heartburn, discomfort, belching, flatulence, loss of appetite, severe pain). Where is the discomfort located (generalized or localized)? Does the discomfort radiate (spread)? If so, to where? Is the discomfort associated with any factors you are aware of (e.g., eating specific types or amounts of food)? When does the discomfort occur (i.e., time of day or night)? Does the discomfort begin gradually or suddenly? What relieves the discomfort (e.g., antacids, rest, activity)? For premenopausal women: Is pregnancy a possibility?

Nausea

Is the nausea associated with vomiting? What factors seem to trigger the nausea (e.g., odors, activities, food intake, time of day)? For premenopausal women: Is pregnancy a possibility?

Vomiting

Describe the emesis (i.e., color, undigested food particles, fresh blood, "coffee ground" appearance). When did the vomiting begin? Is it persistent, or does it come and go? How often do you vomit? How much do you vomit? Can you keep any solids or liquids on your stomach? Is the vomiting associated with any of the following: food intake, anorexia, nausea, diarrhea or constipation, abdominal pain, fever, weight loss, headache, medications? For premenopausal women: Is pregnancy a possibility?

Diarrhea

Describe the stools (i.e., color, presence of blood, mucus, undigested food, fat, odor, volume, consistency). How many diarrheal stools are you having a day? How long have you been having diarrhea? Is the diarrhea related to eating in general, or to eating specific foods? Is the diarrhea related to stress? Is the diarrhea associated with any of the following: abdominal pain or cramping, chills, fever, thirst, weight loss, nausea or vomiting, or fecal incontinence? Have you traveled out of the country recently? How have you been managing the diarrhea?

Constipation

Describe your usual bowel elimination pattern (i.e., frequency of bowel movements and consistency of stool). Has there been a change in the frequency of your bowel movements or in the size and consistency of your stools? When was your last bowel movement? What was the consistency of the stool? Was it painful to pass the stool? Do you alternate between diarrhea and constipation? Are you having abdominal pain or discomfort? Do you have any abdominal swelling? Describe the color of the stool (i.e., brown, streaked with bright blood, dark black or "tarry," clay colored). Has there been any change in your diet or fluid intake? How much fiber do you get in your diet? How have you been managing the constipation?

Fecal Incontinence

Describe your usual bowel elimination pattern (i.e., frequency of bowel movements and consistency of stool). When did you begin having problems with fecal incontinence? Is this a persistent problem, or does it come and go? Do you have voluntary controlled bowel movements also? If yes, how often, and what is the consistency of the stool? How often do the incontinent episodes occur, and what is the consistency of the stool? Does the incontinence occur without warning, or are you aware of rectal filling? Is the incontinence related to intake of specific foods or fluids or to immobility? Is the incontinence associated with use of laxatives or an underlying disease (e.g., inflammatory bowel disease, cancer, diverticular disease, diabetic neuropathy, multiple sclerosis)? How have you been managing the incontinence? How much fiber do you ingest daily? How much fluid do you drink daily?

Rectal Bleeding

When did you first notice rectal bleeding? Was the blood bright red, dark red, or black? Describe the amount of blood (i.e., spotting on toilet paper or active bleeding). Is the bleeding associated with bowel movements? Does the bleeding come and go, or is it persistent? Is there mucus in the stool? Have there been any changes in your stool (e.g., change in color, consistency, size and shape, odor, frequency of bowel movements)? Do you have any of the following symptoms: rectal pain, abdominal pain or cramping, abdominal swelling, weight loss, fever, increased gas, incontinence?

Anal Discomfort

Describe the discomfort (i.e., itching, pain, stinging, burning). Is the discomfort related to position (e.g., standing, sitting, lying) or to bowel movements? Do you pass your stools easily, or do you have to strain to pass the stool? Are you passing mucus or blood through your anus? Does the discomfort interfere with your daily activities or with sleep?

Jaundice

When did you first notice the jaundice? Are you having any abdominal pain, chills, fever, loss of appetite, nausea, vomiting, or abdominal swelling? Describe the color of your stools and urine. Have you been exposed to hepatitis? Have you used intravenous drugs? Have you had any blood transfusions?

MEDICAL HISTORY

In discussing the patient's medical history, the nurse should elicit information about current medications and past illnesses, surgeries, or trauma affecting the gastrointestinal tract or abdominal cavity. A history of abdominal surgery alerts the nurse to the potential for adhesions that may be causing obstruction. Chronic use of aspirin or steroids can cause gastritis or peptic ulcer. Chronic use of laxatives may result in reduced peristaltic activity and constipation. Spinal cord lesions frequently are associated with fecal incontinence as a result of disruption of vital nerve pathways. Episiotomies or fourth-degree lacerations can cause direct damage to the anal sphincter or may damage the nerves controlling rectal sensation and sphincter function.

FAMILY HISTORY

The nurse should explore the patient's family history for evidence of illnesses and conditions affecting the gastrointestinal system that are known or thought to have familial tendencies. Pertinent negatives, as well as positive findings, should be documented. (For example, in documenting the family history of an obese patient, an appropriate note would be: No family history of obesity or metabolic disorder.)

PERSONAL AND SOCIAL HISTORY

The nurse should ask about daily routines and habits that affect gastrointestinal functioning, specifically oral care, nutrient and fluid intake, and exercise patterns. The patient should also be questioned about patterns of alcohol intake, because excessive or frequent alcohol intake can contribute to gastritis, liver disease, and malnutrition. Issues related to alcohol intake are sensitive ones, and the nurse must use a matter-of-fact approach that is nonjudgmental and conveys concern for the patient's well-being.

REVIEW OF GASTROINTESTINAL SYSTEM FUNCTIONING

In completing the systems review, the nurse should ask specific questions about functional status and symptomatology, which may elicit additional information not obtained during the discussion of the patient's current problem. As outlined in the box on page 26, the focus in this review is on patterns of nutrient intake and bowel elimination, and on specific indicators of gastrointestinal dysfunction.

PHYSICAL ASSESSMENT

Physical assessment of gastrointestinal functioning includes attention to nutritional status, the abdomen, the rectum, and anus. Techniques used include inspection, palpation, auscultation, and percussion; required equipment includes a standing platform scale with height attachment, skin fold thickness calipers, measuring tape, stethoscope, examining gloves, and lubricant.

NUTRITIONAL STATUS

Assessment of nutritional status involves anthropometric measurements and inspection for signs of nutritional deficiency.

Anthropometric Measurements

The most commonly used anthropometric measurements are height, weight, triceps skin fold thickness, and midarm muscle circumference.

Height and weight

The patient's height and weight are obtained on a standing platform scale with height attachment. The findings can be used to compute the patient's ideal body weight (see the following box).

Triceps skin fold thickness

The triceps skin fold thickness may be measured when there is concern regarding obesity, because this measurement correlates with the body's fat content. The procedure for measuring triceps skin fold thickness is as follows: (1) The patient is asked to flex the left arm at a right angle. The examiner stands behind the patient and makes a horizontal mark halfway between the olecranon process (shoulder) and the acromion process (elbow) on the posterior aspect of the arm; a vertical line is then drawn to intersect the horizontal line at midpoint (Figure 2-1, *A* and *B*). (2) The patient is instructed to allow the arm to hang down in a relaxed position. Using thumb and forefinger, the examiner grasps the triceps skin fold about 1 cm proximal to the marked "X." The examiner must ensure that the bulk of the triceps muscle can be felt deep to the skin fold. (3) The caliper jaws are placed on each side of the raised skin fold at

---

DETERMINING IDEAL BODY WEIGHT BASED ON HEIGHT*

Women

45 kg (100 lbs) for the first 150 cm (5 ft), plus 2.25 kg (5 lbs) for each additional 2.5 cm (inch)

Men

47.7 kg (106 lbs) for the first 150 cm (5 ft), plus 2.7 kg (6 lbs) for each additional 2.5 cm (inch)

*Yields ideal body weight ± 10%.

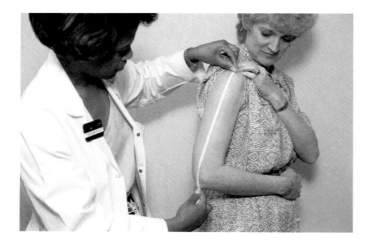

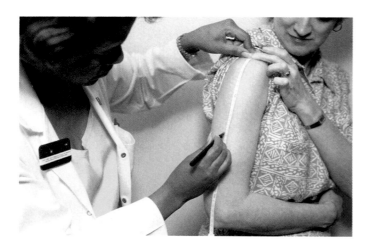

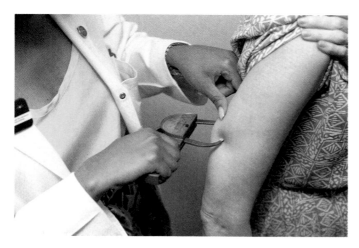

FIGURE 2-1
Placement of calipers for triceps skinfold thickness measurement.

the level of the marked "X" (Figure 2-1 *C*). The calipers should not be tight enough to cause an indentation. (4) Two measurements are taken and averaged.

Midarm muscle circumference. Midarm muscle circumference may be measured when malnutrition is a concern, because this measurement is an indicator of muscle mass and available fat and protein stores. To obtain this measurement, the examiner places a measuring tape around the upper arm midway between the olecranon process and the acromion process (at the point used to measure the triceps skin fold).

Normal findings

Normal findings for anthropometric measurements include: weight normal for height; triceps skin fold measurement under 15 mm in men and 25 mm in women; midarm muscle circumference of above 29.3 cm for men and above 28.5 cm for women.

Variations

Body weight 20% or more over ideal weight with a triceps skin fold measurement over 15 mm in men or 25 mm in women indicates obesity. Body weight 20% or more under ideal weight with a midarm muscle circumference under 20.5 cm in men or 20 cm in women indicates malnutrition.

Inspection

The nurse should inspect the patient's hair, skin, eyes, lips, tongue, mucous membranes, gums, abdomen, and muscles for indicators of nutritional status.

Normal findings

A well-nourished patient has shiny hair; smooth, supple skin; clear eyes; pink, moist mucous membranes with normal papillae evident on the tongue; firm, pink gums; a flat abdomen; and firm, well-developed muscles.

Variations

The following findings indicate malnutrition: dry, easily pluckable hair; dull or dry eyes with conjunctival lesions; swollen, beefy red tongue with fissures and loss of papillae; atrophy of the gums or swollen, bleeding gums; dry, scaly skin; skin ulcerations over pressure points or other areas exposed to friction or maceration; protuberant abdomen; pretibial edema; flaccid or wasted muscles.

ABDOMEN

Most of the organs in the gastrointestinal tract are located in the abdominal cavity (Figure 2-2); therefore the major focus of the physical assessment is on inspection, auscultation, percussion, and palpation of the abdomen. The usual order of physical assessment is inspection, palpation, percussion, and auscultation; the order is altered in abdominal assessment because palpation and percussion can alter the auscultatory findings.

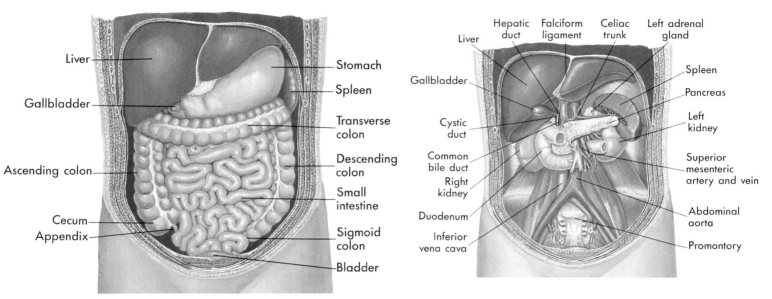

FIGURE 2-2
Organs of the abdominal cavity. (From Seidel.[52])

In conducting and documenting the physical assessment, the abdomen usually is divided into four quadrants or nine regions. The quadrant method is the more common; one imaginary line is drawn from the sternum through the umbilicus to the pubis, and a second imaginary line is drawn horizontally across the abdomen through the umbilicus (Figure 2-3). To divide the abdomen into nine regions, two imaginary horizontal lines are drawn, one across the inferior aspect of the costal margin and the other across the edge of the iliac crest. Two vertical lines are then drawn to intersect the horizontal lines; these lines are drawn bilaterally from the midclavicular line to the center of Poupart's ligament (Figure 2-4). To accurately correlate physical findings with pathologic conditions, the examiner must consistently use one of the two methods and must be able to mentally visualize the organs in each of the anatomic regions. See the following boxes for correlation of abdominal organs and the various regions or quadrants.

Before the physical examination is begun, the patient is asked to empty the bladder. The examiner must ensure the patient's privacy and warmth and should drape the patient to fully expose the abdomen without unnecessarily exposing the breasts or genitalia. The patient is placed in the supine position with arms resting at the sides. Putting a small pillow under the head and another under the slightly flexed knees promotes relax-

Text cont'd. on p. 33.

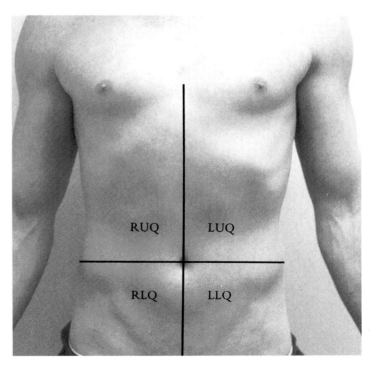

FIGURE 2-3
Four quadrants of the abdomen. **RUQ,** right upper quadrant, **LUQ,** left upper quadrant, **RLQ,** right lower quadrant, **LLQ,** left lower quadrant. (From Seidel.[52])

ANATOMIC CORRELATES OF THE FOUR QUADRANTS OF THE ABDOMEN

Right upper quadrant

Liver and gallbladder
Pylorus
Duodenum
Head of pancreas
Right adrenal gland
Portion of right kidney
Hepatic flexure of colon
Portions of ascending and transverse
  colon

Right lower quadrant

Lower pole of right kidney
Cecum and appendix
Portion of ascending colon
Bladder (if distended)
Ovary and salpinx
Uterus (if enlarged)
Right spermatic cord
Right ureter

(From Malasanos.)

Left upper quadrant

Left lobe of liver
Spleen
Stomach
Body of pancreas
Left adrenal gland
Portion of left kidney
Splenic flexure of colon
Portions of transverse and descend-
  ing colon

Left lower quadrant

Lower pole of left kidney
Sigmoid colon
Portion of descending colon
Bladder (if distended)
Ovary and salpinx
Uterus (if enlarged)
Left spermatic cord
Left ureter

ANATOMIC CORRELATES OF THE NINE REGIONS OF THE ABDOMEN

Right hypochondriac

Right lobe of liver
Gallbladder
Portion of duodenum
Hepatic flexure of colon
Portion of right kidney
Suprarenal gland

Right lumbar

Ascending colon
Lower half of right kidney
Portion of duodenum and
  jejunum

Right inguinal

Cecum
Appendix
Lower end of ileum
Right ureter
Right spermatic cord
Right ovary

(From Malasanos.)

Epigastric

Pyloric end of stomach
Duodenum
Pancreas
Portion of liver

Umbilical

Omentum
Mesentery
Lower part of
  duodenum
Jejunum and ileum

Hypogastric (pubic)

Ileum
Bladder
Uterus (in
  pregnancy)

Left hypochondriac

Stomach
Spleen
Tail of pancreas
Splenic flexure of colon
Upper pole of left kidney
Suprarenal gland

Left lumbar

Descending colon
Lower half of left kidney
Portions of jejunum and
  ileum

Left inguinal

Sigmoid colon
Left ureter
Left spermatic cord
Left ovary

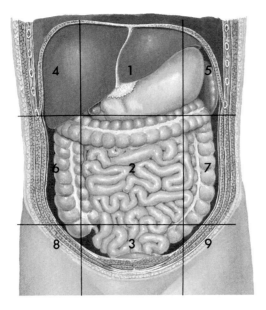

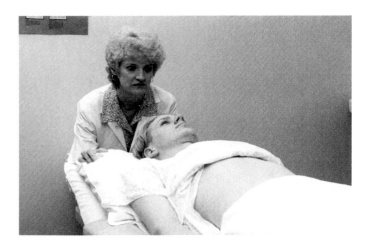

FIGURE 2-4
Nine regions of the abdomen. **1,** Epigastric; **2,** umbilical; **3,** hypogastric (pubic); **4** and **5,** right and left hpochondriac; **6** and **7,** right and left lumbar; **8** and **9,** right and left inquinal. (From Seidel.[52])

ation of the abdominal muscles, which facilitates examination of the underlying organs. The examiner explains the assessment process and has the patient identify any areas of tenderness; these should be examined last.

Inspection

The examiner sits at the patient's side and inspects the abdominal surface for color, lesions, scars, contour, symmetry, and surface motion. The examiner then shifts to a standing position behind the patient's head and again assesses symmetry, carefully observing for distention or asymmetric bulges (Figure 2-5). The patient is asked to take a deep breath and hold it; this lowers the diaphragm and compresses the organs of the abdominal cavity, which may increase visibility of any abdominal masses. The patient is then asked to lift his or her head from the table, which contracts the abdominal muscles; this may cause superficial abdominal wall masses and hernias to become visible, especially in thin or athletic adults.

Normal findings

The color and texture of the abdominal skin usually are comparable to the skin on other parts of the body, although it may be paler than skin exposed to the sun. It is normal to observe a fine venous network; the direction of venous return is toward the head above the umbilicus and toward the feet below the umbilicus

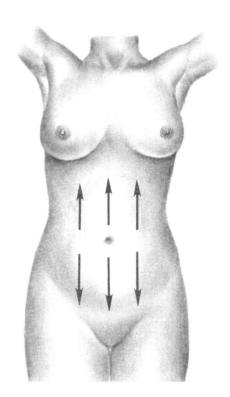

FIGURE 2-6
Normal pattern of abdominal venous flow. (From Seidel.[52])

(Figure 2-6). To evaluate the direction of venous return, the examiner places the index fingers side by side over a vein and then separates the fingers while pressing laterally, which compresses and empties a section of vein. One finger is released, and refill is timed; then the other finger is released, and the refill is timed. The direction of faster refill is the direction of venous return.

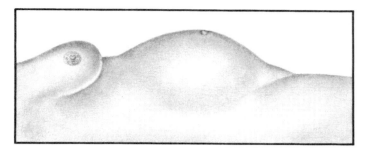

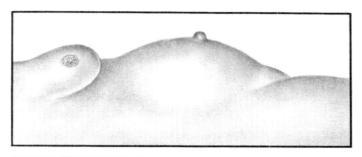

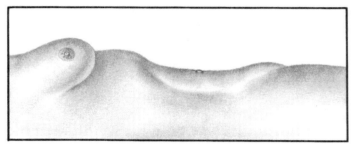

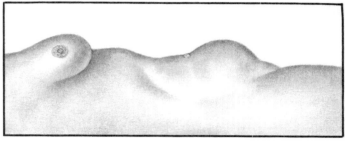

FIGURE 2-7
A, Rounded abdominal contours. **B,** Scaphoid abdominal contours. (From Seidel.[52])

FIGURE 2-8
A, Generalized abdominal distention. **B,** Abdominal distention involving lower one third of abdomen, from umbilicus to symphysis pubis. (From Seidel.[52])

Normally no lesions or nodules are present.

Abdominal contours normally are symmetric and remain so with inspiration and contraction of abdominal muscles. Abdominal contours may be described as flat, rounded, or scaphoid. Flat contours are most commonly seen in athletic adults with good muscle tone. Rounded contours in adults usually indicate excessive subcutaneous fat or poor muscle tone (Figure 2-7, *A*). The scaphoid abdomen is concave and usually seen in thin adults (Figure 2-7, *B*).

The abdomen is inspected for motion occurring with respiration. Normally respiratory movements are smooth and even; women primarily exhibit chest, or costal, movements, whereas men primarily exhibit abdominal movements. In thin adults aortic pulsation may also be visible in the upper midline.

Variations

Variations in color and texture may be generalized or localized. Generalized variations include jaundice, which indicates liver dysfunction or biliary obstruction; cyanosis, which indicates compromised tissue oxygenation; and the taut, shiny appearance commonly seen with ascites. Localized color changes may reflect an intraabdominal pathologic condition. Reddened areas may indicate inflammation; a bluish discoloration around the umbilicus is sometimes seen with intraabdominal bleeding (Cullen's sign). Bruising indicates tissue trauma, which may or may not be associated with internal organ damage and bleeding. Portal hypertension may produce abnormal patterns of venous flow (see Figure 5-2) or venous dilation that is visible through the skin; portal hypertension may also produce a purplish discoloration around an abdominal stoma (caput medusae, see Color Plate 7). Striae may be seen following pregnancy or weight gain, with Cushing's disease, or with ascites or a tumor that causes the skin to stretch. Striae initially are pink or blue; over time they usually become silvery white. The striae associated with Cushing's disease are always purplish.

Any lesions or nodules are abnormal findings and must be carefully evaluated.

Scars must be described in terms of location, size, and configuration and must be investigated as to cause, since they are a clue to previous trauma or surgical intervention. Any previous abdominal surgery may cause internal adhesions.

Probably the most common variation in visual findings is distention, which is present in many pathologic conditions. In assessing a patient with distention, note whether the distention is generalized and symmetric, limited to the upper or lower abdomen, or asymmetric. Symmetric, generalized distention is most commonly caused by obesity, intraabdominal fluid, flatus, or generalized organ enlargement, such as intestinal distention resulting from ileus (Figure 2-8, *A*). Distention confined to a specific region indicates a pathologic con-

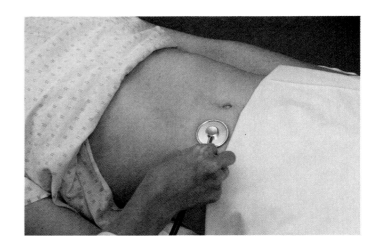

DISTENTION: THE SEVEN MOST COMMON CAUSES

Fat	Fetus
Flatus	Fatal tumor
Fluid	Fibroid
Feces	

dition involving the organs in that region; for example, distention confined to the area between the umbilicus and the symphysis pubis usually indicates bladder distention, pregnancy, ovarian tumors, or uterine fibroids (Figure 2-8, *B*). Localized asymmetry usually is seen as a protrusion or a "bulge" and may be caused by a tumor or cyst, hernia, or organ enlargement.

A variation that may be noted when the patient lifts his or her head from the table is a separation of the abdominal rectus muscles; this condition, known as diastasis recti, may be caused by pregnancy or obesity and is of no clinical significance.

The most common variation in respiratory movements is limitation of abdominal movement, which may be seen in a patient with peritonitis. It is more commonly noted in men, because women usually exhibit costal movements rather than abdominal movements. Occasionally peristaltic waves are visible as a "rippling" motion across the abdominal wall; this always indicates a pathologic condition, usually intestinal obstruction. Markedly pronounced aortic pulsations may indicate an abdominal aortic aneurysm.

Auscultation

The second component of abdominal assessment is auscultation, which provides information about bowel motility and vascular integrity. To assess bowel motility, the examiner places the diaphragm of a warmed stethoscope on the abdomen and holds it in place with light pressure while listening for bowel sounds in each quadrant and for friction rubs over the liver or spleen (Figure 2-9). It is important to warm the stethoscope before placing it on the patient's abdomen, because a cold stethoscope can cause abdominal muscles to contract, which may obscure auscultatory findings. Vascular integrity is best assessed with the stethoscope bell; the examiner listens for bruits in the epigastric area and each of the four quadrants and for a venous hum in the epigastric area and around the umbilicus.

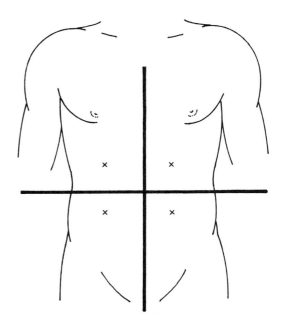

FIGURE 2-9
Auscultation of abdomen. The bottom illustration shows correct placement of stethoscope in each quadrant.

Normal findings

Normal bowel sounds are heard as clicks and gurgles that occur irregularly at the rate of about five to 35 per minute. Friction rubs, bruits, and venous hum should not be heard.

Percussion

The third step in abdominal assessment is percussion, which provides information about the size and density of the abdominal organs and the location of air, fluid, and solid tissue. Percussion may be direct or indirect; with direct percussion, the examiner strikes the hand or finger directly against the body, whereas with indirect percussion the examiner places the middle finger of the nondominant hand against the body surface and then uses the middle finger of the dominant hand to strike the finger on the body surface. The latter is the technique most commonly used for percussion of abdominal organs (Figure 2-10).

General percussion

The examiner begins by systematically percussing all abdominal quadrants (or regions) to identify areas of tympany and dullness (Figure 2-11). Tympany is the note heard over air-filled organs, and dullness is the note produced by solid organs and masses.

Normal findings

Tympany normally is the predominant percussion note because of the air found in the stomach and intes-

Table 2-2

ABDOMINAL AUSCULTATION: ABNORMAL SOUNDS

Sound	Cause
Hyperactive bowel sounds (borborygmi) Loud and prolonged	Hunger, gastroenteritis, or early intestinal obstruction
High-pitched, tinkling sounds	Intestinal air and fluid under pressure; characteristic of early intestinal obstruction
Decreased (hypoactive) bowel sounds Infrequent and abnormally faint	Possible peritonitis or ileus
Absence of bowel sounds (Confirmed only after auscultation of all four quadrants and continuous auscultation for 5 min)	Temporary loss of intestinal motility, as occurs with complete ileus
Friction rubs High-pitched sounds heard over liver and spleen (RUQ and LUQ), synchronous with respiration	Pathologic conditions such as tumors or infection that cause inflammation of organ's peritoneal covering
Bruits Audible swishing sounds that may be heard over aortic, iliac, renal, and femoral arteries	Abnormality of blood flow (requires additional evaluation to determine specific disorder)
Venous hum Low-pitched, continuous sound	Increased collateral circulation between portal and systemic venous systems

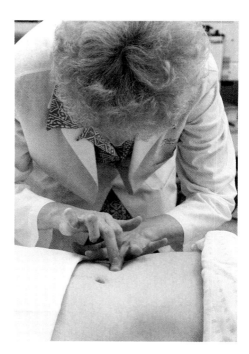

FIGURE 2-10
Indirect percussion of abdomen.

tinal tract. The percussion note changes to dullness over organs and solid masses. Thus dullness is normal in the region of the liver and spleen but not over the central abdominal area, where the note is expected to be tympanic.

Variations

To accurately interpret percussion findings, the examiner must correlate observed percussion notes with the underlying organs and their expected percussion notes. For example, the percussion note in the epigastric area and lower quadrants normally is tympanic; a dull percussion note in these areas would indicate some abnormality. Common causes of dull percussion notes over normally tympanic areas include bladder distention, feces, and solid masses such as tumors. Careful palpation of these areas provides additional data.

Liver percussion

Determining the size of the liver involves the following steps: (1) The examiner begins percussion along the right midclavicular line over an area of tympany and percusses upward until the percussion note changes from tympanic to dull. This point represents the lower border of the liver, which usually is found at or slightly below the costal margin. The lower border of the liver is marked with a marking pen. (2) The examiner then begins percussion along the right midclavicular line over the chest in an area of resonance (the percussion

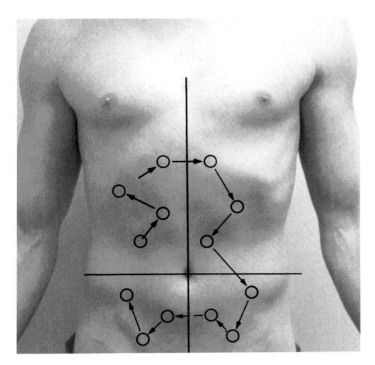

FIGURE 2-11
Systematic route for abdominal percussion. (From Seidel.[52])

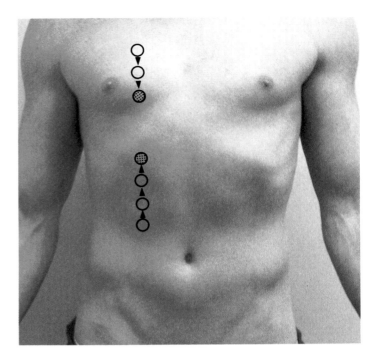

FIGURE 2-12
Route for liver percussion and measurement of liver span. (From Seidel.[52])

note produced by the air-filled lung) and percusses downward until the percussion note changes from resonant to dull (Figure 2-12). This point represents the upper border of the liver, which usually is found at the fifth to seventh intercostal space. The upper border of the liver is also marked. (3) The vertical span of the liver is determined by measuring the space between the two marks. It usually is best to report two indicators of liver size: the projection of liver dullness below the costal margin, and the measured distance between the percussed upper and lower borders of liver dullness.

Liver descent is evaluated by asking the patient to take a deep breath and hold it while the examiner again percusses along the midclavicular line to determine the lower edge of liver dullness. This point is marked and is compared to the original mark of the liver's lower edge to determine the amount of descent.

Additional percussion maneuvers are indicated when liver enlargement is suspected. One maneuver is to percuss along the midaxillary line to determine the point where liver dullness is detected; this point normally is at the fifth to seventh intercostal space. Another maneuver is to percuss along the midsternal line to determine the upper and lower borders of liver dullness and then to measure the distance between the two points.

Normal findings

The vertical span of the liver, as percussed along the midclavicular line, is about 6 to 12 cm in adults.

The span usually is greater in men and tall individuals. The vertical span of the liver at the midsternal line usually is 4 to 8 cm. The normal descent of the liver with inspiration (as measured by percussion during a held breath compared to percussion following expiration) is 2 to 3 cm.

Variations

Hypertrophy of the liver is indicated by a vertical span exceeding 12 cm in the midclavicular line and 8 cm in the midsternal line (Figure 2-13). However, the examiner must remember that liver span can be overestimated in a patient with pleural effusion or lung consolidation; the dullness produced by these conditions can obscure the upper border of the liver. Atrophy of the liver is suggested by a midclavicular vertical span of less than 6 cm and a midsternal vertical span of less than 4 cm; again, the examiner should be aware that gas in the colon may produce a tympanic percussion note in the right upper quadrant, obscuring the dullness of the liver and leading to underestimation of liver size. Thus percussion findings must be correlated with historical data and other findings from the physical assessment.

Stomach percussion

Percussion of the stomach is focused on the left epigastric region and the left lower anterior rib cage; the air-filled stomach produces a tympanic note that is lower in pitch than the tympany produced by the intestine.

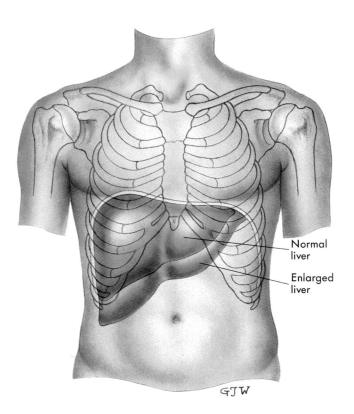

FIGURE 2-13
Normal and enlarged liver. (From Mudge.[41])

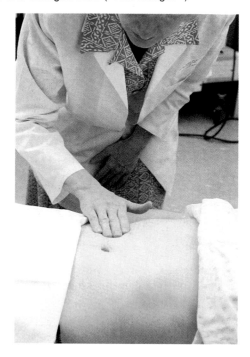

FIGURE 2-14
Technique for light palpation of abdomen.

Palpation

Palpation involves the use of light and deep touch to determine the size, shape, mobility, consistency, and tension of the abdominal organs. Palpation is also used to detect masses, areas of tenderness, muscle spasm, and fluid accumulation. Palpation can be classified as light, moderate, or deep, depending on the depth of palpation and the amount of pressure applied.

Light palpation

The examiner should begin by lightly and systematically palpating all four quadrants. Any areas identified during the interview or during percussion as being sensitive or tender should be avoided during initial palpation. Light palpation is performed by placing the palm of the hand lightly on the abdomen with the fingers approximated; the examiner then uses the fingers to gently depress the abdominal wall no more than 1 cm, using even pressure (Figure 2-14). Light palpation is particularly helpful in determining muscular resistance and areas of tenderness. If an area of resistance is encountered, the examiner should assess further as to the cause (i.e., voluntary or involuntary). A pillow is placed under the patient's knees, and the patient is instructed to breathe slowly through the mouth. The examiner then feels for relaxation of the abdominal muscles, which normally occurs with expiration. If this relaxation does not occur, the resistance is involuntary and probably related to an underlying intraabdominal pathologic condition.

Cutaneous hypersensitivity testing. The examiner may also use the cutaneous hypersensitivity maneuver to test for areas of peritoneal irritation. To perform this test, the examiner lifts the abdominal skin away from the underlying muscle or stimulates the skin with a pin and asks the patient to describe the sensation. If the underlying peritoneum is irritated, the patient will show an exaggerated response to this stimulus (Figure 2-15).

Moderate palpation

Moderate palpation follows light palpation and is a transition to deep palpation. The examiner uses the same hand position and approach as for light palpation but exerts greater pressure. Moderate palpation may reveal tenderness that was not evident with light palpation. The examiner may also use moderate palpation with the side of the hand to identify the borders of organs that move with respiration (Figure 2-16). The examiner must palpate the area throughout the respiratory cycle; inspiration causes downward displacement of the organ, which may be felt as a bump against the examining hand.

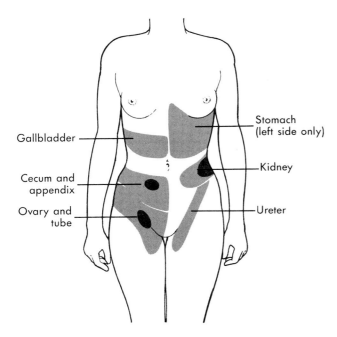

FIGURE 2-15
Areas of cutaneous hypersensitivity. (From Seidel.[52])

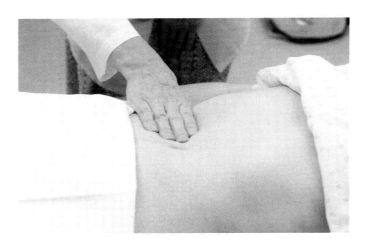

FIGURE 2-16
Technique for moderate palpation using the side of the hand.

Deep palpation

The examiner then moves on to deep palpation, which is used to determine organ size and to detect less obvious masses. The examiner uses the same hand position as for light and moderate palpation, but the fingers are now pressed deeply and evenly into the abdominal wall (Figure 2-17). For obese patients or in the instance of muscular resistance, the examiner may choose to use a bimanual palpation technique; this involves placing one hand on top of the other and using the top hand to exert pressure while the bottom hand detects palpatory findings. Deep palpation may reveal areas of tenderness not previously elicited and may also identify specific anatomic structures such as the borders of the abdominal rectus muscles, the aorta, and portions of the colon. The examiner should be aware that deep palpation may cause tenderness even in a healthy individual in certain locations (e.g., xiphoid process, cecum, sigmoid colon, and aorta).

In performing deep palpation, the examiner should note any masses and describe them in terms of location, size, shape, consistency, tenderness, mobility, pulsation, and movement with respiration. The examiner should attempt to distinguish between intraabdominal masses and masses located in the abdominal wall. To do this, the patient is asked to lift his or her head from the table, which causes the abdominal muscles to contract; this will obscure the outlines of intraabdominal masses,

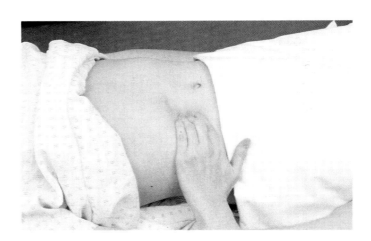

FIGURE 2-17
Technique for deep palpation.

but masses within the abdominal wall will still be palpable. In palpating for masses, the examiner should be aware of normal structures that commonly are mistaken for masses (Figure 2-18). To avoid mistaking normal structures for masses, the examiner must have a clear picture of the location of intraabdominal organs and must be aware of normal variations associated with each organ (such as stool in the colon).

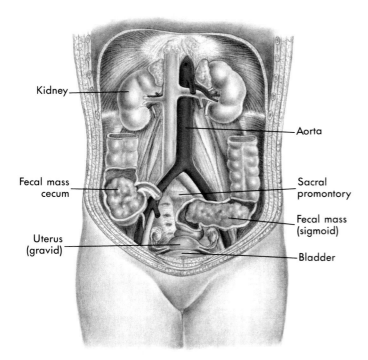

FIGURE 2-18
Abdominal structures frequently felt as "masses". (From Seidel.[52])

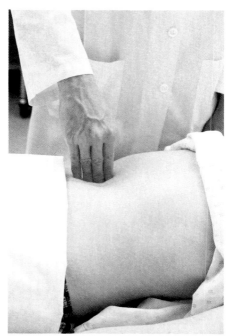

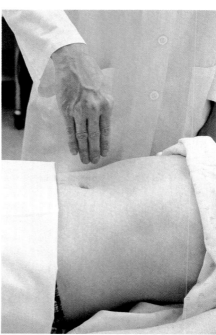

FIGURE 2-19
Technique for eliciting rebound tenderness.

Deep palpation should include evaluation of the periumbilical area; the examiner determines the integrity of the umbilical ring and feels for any nodules or bulges.

Normal findings

A healthy abdomen has no tenderness or masses. On light palpation the abdomen should feel consistently smooth and soft, without resistance. With deep palpation the examiner usually can identify the aorta, the borders of the rectus muscle, and portions of the colon. The umbilical ring should be intact and free of irregularities. Deep palpation may elicit slight tenderness over the cecum, sigmoid colon, aorta, and xiphoid process, even in a healthy individual; marked tenderness or guarding is always abnormal.

Variations

Muscular resistance is a common variation. It may result from voluntary guarding by the patient or may indicate peritoneal irritation. A rigid abdominal wall is seen over areas of peritonitis. Tenderness in response to palpation also indicates an underlying pathologic condition and peritoneal irritation; tenderness is particularly evident with deep palpation. Peritoneal irritation can be further confirmed by the cutaneous hypersensitivity test; with peritoneal irritation, the patient will experience pain. Another maneuver sometimes used to confirm peritoneal irritation is the test for rebound tenderness (Figure 2-19). For this test the patient is placed in the supine position. The examiner holds her hand at a 90-degree angle to the patient's abdomen with fingers extended, and then presses the fingers gently and deeply into an area far removed from the site of tenderness. The fingers are then rapidly withdrawn, allowing the abdominal organs to "rebound" to their normal position; this causes sharp pain at the site of peritoneal irritation. If this test is done, it should be deferred until

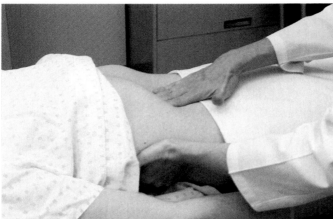

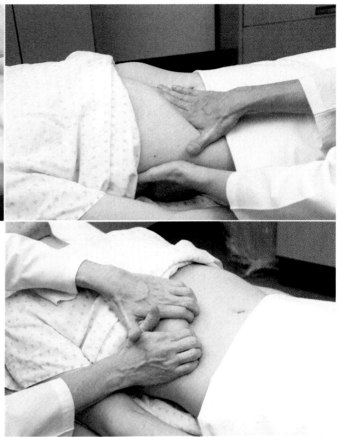

FIGURE 2-20
A, Technique for liver palpation. **B,** Alternate technique. **C,**
Palpating the liver with fingers hooked over the costal margin.

the end of the examination, since the pain and muscle
spasm induced by the maneuver will interfere with further examination. Some examiners feel that this test is
unnecessary, because light percussion can be used to
elicit a mild localized response in areas of peritoneal irritation. Since the test for rebound tenderness can
cause severe pain, it should be used only when necessary to clarify other findings.

Another variation in palpatory findings is the detection of masses. Masses are most likely to be felt on
deep palpation, although light palpation may detect
some sense of resistance.

A defect in the umbilical ring is significant in that it
may increase the patient's potential for herniation.

Liver palpation

The liver is palpated to detect any tenderness or enlargement. The technique for a right-handed examiner
is described; the examiner's position and hand positions
are reversed for left-handed examiners. The examiner
stands on the patient's right side, places her left hand
under the patient's back at the level of the eleventh and
twelfth ribs, and presses upward to push the liver toward the abdominal wall. The right hand is then placed
on the abdomen with the fingers pointing toward the
patient's head and the fingertips resting on the midclavicular line below the level of liver dullness (as determined by palpation) (Figure 2-20, *A*). The right hand is
pressed firmly in and up; this hand position is maintained while the patient is instructed to breathe normally and then to take a deep breath. Deep inspiration
causes the liver to descend, and the examiner may be
able to feel the edge of the liver bump her fingertips. If
the liver is palpable, the examiner should note any nod-

ules, irregularities, or tenderness and should repeat
palpation medially and laterally to assess the liver's contours and surface.

A variation of the above technique is to use both
hands on the abdominal surface, as opposed to one
hand under the patient's posterior rib cage and one
hand on the abdomen. This bimanual approach enables
the examiner to use greater pressure on the abdominal
wall, but the posterior support is lost. Either approach
is appropriate. Another variation of the standard technique is to place the right hand parallel to the right costal margin, as shown in Figure 2-20, *B*. The examiner
pushes the hand in and up and then instructs the patient to take a deep breath. If the liver is palpable, the
examiner will feel the edge of the liver brush against
the side of her hand.

Another approach is the "hook" technique, in which
the examiner stands at the patient's right side facing the
patient's feet and "hooks" the fingertips over the right
costal margin below the level of liver dullness (Figure
2-20, *C*). The examiner pushes in and up with the fingertips and then asks the patient to take a deep breath;
the examiner may be able to feel the edge of the liver
as it descends with inspiration.

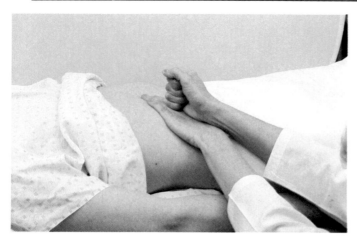

FIGURE 2-21
Fist percussion of the liver.

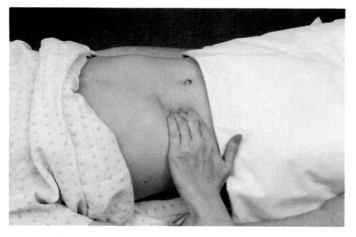

FIGURE 2-22
Palpation of the gallbladder.

Fist percussion may be used to check for liver tenderness when the liver is not palpable. The examiner places one hand along the right costal margin and then strikes this hand with the ulnar surface of the fist of the other hand (Figure 2-21); this elicits a sensation of pain when the liver is inflamed.

Gallbladder palpation

The gallbladder normally is not palpable. To detect an enlarged gallbladder, the examiner palpates below the margin of the liver at the lateral border of the rectus muscle. To detect gallbladder tenderness, the examiner asks the patient to take a deep breath during deep palpation of this area (Figure 2-22).

Normal findings

The liver and gallbladder usually are not palpable.

Variations

If the liver or gallbladder can be palpated, the organ may be enlarged. Palpatory findings must be correlated with percussion findings and the patient's history. Tenderness of any of these organs suggests inflammation. For example, an enlarged gallbladder suggests obstruction of the common bile duct, whereas tenderness suggests cholecystitis. (Tenderness is elicited by asking the patient to take a deep breath during deep palpation; when the inflamed gallbladder comes into contact with the examiner's fingers, the patient experiences sudden pain and halts the inspiration—this is known as Murphy's sign.)

SPECIFIC ASSESSMENT MANEUVERS

In addition to the standard components of abdominal assessment described above, specific maneuvers are used to assess for ascites and abdominal pain.

Ascites

Ascites should be suspected when the patient has abdominal distention or flanks that bulge in the supine position, especially if the patient also has a history of liver disease. Various percussion techniques can be used to determine the amount of ascites present; serial evaluations can then reflect increases or decreases in the volume of ascitic fluid. The first percussion technique is performed with the patient in the supine position. The examiner percusses for areas of dullness and tympany and marks the border between the two percussion notes. (The ascitic fluid settles in dependent areas and produces a dull percussion note, whereas the air-filled bowel superior to the ascitic fluid produces a tympanic note.) The fluid line usually assumes a U-shape, as shown in Figure 2-23. It is helpful to record the distance between the umbilicus and the midpoint of the fluid line (inferior to the umbilicus). Serial measurements then document changes in the levels of ascitic fluid.

Another approach is to have the patient turn to the side and then to perform percussion and note the point where tympany changes to dullness. If ascitic fluid is present, it will settle and produce a dull percussion note in the dependent area of the abdomen. The patient can then be repositioned to determine shifting patterns of dullness, which are consistent with ascites.

Abdominal Pain

Accurate assessment of a patient with abdominal pain requires careful attention to the patient's nonverbal responses as well as verbal statements. While palpating the abdomen, the examiner should always watch the patient's face to detect signs of discomfort or pain. Facial indications of distress accompanied by involuntary muscle guarding indicate pain. If there is any suspicion

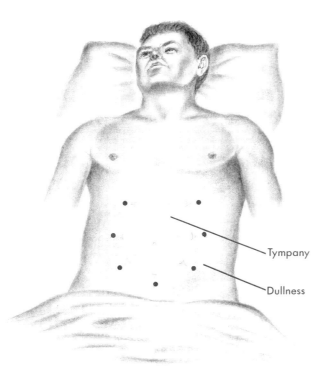

FIGURE 2-23
Percussion pattern produced by ascites. (From Seidel.[52])

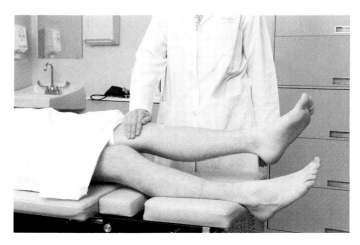

FIGURE 2-24
Iliopsoas muscle test.

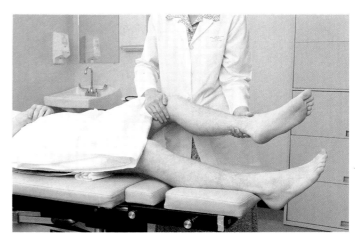

FIGURE 2-25
Obturator muscle test.

of psychosomatic pain, the examiner may apply light pressure with the diaphragm of the stethoscope while auscultating the four quadrants. This should elicit the same response as light palpation. If the patient showed signs of pain with light palpation but not with stethoscope pressure, psychogenic causes for the pain should be considered.

Specific maneuvers are sometimes used to assess for peritoneal irritation. The rebound tenderness maneuver has already been described. Another technique is the iliopsoas muscle test, which may be performed when appendicitis is suspected, because appendicitis may cause irritation of the iliopsoas muscle. This test can be done in three ways: (1) With the patient in the supine position, the examiner places her hand over the lower thigh and asks the patient to raise the leg by flexing at the hip while the examiner exerts downward pressure on the leg (Figure 2-24); (2) the patient is positioned on the left side and asked to raise the right leg from the hip while the examiner presses against the leg; (3) with the patient on the right side, the right leg is hyperextended by pulling it backward. If any of the three forms of this test causes lower quadrant pain, it is said to be a positive iliopsoas sign.

The obturator muscle test is performed when a ruptured appendix or pelvic abscess is suspected, since both of these conditions can irritate the obturator mus-

cle. For this test the patient is placed in the supine position and asked to flex the right leg at the hip and knee to 90 degrees. The examiner holds the leg just above the knee, grasps the ankle, and rotates the leg laterally and medially (Figure 2-25). If this maneuver elicits pain in the hypogastric area, the test result is considered positive.

The Markle heel jar test is another technique for detecting peritoneal irritation. The patient is instructed to stand with straight knees and then to raise up on the toes, relax, and allow the heels to hit the floor. This motion jars the body and causes abdominal pain if peritoneal irritation is present.

Table 2-1 on page 27 correlates common pathologic states with pain characteristics and associated findings.

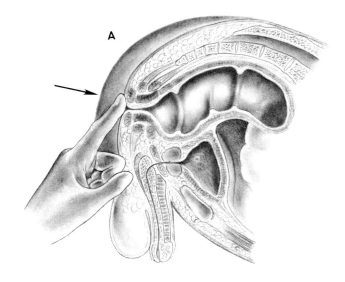

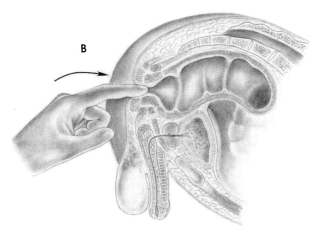

FIGURE 2-26
Correct technique for introducing finger into rectum. **A,** Pad of finger is pressed against the anal opening. **B,** As external sphincter relaxes, fingertip is slipped into the anal canal. (From Seidel.[52])

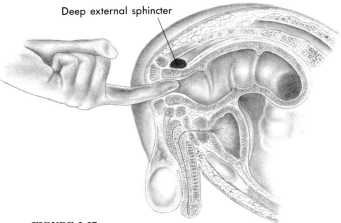

Deep external sphincter

FIGURE 2-27
Rotating of examining finger to examine muscular anal ring (external sphincter). (From Seidel.[52])

RECTUM AND ANUS

The anorectal examination may be uncomfortable and embarrassing to the patient, and it frequently is deferred. However, it provides critical information for evaluation of intestinal tract functioning and should be included in any thorough physical examination. For a patient with a gastrointestinal disorder, the anorectal examination is mandatory.

It is very important to ensure privacy and to explain each step of the examination. The patient is then placed in the examining position most comfortable to him and is draped to provide good visualization of the anorectal area without unnecessary exposure of the genitalia. (Acceptable positions include knee-chest, left side-lying with hips and knees flexed, and bending over an examination table with hips flexed and upper body supported by the table. In women the examination may be done in the lithotomy position in conjunction with the pelvic examination.)

Inspection

The examiner dons gloves and begins with inspection of the perianal and sacrococcygeal areas, looking for dimples or tufts of hair in the sacrococcygeal region and for rashes, skin irritation, inflammatory changes, lumps, or scars anywhere in the area. The examiner then palpates the perianal and sacrococcygeal regions to detect areas of tenderness. The buttocks are spread to facilitate inspection of the anus; the examiner looks for skin lesions, warts or skin tags, external hemorrhoids, fissures, and fistulas. The patient is asked to bear down, which improves visualization of any fistulas, fissures, rectal prolapse, internal hemorrhoids, and polyps. In documenting any findings, the face of a clock is used as a reference point, with 6 o'clock representing the midline on the dorsal surface and 12 o'clock representing the midline on the ventral surface.

Palpation

The examiner then palpates the anal opening and rectal walls. The gloved index finger is lubricated and pressed against the anal opening. The patient is asked to bear down as if trying to have a bowel movement; this maneuver causes sphincter relaxation, which allows the examiner to slide the examining finger into the anal canal, as illustrated in Figure 2-26, *A* and *B*. (It is important to reassure the patient that a feeling of fecal urgency is normal, and that he is not likely to have a bowel movement.) The patient is asked to tighten the sphincter as if trying to prevent a bowel movement, and the examiner notes the integrity and strength of the external sphincter. The examiner then rotates the finger to examine the muscular anal ring (Figure 2-27), noting integrity and any irregularities. The examining finger is then advanced into the rectum, and the rectal walls are palpated according to the following sequence: lateral walls, posterior wall, anterior wall. Bidigital palpation sometimes provides additional information; it is performed by pressing the thumb lightly against the perianal tissue and bringing the index finger toward the thumb. After all rectal walls have been palpated, the patient is asked to bear down; this allows the examiner to reach a few more centimeters into the rectum. Normally the examiner can palpate the most distal 6 to 10 cm of the rectum. When palpation has been completed, the examiner withdraws the gloved finger and examines it for fecal material; if stool is obtained, it should be routinely tested with guaiac.

Normal findings

The perianal and sacrococcygeal skin should be smooth and free of rashes, skin irritation, inflammatory changes, lumps, and dimpling or tufts of hair in the sacrococcygeal (pilonidal) area. It is normal for the skin around the anus to appear coarser and more darkly pigmented; the anal area should be free of lesions, skin tags, warts, fissures, fistulas, and hemorrhoids. The external sphincter should be closed.

Palpation of the perianal area and rectal walls normally elicits no tenderness. Normal sphincter function is demonstrated by relaxation of the external sphincter when the patient is asked to bear down as if having a bowel movement and by even contraction of the external sphincter around the examining finger when the patient is asked to tighten. The rectal vault normally is empty. The anorectal ring should feel smooth and should exert even pressure on the examining finger; the rectal walls should also feel smooth, without lesions, lumps, or irregularities. Any stool obtained during the digital examination normally is soft, brown, and guaiac negative.

Common variations

Dimpling with a sinus tract opening in the sacrococcygeal area may indicate a pilonidal cyst or sinus; there may also be a tuft of hair seen in the sinus tract. Erythema and tenderness in the area indicate an infection.

Perianal irritation may be seen as a result of pruritic conditions, such as pinworms in children or fungal infections in adults. Perianal irritation may also result from fecal incontinence. Skin tags may be seen with fissures and resolved hemorrhoids, and warts may be seen in some sexually transmitted diseases. A fissure is seen as a tear in the anal mucosa; fissures are commonly caused by difficult elimination of hard stool and are associated with pain, itching, and bleeding. If the area is very tender, a local anesthetic may be required before the digital examination. An anorectal fistula is a tract resulting from an inflammatory process that extends from the anus or rectum to the perianal skin or other tissue; the external opening usually appears elevated and red, and palpation of the area may produce a serosanguineous or purulent exudate.

External hemorrhoids are not usually visible at rest unless they are thrombosed, in which case they appear as blue, shiny masses around the anus. Internal hemorrhoids are not visible unless they prolapse through the anus, are not normally palpable, and do not usually produce symptoms unless they become thrombosed, infected, or prolapsed. However, internal hemorrhoids may cause bleeding, with or without defecation and with or without other symptoms.

Anorectal masses may be identified by inspection but are more commonly discovered during palpation. Polyps and carcinomas are the most common types of anorectal masses. Polyps may be seen protruding through the anus or may be palpated, when they are felt as soft nodules that are either pedunculated (attached by a stalk) or closely adherent to the intestinal wall (sessile). Cancerous lesions usually are felt as adherent (sessile) masses with nodular raised edges, irregular contours, and a stony consistency. Biopsy is required to differentiate malignant lesions from benign polyps.

Tenderness on palpation usually is associated with an inflammation such as a fissure, fistula, perianal abscess, or infected pilonidal cyst.

Hard stool in the rectal vault is seen with constipation. Damage to the sphincter musculature may be evidenced by uneven contraction of the sphincter or by irregularities in the anorectal ring. Loss of innervation to the sphincter musculature is evidenced by a lax external sphincter and the patient's inability to voluntarily tighten or relax the sphincter muscles.

Abnormalities in the stool itself are diagnostically significant. Blood-streaked stools indicate a lower GI pathologic condition, whereas tarry, black stools signal upper intestinal bleeding. Microscopic bleeding can be detected by guaiac testing, and positive results require further diagnostic workup to determine the cause of the bleeding. Light tan or clay-colored stools are seen with obstruction of the biliary tree.

CHAPTER 3

Diagnostic Procedures

ABDOMINAL X-RAY EXAMINATION

Plain film x-rays are noninvasive studies that provide considerable information about the gastrointestinal system. Beams of radiation are passed through the body to produce films that contrast structures of greater and lesser density. Plain films are used to determine the distribution of intestinal gas, fluid, masses, calcifications, and the size and position of solid organs (Figure 3-1). The erect position is preferred, but the lateral position can be used if the patient cannot stand (Figure 3-2).

INDICATIONS

To diagnose:
    Perforated viscus
    Paralytic ileus
    Mechanical obstruction
    Intraabdominal mass

To evaluate:
    Distribution of
      visceral gas
    Organ size

CONTRAINDICATION Pregnancy

NURSING CARE

No preparation is required. The patient is given a hospital gown to wear for the test and is instructed to assume the desired position. A very ill patient may need to be supported in the correct position. The patient is instructed to hold his breath when the film is taken. Several films may be required, and the patient may be asked to assume various positions. The patient may be

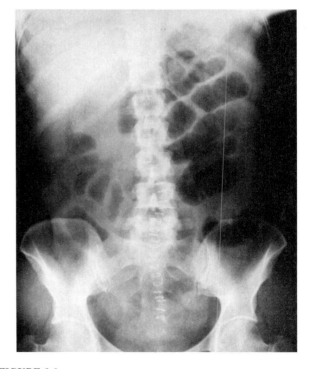

FIGURE 3-1
Flat plate of abdomen depicting multiple, somewhat dilated loops of small bowel consistent with postoperative ileus.

asked to remain in the radiology department until the films have been reviewed and the need for additional films has been ruled out.

PATIENT TEACHING

Explain the purpose of the x-ray and the procedure itself, emphasizing that it is noninvasive and painless. Explain that several films may be taken and that different positions may be required.

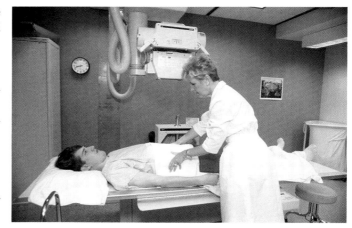

FIGURE 3-2
Patient undergoing abdominal x-ray.

ULTRASONOGRAPHY

Ultrasonography uses sound waves to produce images of the structures in the abdominal cavity. A microphone transducer, which can both emit and receive sound waves, is moved slowly over the skin surface overlying the structure to be studied. The underlying structures are bombarded with sound waves, which are reflected as "echoes" or vibrations; tissues of different densities produce varying vibrations. These vibrations are picked up by the transducer and converted into electrical signals that are displayed as visual images on a screen (Figure 3-3). The advantages of ultrasonography are that it is noninvasive and requires no ionizing radiation. The disadvantages are that intestinal gas, ascites, and extreme obesity can interfere with the sound waves, and ultrasound cannot identify all lesions and therefore cannot be used as the sole diagnostic measure.

The examination itself involves repeated movement of a lubricated microphone transducer over the skin surface in both horizontal and vertical planes (the transducer is lubricated to reduce discomfort and to maintain an air-free connection between the transducer and the skin). An endorectal ultrasound scan can be accomplished by introducing a transducer through the anus and into the rectum. The passage of the sound waves through various tissues produces contrasting images, which are projected onto a screen. Photographs of the screen are taken as a permanent record of the study results.

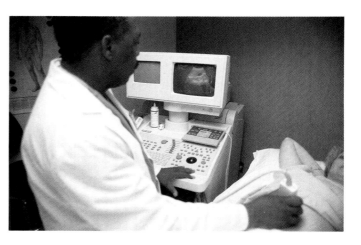

FIGURE 3-3
Patient undergoing abdominal ultrasonography.

INDICATIONS

To evaluate:
    Pancreas
    Biliary ducts
    Gallbladder
    Liver
Limitations:
    Ascites
    Obesity

To diagnose:
    Stage of rectal cancer
    Abdominal abscesses

CONTRAINDICATIONS None

NURSING CARE

Because barium interferes with ultrasonography, any barium studies are scheduled to be done after the ultrasound scan; if barium studies have already been done, the ultrasound should be delayed for at least 48 hours. Any dietary or fluid restrictions are explained to the patient.

PATIENT TEACHING

Explain the purpose of the test and the procedure. Instruct the patient in any dietary and fluid restrictions (e.g., NPO for 8 to 12 hours before the examination). Explain that the test involves rubbing a lubricated transducer against the skin overlying the structure to be tested; tell the patient that this is painless but may cause a tickling sensation. Explain to the patient that she must lie still during the procedure and that the entire test usually takes about 20 to 30 minutes.

COMPUTED TOMOGRAPHY

A computed tomography (CT) scan involves multiple x-rays taken at numerous angles; these films are synthesized by a computer to produce very clear and accurate images of the structures being studied. CT scans are safe and painless, involve only low amounts of radiation, and provide considerable diagnostic data.

In preparation for an abdominal CT scan, the patient is kept NPO for 8 to 12 hours before the procedure and is given 300 to 500 ml of oral contrast medium 4 to 6 hours before the scan. Commonly used contrast agents include sweetened water-soluble contrast and a 1% barium solution. A small amount of water-soluble contrast may also be given rectally to provide clearer images of the sigmoid colon and rectum. Occasionally intravenous contrast is given to delineate the blood vessels more clearly.

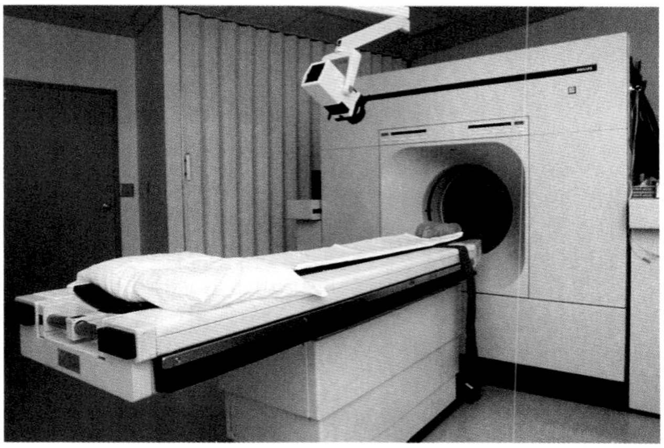

FIGURE 3-4
Computed tomography (CT) equipment. (From Brundage.[7a])

INDICATIONS

To diagnose:
  Tumors
  Pancreatic carcinoma
  Pancreatitis
  Biliary tract disorders
  Obstructive vs. nonobstructive jaundice
  Liver metastases
  Lymph node metastases
To evaluate:
  Vasculature
  Focal points found on nuclear scans (i.e., cystic, solid, inflammatory, or vascular)
To direct:
  Biopsy of tumors
  Aspiration of abscesses

CONTRAINDICATION Pregnancy

The patient is placed on a table with the area to be scanned inside the scanner's opening (Figure 3-4). The scanner rotates slowly around the patient's body, and numerous films are taken from different angles. These cross-sectional images are synthesized by a computer and displayed on a computer printout. Film prints of the computer images are also obtained.

CAUTION

Sensitivity to iodine (if iodine-based contrast is used)

NURSING CARE

Any barium studies should be scheduled to follow the CT scan, since barium can obscure visualization of intraabdominal structures. If the patient has already had barium studies done, the CT scan should be delayed for 4 days. Also, because oral dyes used for biliary studies can interfere with visualization of the biliary tree on a CT scan, the CT should be delayed if the patient has had these studies done.

PATIENT TEACHING

Explain the purpose of the test and the procedure. Explain to the patient that he will be positioned on a table surrounded by a "scanning" machine and that the machine will move around (or up and down) his body, taking a number of x-rays from different angles. Tell the patient that a "clicking" sound is normal as the scanner moves to different positions. Explain that the scan usually takes about 10 to 60 minutes and that it is important for him to remain as still as possible.

Instruct the patient not to eat or drink anything for at least 8 hours before the examination. Tell him that an oral contrast medium may be given to enhance visualization of the intestinal tract. Explain that he may also be given intravenous contrast to improve visualization of the blood vessels and that dye occasionally is given rectally. Patients who are to receive water-soluble oral contrast should be told that they may have temporary diarrhea (because of the osmotic effect of the contrast in the intestinal tract).

MAGNETIC RESONANCE IMAGING

Magnetic resonance imaging (MRI) uses radiofrequency waves and a strong magnetic field to produce clear images of soft tissues and blood vessels. The advantages of MRI are that it is noninvasive, does not involve radiation, provides superior images of soft tissues and blood vessels, and can provide images of structures bounded by bony structures because bone does not distort the images.

MRI works on the following principles: (1) Some atoms in the body's molecules have magnetic properties; when the patient is placed in a strong magnetic field, these atoms align themselves with the magnetic force. (2) If these "aligned" atoms are subjected to radiofrequency waves, some of the nuclei absorb energy and change directions, or "flip," a process called resonance. (3) When the radiofrequency waves are turned off, the absorbed energy is released in a process known as relaxation. (4) The absorption and release of energy produce signals that can be measured and used by the computer to produce images. (5) Different tissues produce different signals, which in turn produce the contrasting images provided by the MRI computer. The strength of the signal a particular tissue produces is determined in large part by the amount of water in that tissue, because each water molecule has two hydrogen atoms, and hydrogen atoms demonstrate magnetic activity. This means that tissues with a large amount of water, such as blood vessels, produce very strong signals, whereas tissues with minimal water, such as bone, produce weak signals. This explains why MRI is a superior tool for diagnosing abnormalities in soft tissues or blood flow, and why it can be used to image structures bordered by bone, where CT scanning and regular x-ray films are inadequate.

INDICATIONS

To diagnose:
   Hepatic metastases
To evaluate:
   Complex abscesses, fistulas, and sinus tracts
   Staging for colorectal cancer
   Source of gastrointestinal bleeding

CONTRAINDICATIONS

   Pregnancy
   Marked obesity (because an obese patient may not fit in the narrow scanner tunnel)
   Metal implants or objects in the body that could be dislodged by the magnet (e.g., metal-containing heart valves, stainless steel vascular clips, shrapnel)
   Permanent pacemaker
   Implanted insulin pump or transcutaneous electric nerve stimulation (TENS) device
   Patient needing life-support equipment

NURSING CARE

Patients are kept NPO for up to 6 hours before an abdominal or pelvic MRI scan to reduce peristaltic activity; no additional preparation is required. The nurse should question the patient about any metallic agents or implants such as heart valves or pacemakers. Some metal-containing implants may not be contraindications for MRI scanning; hip prostheses, dental fillings, orthodontic braces, sternal wire sutures, and intrauterine devices are among implants that do not present strict contraindications to MRI. However, *any* metal-containing implant should be reported to the radiology department. All metallic items must be removed before the patient enters the scanning room.

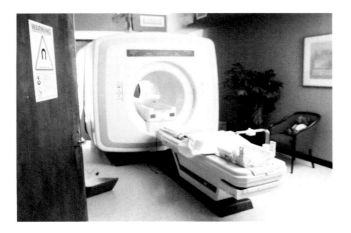

FIGURE 3-5
Magnetic resonance imaging (MRI) equipment. (From Brundage.[7a])

The nurse should assess the patient's degree of anxiety about the procedure; if the patient is very anxious, the nurse should contact the physician about a mild sedative.

PATIENT TEACHING

Explain the purpose of the test and the procedure. Tell the patient that she will be positioned on a narrow, padded stretcher that fits into the scanner tunnel (Figure 3-5), and explain that the close fit of the tunnel helps ensure accurate test results. Explain that the scanner tunnel is equipped with fans and mirrors and that the scanner operator will constantly monitor the patient through the mirrors. The scanner is also equipped with an intercom system or a call button, so that the patient can contact the scanner operator. Tell the patient that the machine makes metallic thumping sounds, which sound like the beating of a drum.

Reassure the patient that the MRI procedure is painless, but explain that she may be uncomfortable because of the fixed position in a very narrow space. Teach the patient relaxation exercises that she can use to reduce anxiety, such as visual imagery and slow deep breathing. Explain that the entire scan can take as long as 1½ hours, and encourage her to go to the bathroom before entering the scanning room. Tell her that no follow-up care is required.

ESOPHAGOGASTRODUODENOSCOPY

Esophagogastroduodenoscopy involves the insertion of an endoscopic instrument through the oral cavity and esophagus into the stomach and duodenum (Figure 3-6). Esophagogastroduodenoscopy usually is performed with a flexible endoscope. This procedure permits visualization of the esophageal, gastric, and duodenal mucosa; inflammatory changes and lesions too small or too shallow to be detected by x-ray examination can be seen, and bleeding sources can be identified and controlled. Esophageal and gastric motility can also be evaluated, and films can be taken for comparison with earlier or later examinations.

INDICATIONS

To diagnose:

Esophagitis	Gastric ulcers
Esophageal ulcers	Pyloric obstruction
Esophageal strictures	Pernicious anemia
Esophageal varices	Foreign bodies in the esophagus and stomach
Hiatal hernia	
Gastritis	Duodenal inflammation or ulcers

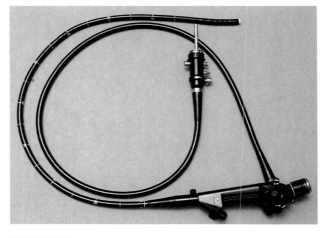

FIGURE 3-6
Endoscope used to perform esophagogastroduodenoscopy.

To evaluate:
Esophageal and gastric motility
Esophageal or gastric bleeding
Esophageal or gastric lesions (biopsy)
Status of surgical anastomoses

CONTRAINDICATIONS None

CAUTIONS

Obstructive lesions
Aortic aneurysm
Severe inflammation (esophagogastroduodenitis)
Esophageal varices
Recent perforation of esophagus, stomach, or duodenum
Severe cardiovascular or pulmonary disease

NURSING CARE

The patient is maintained in a fasting state for 4 to 6 hours before the examination to ensure an empty stomach and thus reduce the risk of vomiting and aspiration. Atropine is administered if ordered to reduce the volume of secretions. The patient is instructed to remove any dentures or removable bridges before the examination. After the examination, the patient is kept NPO until the gag reflex returns; the nurse tests for the gag reflex by touching the oropharynx with a tongue depressor or cotton swab. The gag reflex usually returns within 2 to 4 hours. The patient is monitored for evidence of perforation (bleeding, fever, dysphagia, crepitus of the neck tissues, and pain are common indicators of perforation). The location of the pain varies with the site of perforation. Perforation in the cervical area causes neck and throat pain that is aggravated by swallowing or moving the cervical spine; thoracic perforation causes substernal or epigastric pain that is worsened by breathing or trunk movements and possibly accompanied by cyanosis and back pain. Perforation of the distal esophagus causes shoulder pain and dyspnea. If vomiting occurred during the examination, the patient must also be monitored for signs of aspiration pneumonia (e.g., fever, dyspnea, diminished breath sounds or rales, tachycardia, confusion, diaphoresis).

Patients who were sedated for the examination are maintained on bed rest until they are alert and able to ambulate independently.

ENDOSCOPY

Endoscopy involves insertion of a hollow tube, or endoscope, into the gastrointestinal tract. Endoscopes are available in both rigid metal and flexible fiberoptic forms. All endoscopes include a light source, a power source and cord, a lens system that permits multidirectional viewing, and accessories for suction and biopsy. Endoscopy allows direct visualization of gastrointestinal structures and collection of secretions and tissue specimens for further analysis.

All endoscopic procedures require a signed consent and some preparation for the examination. Because most endoscopic procedures are done using some type of anesthesia or sedation, ongoing assessment of the patient is necessary during and after the procedure, and the patient must be informed about postprocedural care and monitoring.

PATIENT TEACHING

Explain the procedure and its purpose. Explain that sedation is given as needed and that a topical anesthetic is applied to the throat before the endoscope is inserted. Explain the importance of an empty stomach and the need to forgo food and fluids for the specified time before the examination. If the procedure is to be done on an outpatient basis, explain to the patient that she will not be able to drive for at least 12 hours after the procedure (because of the sedative), and instruct her to bring an adult who will be able to drive her home.

Explain to the patient that the topical anesthetic blocks the gag reflex and that she will not be allowed food or fluids until the gag reflex returns to eliminate the risk of choking. Once the gag reflex has returned, explain to the patient that any throat irritation can be treated with saline gargles or throat lozenges. Instruct the patient to report any of the following symptoms promptly: fever, difficulty swallowing, bleeding, shortness of breath, or pain in the throat, chest, or shoulder area.

PROCTOSIGMOIDOSCOPY

Proctosigmoidoscopy involves direct inspection of the rectal mucosa and sigmoid colon with a sigmoidoscope. Proctosigmoidoscopy may be performed with a rigid metal tube and with the patient in a knee-chest position or on the left side with the knees flexed to straighten the colon and facilitate passage of the sigmoidoscope. More commonly a flexible fiberoptic sigmoidoscope is used (Figure 3-7); this instrument is more comfortable for the patient and also allows examination of more of the descending colon. Air may be introduced into the colon during the study to distend the bowel and improve visualization, and suction may be used to remove

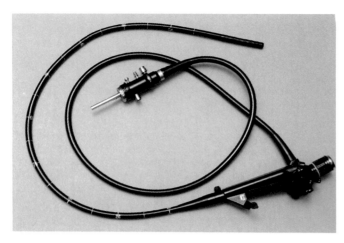

FIGURE 3-7
Flexible scope used to perform proctosigmoidoscopy.

secretions. Lesions can be biopsied through the endoscope, because there are no sensory nerve endings in the bowel wall. Sedation is not usually required for the proctosigmoidoscopic examination.

INDICATIONS

To diagnose:
   Rectosigmoid cancer
   Rectosigmoid strictures
   Rectosigmoid polyps
   Inflammatory process (Crohn's disease, ulcerative colitis, pseudomembranous colitis)
   Internal hemorrhoids
To evaluate:
   Bleeding from rectosigmoid
   Surgical anastomoses

CONTRAINDICATIONS

Pregnancy
Toxic megacolon
Severe stricture of anus, rectum, or sigmoid

Preparation for proctosigmoidoscopy most commonly involves a low-volume enema, such as a Fleet enema, to cleanse the distal colon and the rectum. In some cases the patient is placed on a restricted-residue diet the day before the study, and he may be given an enema the evening before the examination as well as one just before the procedure.

NURSING CARE

The nurse is responsible for administering the bowel preparation or for instructing the patient in the preparation procedure (when done on an outpatient basis). After the procedure, the patient is monitored for rectal bleeding and signs of perforation (fever, purulent rectal drainage, abdominal distention, abdominal pain, and tenesmus).

PATIENT TEACHING

Explain the procedure and its purpose. Explain the reason for the bowel preparation and the specifics of that regimen. Explain the position that the patient will be asked to assume (usually a supported knee-chest position or a left side-lying position with knees flexed), and explain that the position helps straighten the lower colon and facilitates passage of the sigmoidoscope. Explain that the test is not painful but that the scope may feel cool and insertion of the sigmoidoscope may cause a strong urge to defecate. Instruct the patient in relaxation techniques he can use to control the urge to defecate and to reduce the cramping that may result from introduction of air; breathing slowly and deeply through the mouth usually is an effective technique.

When the test has been completed, tell the patient he may resume his usual diet and activities unless instructed otherwise by his physician. Explain that the procedure normally causes no adverse effects, and instruct the patient to report any unusual symptoms (e.g., fever, pain, abdominal swelling, rectal bleeding, or tenesmus) to his physician.

COLONOSCOPY

Colonoscopy involves passage of a flexible fiberoptic scope the length of the colon and into the cecum. Colonoscopy plays an important role in surveillance for colonic neoplasms, since it allows visualization of the entire colonic mucosa.

Adequate preparation is essential, and various protocols for bowel cleansing have been established. One regimen calls for a clear liquid diet the day before the examination, metoclopramide 10 mg PO the afternoon before the procedure, and 4 L of a polyethylene glycol–electrolyte solution consumed at the rate of one glass every 10 minutes. Oral laxatives and tap water enemas may be used as an alternative to the metoclopramide and polyethylene glycol-electrolyte solution. The preparation regimen is modified for patients with an acute abdominal disorder, intestinal obstruction, or diarrhea.

Prophylactic antibiotics are recommended for some patients, especially if polypectomy is anticipated (e.g., patients with cardiac valve prostheses, valvular heart disease, pacemakers, history of endocarditis, implanted orthopedic prostheses, and ventricular shunts).

Colonoscopy usually is performed using light sedation; medications commonly used include meperidine (25-100 mg IV), diazepam (2.5-15 mg IV), or midazolam (1-2.5 mg IV). Glucagon (1 mg IV) sometimes is given to relax the colonic musculature. If needed, air or carbon dioxide may be used to distend the colon walls and improve visualization. Colonoscopy includes snare polypectomy (removal of polyps with an endoscopic snare) and biopsy of any lesions with biopsy forceps.

INDICATIONS

To diagnose:

Diverticular disease	Polyps
Obstruction	Neoplasms
Strictures	Bleeding
Radiation injury	Ischemia
Inflammatory bowel disease	

To treat:

Bleeding	Strictures
Polyps	

CONTRAINDICATIONS

Suspected perforation
Recent colonic anastomosis
Uncooperative patient

CAUTION

Fulminant colitis

NURSING CARE

The nurse administers the bowel preparation, evaluates its effectiveness, and monitors the patient's fluid-electrolyte balance. After the procedure, the nurse monitors the patient for evidence of complications (bleeding, fever, abdominal pain, abdominal distention, and abdominal rigidity).

PATIENT TEACHING

Explain that colonoscopy involves insertion of a long, flexible instrument throughout the length of the colon, allowing direct inspection of the entire large intestine. Explain that the bowel must be cleansed of all fecal material, and then explain the specifics of the bowel preparation procedure. If the patient is to receive prophylactic antibiotics or to undergo preprocedural sedation, explain the purpose of the medications and instruct the patient to remain in bed after he has been given the sedating medication. If no sedation is to be used, explain to the patient that the procedure may be uncomfortable at times, but not painful. Teach the patient relaxation exercises that may be used to promote relaxation and reduce discomfort, such as slow deep breathing.

After the procedure, instruct the patient in any restrictions on activity (e.g., an outpatient who has been sedated should not drive for at least 12 hours), and instruct the patient to report any unusual symptoms such as fever, abdominal pain, or rectal bleeding.

ENDOSCOPIC RETROGRADE CHOLANGIOPANCREATOGRAPHY

Endoscopic retrograde cholangiopancreatography (ERCP) involves insertion of an endoscope (duodenoscope) through the stomach into the duodenum, injection of dye into the pancreatic and common bile ducts, and serial x-rays of the pancreas, gallbladder, liver, and biliary ducts. The endoscopy is performed primarily to provide access to the pancreatic and biliary ducts for injection of contrast medium; however, the endoscopy also allows direct visualization of the esophageal, gastric, and duodenal mucosa (as described under esophagogastroduodenoscopy).

Patient preparation for ERCP is the same as for esophagogastroduodenoscopy (i.e., the patient is kept NPO for up to 6 hours before the procedure). Light sedation is provided by intravenous injection of sedatives such as midazolam or meperidine, and a topical anesthetic is applied to the oropharynx before insertion of the duodenoscope. Glucagon or a similar agent usually is administered intravenously to suppress duodenal peristalsis and promote visualization of Vater's ampulla, and atropine may be given to reduce oral secretions.

The major complications associated with ERCP are pancreatitis and sepsis. Because the duodenoscope is passed through the oral cavity, ERCP is not a sterile procedure, and contamination of the pancreas and biliary system is possible. The potential for contamination is particularly significant in a patient with biliary or pancreatic stasis, because pathogens can proliferate rapidly in a stagnant system.

INDICATIONS

To diagnose:
   Biliary stones
   Ductal stricture
   Ductal compression
   Neoplasms of the pancreas and biliary system
To evaluate:
   Patency of biliary and pancreatic ducts
   Jaundice (intrahepatic or extrahepatic)
   Pancreatitis
   Cholecystitis
   Hepatitis

CONTRAINDICATIONS

   Uncooperative patient
   Severe pulmonary or cardiac disease

COMPLICATIONS

Pancreatitis
Ascending cholangitis
Sepsis

NURSING CARE

The patient is kept NPO for 6 hours before the examination to ensure an empty stomach and thus reduce the risk of vomiting and aspiration. Medications are administered as ordered; patients are kept on bed rest after administration of sedatives or narcotics. All dentures and removable bridges must be removed before the procedure.

After the procedure, the patient is kept NPO until the gag reflex returns, which usually occurs within 2 to 4 hours. The nurse checks the gag reflex by touching the oropharynx with a tongue depressor or cotton swab.

The patient is monitored for signs of perforation (described under esophagogastroduodenoscopy) and of ascending cholangitis, pancreatitis, or sepsis. Fever, abdominal pain, nausea and vomiting, and abdominal tenderness or rigidity are indicators of ascending cholangitis and pancreatitis; sepsis is evidenced by these signs and symptoms accompanied by hypotension.

Patients are maintained on bed rest until they are alert and able to ambulate independently.

PATIENT TEACHING

Explain the procedure and its purpose. Explain that a flexible tube is passed through the mouth into the small intestine to the point where the pancreatic and biliary ducts empty into the intestinal tract, and dye is then injected into the ducts draining the gallbladder and pancreas so that x-rays can be taken. Explain that the back of the throat is anesthetized to prevent gagging and discomfort when the tube is passed, and that medication is given to promote relaxation and prevent discomfort. If the examination is to be done on an outpatient basis, tell the patient that she will be unable to drive for 12 hours after the procedure (because of the sedatives), and instruct her to come with an adult who can drive her home after the examination.

After the examination, explain to the patient that she must not drink fluids or attempt to eat until the gag reflex has returned, to prevent choking. After the gag reflex has returned and fluids are permitted, teach the patient how to use saline gargles or anesthetic lozenges to reduce throat irritation. Explain to the patient that she may have a mildly elevated temperature and slight sore throat for a day or two after the procedure; instruct her to report any other symptoms immediately (e.g., chest or abdominal pain, difficulty swallowing, high fever, nausea or vomiting, abdominal tenderness).

BARIUM SWALLOW (UPPER GASTROINTESTINAL SERIES)

With a barium swallow the patient is asked to swallow a thick barium solution or to eat a "barium burger" (barium is a chalky, radiopaque substance that coats the mucosal surface and is used to provide a radiographic outline of the structures of the alimentary canal). After ingesting the barium, the patient is asked to assume a number of positions on the x-ray table, and serial films are taken as the barium passes through the alimentary canal. Because of the rapid esophageal transit time, the patient is given a single swallow of thick barium and placed in the supine position while esophageal films are obtained; the Trendelenburg position may be required to evaluate the patient accurately for gastric reflux or hiatal hernia. The patient is then asked to assume different positions so that the gastric mucosa is effectively coated and visualized. In some instances abdominal palpation may be performed to promote contact of the barium with all regions of the gastric wall. If a small bowel disorder is a possibility, sequential films of the small intestine are taken as the barium traverses the length of the small bowel; this may take up to 6 hours, even with normal motility. Additional follow-up films may be taken to demonstrate passage of the barium into and through the large intestine.

INDICATIONS

To diagnose:

Esophageal lesions (strictures, varices, polyps, diverticula, ulcers, tumors, hiatal hernia)
Esophageal motility disorders
Gastric ulcers and tumors
Small bowel obstruction
Small bowel lesions (polyps, diverticula, tumors)
Crohn's disease

To evaluate:

Gastric and small bowel motility

CONTRAINDICATIONS Pregnancy, perforated viscus

CAUTION

With suspected obstruction, could cause perforation

NURSING CARE

An empty stomach and small bowel ensure good contact between the barium and the mucosal surface; thus a limited bowel preparation is required to obtain the most accurate results. The patient may be placed on a low-residue diet for 1 to 3 days before the procedure, and he is made NPO at midnight on the day before the test. It is best to avoid using anticholinergics or narcotics for the 24 hours preceding the test, since these substances alter small bowel motility. Antacids should not be given for several hours preceding the test, especially if the patient is being evaluated for esophageal reflux.

Follow-up care is required to ensure complete elimination of the barium. Stools are monitored for frequency, consistency, and color until the barium has been eliminated and the stools have returned to normal. Barium can turn into a hard mass that can cause constipation or obstruction; failure to eliminate the barium promptly (within 1 to 3 days) requires intervention (i.e., administration of a laxative or enema). In some facilities standing orders for the patient who has had a barium swallow include administration of a laxative or enema.

PATIENT TEACHING

Explain the reason for the test and the procedure itself. Explain that the patient will be asked to ingest barium in the form of a thick (flavored) solution or a "burger" and then will be asked to assume various positions on the x-ray table while a series of x-rays is taken. Explain that the barium outlines the walls of the esophagus, stomach, and small intestine, and that several x-rays are required to obtain accurate films of each section as the barium reaches it. Explain that the test may take as long as 6 hours and that follow-up films may be required. Explain the preparatory diet and fluid restrictions and the reason for them. Explain that the barium will be eliminated through the stool and that it is important to drink additional fluids to promote the elimination of barium. Instruct the patient to monitor the color of his stools, and explain that a "chalky" appearance is normal for 1 to 3 days. Instruct the patient to notify the nurse or physician if he does not eliminate the barium promptly (within 1 to 3 days) or if he feels constipated.

BARIUM ENEMA (LOWER GASTROINTESTINAL SERIES)

A barium enema is one of the most commonly performed diagnostic procedures for a patient with a disorder of the colon. The procedure is safe and when properly done provides accurate information about the structure of the large intestine and any lesions. The patient is given barium through an enema; for the patient with poor sphincter control, a rectal catheter with an inflatable balloon may be used to promote retention of the barium. The patient is then asked to assume various positions to assure good contact between the barium and the colonic mucosa, or the x-ray table is manipulated to achieve the same results. Films of the colon are then taken, and the patient is allowed to expel the barium.

The barium enema may be administered as a single-contrast or double-contrast study (Figure 3-8, *A* and *B*). In the single-contrast study, low-density barium is the only contrast agent used. In the double-contrast study, a high-density barium solution is used in combination with air insufflation of the colon; this provides excellent contrast between the air-filled lumen and the barium-coated mucosa. The double-contrast study is the standard in many institutions for the average adult, since it provides more mucosal detail, detects smaller lesions, and allows more accurate evaluation of the rectum. However, it involves more discomfort for the patient and may be very poorly tolerated by some patients, especially those who are debilitated; it also is a lengthier and more expensive procedure than the single-contrast

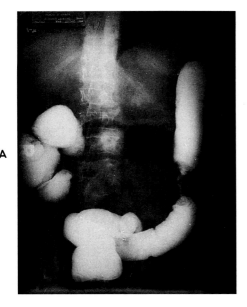

A

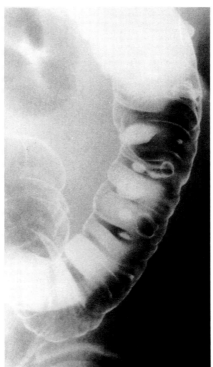

B

FIGURE 3-8
A, Single-contrast barium enema illustrating obstructing circumferential carcinoma of the sigmoid colon.
B, Double-contrast barium enema showing multiple colonic diverticula. (Diverticula on dependent surfaces are barium-filled; diverticula on nondependent surfaces are seen as ring shadows.)

study. In addition, the single-contrast study provides more accurate data in patients with suspected colonic obstruction or fistulas.

INDICATIONS

To diagnose:
  Colorectal lesions (e.g., polyps, carcinomas)
  Diverticulosis
  Inflammatory bowel disease of the colon
  Strictures
  Fistulas and sinus tracts
To evaluate:
  Colon size and length
  Patency of colonic lumen

CONTRAINDICATIONS

  Pregnancy
  Toxic megacolon/fulminant inflammatory bowel disease
  Perforation
  Obstruction
  Acute diverticulitis

COMPLICATION

Perforation of colon or rectum with leakage of barium into retroperitoneum or peritoneal cavity

NURSING CARE

If the patient is to have both a barium swallow and a barium enema, the barium enema should be scheduled *before* the barium swallow, because elimination of the barium from the upper intestinal tract takes several days. An adequate bowel preparation is critical for diagnostic accuracy; the lumen must be free of stool. A standard "prep" for the barium enema includes a clear liquid diet for 24 hours preceding the study, and laxatives or enemas (or both) to cleanse the colon of stool. It is essential that the nurse monitor the results of the ordered preparation and that the physician be notified of inadequate results (e.g., failure to obtain "clear" results with the final enema or suppository). After the test the patient must be monitored for elimination of the barium, which can cause an obstruction if not eliminated completely. The nurse must monitor the patient's stools and obtain an order for a laxative or enema if the barium is not completely eliminated within 2 days. In some institutions, laxatives or enemas are routinely administered after the barium enema.

PATIENT TEACHING

Explain the reason for the procedure (i.e., to evaluate the large intestine and rectum and identify any abnormalities). Tell the patient barium will be given as an enema, and she will be asked to assume different positions to help coat the colon and rectal walls with the barium; then a number of x-rays will be taken to provide a clear picture of the colon and rectum. Tell the patient that the barium may cause a strong urge to defecate, and explain the importance of retaining the barium until the study has been completed. Explain the importance of cleansing the colon and rectum of all fecal material before the study, and explain the steps of the bowel preparation regimen. Patients are instructed to have their stools checked by a nurse during the course of the bowel preparation; patients completing the regimen on an outpatient basis are instructed to monitor their stools and to notify the physician or radiology department if the regimen fails to produce clear returns. Explain to the patient the importance of adequate fluid intake after the study to facilitate elimina-

tion of the barium. Explain that it is normal for the stools to appear chalky for 1 to 2 days, until the barium has been eliminated. Instruct the patient to monitor the stools and to notify the nurse if they do not return to normal within 3 days or if she begins to feel constipated. Stress that this is very important, because the barium can harden and cause a blockage. (If laxatives or enemas are routinely given after the study, this should be explained as well.)

If the patient is scheduled for a double-contrast study, it is important to explain that it is normal to feel cramping and discomfort when the air is introduced into the colon. The patient should be told that this discomfort is temporary and that the air is necessary to ensure good visualization of the colon and rectal walls.

WATER-SOLUBLE CONTRAST STUDY

Water-soluble iodinated contrast studies, such as Gastrografin (meglumine diatrizoate and diatrizoate sodium solution), are an alternative to barium studies for patients with suspected perforation of the colon (barium studies are contraindicated in these patients because of the risk of peritoneal contamination). Water-soluble contrast may also be preferred for the study of fistulas or sinus tracts. (Besides the potential for peritoneal contamination with barium, there is the risk that the barium will become hardened and impacted in the sinus tract or fistula.) Water-soluble contrast may also be used for its ability to soften and dissolve impacted stool.

Water-soluble contrast studies are performed in the same manner as barium studies; the difference is in the contrast solution.

INDICATIONS

To diagnose: *To evaluate:*
  Colonic perforation   Fistulas or sinus tracts
To treat:
  Fecal impaction

CONTRAINDICATION Pregnancy

CAUTION

History of sensitivity to iodine or other contrast media

NURSING CARE

Because iodinated contrast solutions may alter the results of thyroid function tests, such tests should be

completed before the water-soluble contrast medium is administered. The patient is questioned about any allergies to iodine or to contrast solutions, and the physician and radiology department are notified accordingly. The amount of bowel preparation depends on the patient's underlying condition and the reason for the study. For optimum results the patient undergoes bowel preparation as for a barium study; however, this step may be omitted when perforation is suspected or when the patient has a fistula. The contrast is readily eliminated, so no postprocedural laxative or enema is required; however the patient may have some diarrhea as a result of the osmotic effect of the contrast solution. Patients at risk for fluid volume deficit should be monitored and fluid replacement provided as needed.

PATIENT TEACHING

Explain the purpose of the procedure, and the purpose and procedure for any bowel preparation. Explain how the contrast medium is to be administered. If the contrast is to be administered per rectum, explain to the patient that he may feel an urgency to defecate. Explain that this sensation is caused by stretching of the rectal walls as the rectum fills with the contrast solution, that the feeling is usually temporary, and that he will be allowed to expel the contrast as soon as the films are obtained. Explain that he may be asked to assume different positions on the x-ray table so that the contrast material coats the walls of the intestine. Tell the patient that he may have some diarrhea after the procedure, which is normal and temporary. Encourage the patient to increase his fluid intake after the procedure (unless this is contraindicated).

ORAL CHOLECYSTOGRAPHY

Oral cholecystography involves radiologic examination of the gallbladder after oral ingestion of a radiopaque dye. The patient is given an oral dye suspension or a series of six dye capsules about 12 hours before the test. In some facilities the patient is given a double dose of the oral dye (two packets of granules mixed with water to form a suspension, or 12 capsules); this is done to reduce the incidence of "nonvisualization," which sometimes occurs when the standard dose is given. Normally the dye is absorbed in the intestine, removed from the bloodstream by the liver and excreted in the bile, and then concentrated and stored in the gallbladder. Concentration of the dye in the gallbladder permits radiographic visualization of the gallbladder (Figure 3-9). After x-ray examination of the gallbladder, the patient may be given a fatty meal to stimulate contraction of the gallbladder; follow-up films may then be taken to evaluate emptying of the gallbladder and the patency of the bile ducts.

INDICATIONS

To diagnose:
  Cholecystitis
  Cholelithiasis
  Ductal obstruction (e.g., ductal stones, ductal stricture, compression)
To evaluate:
  Gallbladder function
  Ductal system

CONTRAINDICATIONS

  Pregnancy
  Hypersensitivity to iodine

CAUTION

  Renal and hepatic damage

NURSING CARE

Because the dye used for the oral cholecystogram is iodine based, the patient must be questioned about allergies to iodine products. In addition, it is important to schedule tests such as protein-bound iodine or iodine uptake before the oral cholecystogram (or any other studies involving iodine-based dyes); once the patient has received the dye, a delay of several months is required before the protein-bound iodine or iodine uptake study can be performed.

The nurse should also be aware that the dye is excreted by the liver and kidneys; if the patient has significant renal or hepatic damage, or both, the nurse should consult with the physician about the safety of using the dye.

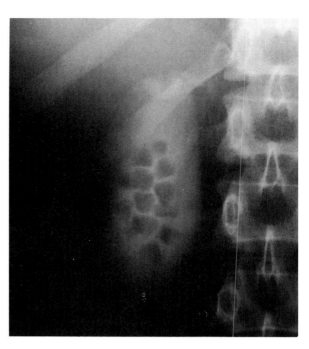

FIGURE 3-9
Oral cholecystogram; stones are visualized as negative filling defects (gallstone disease).

Adequate preparation for the test is critical. It is important to administer the dye suspension or dye capsules as ordered approximately 12 hours before the test, with only a small amount of water, and to monitor tolerance to the dye. Intolerance to the dye is evidenced by side effects such as urticaria, flushing, abdominal cramping, vomiting, and diarrhea; these side effects are more common when a double dose of dye is given. Any intolerance to the dye should be promptly reported to the physician and radiology department; prompt notification is particularly important when there is the potential for an allergic reaction (as indicated by urticaria) or for dye loss (as may occur with vomiting and diarrhea).

On the day before the test, the patient usually is given (or instructed to consume) a meal containing fats; the evening meal should be fat free. The patient may be given a cleansing enema before the examination to ensure clear visualization of the biliary tree. After the dye has been administered, the patient is kept NPO until the test is completed. The nurse must ensure that the study is finished before the patient is allowed to resume usual oral intake.

PATIENT TEACHING

Explain the purpose of the test, and ask the patient about any sensitivity to iodine. Explain any dietary guidelines to be followed the day before the test and the importance of remaining NPO after midnight the night before the test. Explain how to take the oral dye, and instruct the patient to report any side effects such as rash, vomiting, or diarrhea. Explain the importance of taking the dye on time, since the x-rays are scheduled according to the intake of the dye. If a cleansing enema is to be given, explain the purpose and the procedure.

Explain that a special meal may be served after the initial films and that this meal is high in fat to make the gallbladder contract and empty. Explain that additional films may be taken after the "fat meal" to determine how well the gallbladder empties.

PERCUTANEOUS TRANSHEPATIC CHOLANGIOGRAPHY

Percutaneous transhepatic cholangiography (PTC) involves percutaneous insertion of a long, flexible needle (Chiba needle) into the liver; suction is applied while the needle is slowly withdrawn until a bile duct is entered. Bile is then aspirated through the needle, and contrast medium is injected. Serial x-rays are taken as the biliary ducts are visualized.

After the procedure the patient must be carefully monitored for evidence of hemorrhage or biliary leakage into the peritoneal cavity.

INDICATIONS

To diagnose:
 Extrahepatic or intrahepatic jaundice
 Biliary calculi
 Bile duct obstruction caused by tumors, stricture, stenosis, or inflammation
 Injury to common bile duct
To evaluate:
 Patency of ductal system

CONTRAINDICATIONS

Uncorrectable coagulopathy   Cholangitis
Hypersensitivity to iodine   Severe ascites

NURSING CARE

Because the contrast medium is iodine based, the patient must be questioned about allergy to iodine or contrast medium, and any sensitivities must be reported to the radiology department. Bleeding is a common complication after liver puncture and can be massive; thus it is important to evaluate the patient for any clotting disorder before the procedure. Studies commonly done include prothrombin time, bleeding time, clotting time, and platelet count.

After the procedure the patient is maintained on bed rest for at least 6 hours. Vital signs are monitored for evidence of bleeding (q 15 min for 1 hour, q 30 min for 2 hours, then qh for 4 hours), and the injection site is checked for bleeding, swelling, or tenderness. The patient must be monitored for signs of peritonitis as well as hemorrhage; abdominal pain, fever, chills, tenderness, and distention are promptly reported.

PATIENT TEACHING

Explain the purpose of the test and the procedure. Tell the patient that she will be positioned on her left side and that a local anesthetic is used to numb the area before the needle is inserted. Explain that dye is injected and a series of x-rays is taken as the bile ducts are visualized.

ARTERIOGRAPHY

Arteriography involves injection of contrast medium into the celiac or mesenteric arteries to provide visualization of the vasculature supplying the intestinal tract and biliary tree (Figure 3-10). A needle is inserted into the femoral artery, and a guidewire is advanced through the needle into the aorta. The needle is re-

moved, and an arteriographic catheter is advanced over the guidewire under fluoroscopic guidance. When the catheter's position has been confirmed, the guidewire is removed and the catheter is again advanced, under fluoroscopy, into the vessel to be studied. Contrast medium is then injected, and serial films are taken as the vessels are visualized during the phases of arterial perfusion and venous drainage.

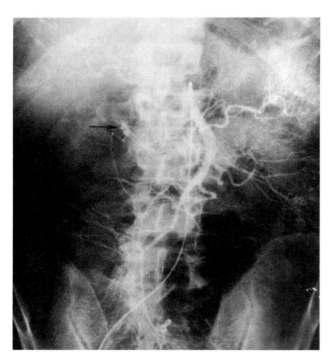

FIGURE 3-10
Arteriogram of superior mesenteric artery showing diverticular bleeding (note area of contrast extravasation).

INDICATIONS

To diagnose:
   Source of gastrointestinal bleeding
To evaluate:
   Cirrhosis
   Portal hypertension
   Vascular damage resulting from trauma
   Intestinal ischemia
   Vascular abnormalities
   Benign or malignant tumors
To treat:
   Gastrointestinal bleeding with vasopressin or embolic material

CONTRAINDICATIONS None

CAUTIONS

   Pregnancy
   Clotting abnormalities
   Allergy to iodine or contrast medium

NURSING CARE

The patient is questioned about any allergies to iodine or contrast agents, and the radiology department is notified if any sensitivities exist. Laboratory studies of clotting parameters should be obtained and reviewed before the procedure; any abnormalities in platelet count, clotting time, prothrombin time, or activated partial thromboplastin time are promptly reported, as are abnormalities in hemoglobin and hematocrit.

After the procedure the patient must be maintained on bed rest in the supine position for at least 12 hours. A sandbag or ice bag may be placed over the puncture site for 2 to 4 hours to reduce the risk of bleeding and hematoma formation. The puncture site is monitored for bleeding and hematoma formation, and the involved leg is monitored for any evidence of circulatory impairment (e.g., coolness, pallor, pain, reduced pulses compared to uninvolved extremity). The patient's vital signs are also monitored. Any evidence of bleeding or circulatory compromise is reported promptly to the physician.

PATIENT TEACHING

Explain the purpose of the test and the procedure. Explain that a venipuncture is performed, using the femoral artery, and that a catheter is threaded through this artery into the arteries to be studied. Explain that continuous x-rays are used to guide the catheter to the correct vessel. Tell the patient that dye is injected through the catheter into the vessel to be studied, and x-rays are taken as the dye passes into the arteries and then the veins. Tell the patient that some individuals experience a flushing, warm sensation when the dye is injected and that this is temporary.

STOOL ANALYSIS

Stool samples may be analyzed for abnormal constituents such as occult blood, pathogens, or excessive fats. Stool may also be analyzed to determine whether expected constituents, such as urobilinogen, are present.

Stool samples may be collected on a random base for qualitative studies or on a continual base (24-hour or 72-hour collection) for quantitative studies. When testing for fecal fat, the stool must be collected in a wax-free container to prevent altered test results. When testing for urobilinogen, the stool must be collected in a light-resistant container to prevent breakdown of the urobilinogen. All stool samples should be transported promptly to the laboratory or stored in the refrigerator to prevent distortion of test results.

Preparatory diet and medication restrictions may be required.

INDICATIONS

To diagnose:
    Gastrointestinal bleeding (blood)
    Bacterial diarrhea (culture)
    Malabsorption syndrome (fat)
To evaluate:
    Jaundice and hepatobiliary disorders

CONTRAINDICATIONS None

NURSING CARE

Some fecal studies require dietary modifications or omission of certain medications, and some analyses require that specific guidelines be followed in obtaining the stool sample.

Stool for occult blood (e.g., Hemoccult, Colo-Screen). Patients should forgo red meat, turnips, and horseradish and should consume a high-fiber diet for 48 to 72 hours before the test and throughout the test period. Patients are also advised to omit iron preparations and ascorbic acid for 48 hours before the test and throughout the testing period. These guidelines are designed to minimize false-positive and false-negative results.

The patient is instructed to obtain three separate stool specimens and to apply a small smear of stool to the test pad. The test envelope should be promptly returned to the laboratory and processed to reduce the incidence of false-negative results.

Stool for fecal fat. The patient is instructed to forgo alcohol and to follow a high-fat diet (100 g/day) for 72 hours before the test and during the test period. The following drugs should be omitted, because they affect fat absorption or the digestive process and thus would

alter the test results: azathioprine, kanamycin, bisacodyl, cholestyramine, neomycin, colchicine, aluminum hydroxide, calcium carbonate, potassium chloride, and mineral oil.

Analysis of fecal fat may be performed as a random study on a single stool specimen or may involve a 72-hour stool collection. The random study involves identification of muscle fibers and various fats; fecal lipids normally constitute less than 20% of the excreted solids. The 72-hour study involves quantification of the amount of fats excreted into the stool; fecal lipids are normally less than 7 g/24 h. Stool specimens should be collected in unwaxed containers and must be refrigerated until they can be taken to the laboratory.

Fecal urobilinogen. For optimum results antibiotics, sulfonamides, and salicylates should be avoided for the 2 weeks preceding the test, because they can affect fecal urobilinogen levels or can alter test results. The stool may be collected as a random specimen or as a 24-hour collection; the stool should be collected in a light-resistant container, since exposure to light causes urobilinogen to convert to urobilin. Normal values are 50 to 300 mg/24 h. Low levels may be seen with liver dysfunction or obstructive jaundice; elevated levels may be seen with hemolytic conditions.

Stool for culture. A freshly passed stool specimen is collected and sent immediately to the laboratory; if immediate transport cannot be arranged, the laboratory should be contacted about storage requirements. (Many organisms die if exposed to cold, so refrigeration is not usually recommended.) Cultures for *Salmonella* and *Shigella* organisms should be obtained before antibiotic therapy.

PATIENT TEACHING

Explain to the patient the purpose of the stool analysis and the procedure for stool collection. Explain any dietary and medication restrictions, as described in the section on Nursing Care.

ANORECTAL MANOMETRY

Anorectal manometry measures the resting tone of the internal sphincter, the contractility of the external sphincter, and the length of the anal canal by means of a rectoanal catheter connected to a transducer and a recorder or computer. The rectoanal catheter has three balloons: an intrarectal balloon, which can be inflated to

cause rectal distention; a proximal intraanal balloon, which reflects internal sphincter activity; and a distal intraanal balloon, which reflects external sphincter activity (Figure 3-11). Changes in the intrarectal and anal canal pressures produce changes in the balloon pressures, which are reflected on the recorder or computer.

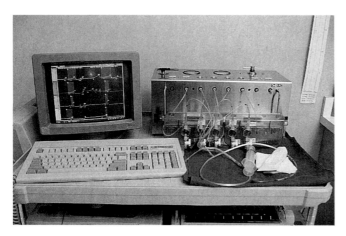

FIGURE 3-11
Anorectal manometry equipment and recording.

INDICATIONS

To evaluate:
Internal and external anal sphincter function
Chronic constipation
Fecal incontinence
To diagnose:
Reduced contractility of anal sphincter

Increased contractility of anal sphincter
Denervation of anal sphincter

CONTRAINDICATION

Unhealed anorectal anastomoses

NURSING CARE

A low-volume rectal enema may be ordered to cleanse the rectal vault before the procedure. No postprocedural care is required.

PATIENT TEACHING

Explain the purpose of the test and the procedure. Explain to the patient that a special pressure-sensitive catheter is inserted into the rectum and connected to a pressure transducer and a recording device. Explain that the portion of the catheter in the rectum is filled with air or water to simulate the rectum filling with stool and that the pressure-sensitive areas in the anal canal will reflect sphincter activity. Explain that this enables the physician to determine whether the sphincters are working correctly. Tell the patient that insertion of the catheter and instillation of air or water into the rectum may cause temporary discomfort or a need to defecate, but this will pass; instruct the patient to breathe slowly and deeply to facilitate relaxation.

COLONIC TRANSIT STUDY

In a colonic transit study, the patient is given a capsule containing 20 radiopaque markers, and a plain x-ray of the abdomen is obtained 5 days later. Normally all of the markers will have been eliminated by this time; transit time varies from person to person but averages 33 hours in men and 47 hours in women. Follow-up films revealing a number of the markers scattered throughout the colon indicate motility disorders; films revealing a number of the markers clustered in the rectum indicate an obstructive defecation syndrome.

INDICATIONS

To evaluate:
Colonic motility

To diagnose:
Chronic constipation
Colonic motility disorders
Obstructive defecation syndromes

CONTRAINDICATION

Pregnancy

PATIENT TEACHING

Explain the procedure and its purpose. Explain that the radiopaque markers are not harmful in any way and that they do not make the patient "radioactive." Tell the patient to follow her regular diet and activity patterns. With outpatients, reinforce the importance of returning for the x-ray on the scheduled day.

RECTAL SENSORY FUNCTION TEST

In the rectal sensory function test, a catheter with a balloon is passed into the rectum, and the balloon is gradually inflated with air until the patient senses rectal distention (normally at about 15 ml).

INDICATIONS

To evaluate:
   Rectal sensory function

To diagnose:
   Rectal sensory neuropathy

CONTRAINDICATION

Unhealed anorectal anastomoses

PATIENT TEACHING

Explain the purpose of the test and the procedure. Explain to the patient that she will be asked to indicate when she first feels rectal distention.

HYDROGEN BREATH TEST

The hydrogen breath test is used to evaluate carbohydrate absorption (Figure 3-12). Normally all carbohydrates are absorbed in the jejunum; carbohydrates that are not absorbed are subjected to bacterial action, which produces carbon dioxide and hydrogen. Carbohydrate malabsorption can be detected by the marked increase in hydrogen in exhaled breath.

The hydrogen breath test involves administration of a measured amount of carbohydrate, usually lactose or D-glucose, followed by collection and analysis of exhaled gases after a specific period, usually about 90 minutes. The test is noninvasive, simple, and inexpensive.

INDICATIONS

To diagnose:
   Malabsorption caused by bacterial overgrowth in small intestine (e.g., blind loop syndrome, Crohn's disease, distal ileal disease)
   Malabsorption caused by enzyme deficiency (e.g., lactase or galactase deficiency)

CONTRAINDICATIONS None

NURSING CARE

Foods and carbohydrate beverages may be withheld for 8 hours preceding the test. If the nurse is responsible for giving the test substance, the time and amount are recorded and reported to the testing department. No aftercare is required.

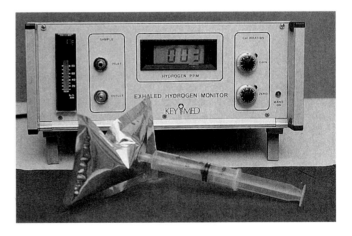

FIGURE 3-12
Equipment used for hydrogen breath test.

PATIENT TEACHING

Explain the purpose of the test and the procedure. Instruct the patient in any food or fluid restrictions to be followed before the test. Explain the importance of ingesting the test substance at the specified time. Tell the patient that she may resume her normal diet after the study.

S CHILLING TEST

The Schilling test is done to evaluate small bowel absorption of vitamin B_{12}. Adequate absorption of this vitamin depends on production of intrinsic factor by the stomach and adequate absorption of the intrinsic factor–vitamin B_{12} complex, which occurs only in the distal ileum.

The Schilling test involves intramuscular administration of vitamin B_{12} (1,000 μg), followed by oral administration of radioactive cobalt–labeled vitamin B_{12}. (The vitamin B_{12} administered intramuscularly ensures saturation of all storage sites in the liver; the radioactive vitamin B_{12} administered orally should then be excreted through the urine, assuming absorption into the bloodstream.) The patient's urine is collected for 24 hours after the radioactive vitamin B_{12} is taken, and the urine is analyzed for excreted vitamin B_{12}. Normally more than 7% of the orally administered radioactive vitamin B_{12} is excreted within 24 hours.

INDICATIONS

To evaluate:
   Ileal absorption of vitamin B_{12}
To diagnose:
   Pernicious anemia caused by loss of intrinsic factor or inadequate ileal absorption of intrinsic factor–vitamin B_{12} complex

CONTRAINDICATIONS None

NURSING CARE

The nurse administers the intramuscular vitamin B_{12} and may be asked to give the radioactive oral dose. All urine must be carefully collected for the 24 hours following oral administration of radioactive vitamin B_{12}. The nurse should use universal precautions in handling the patient's urine and other bodily fluids; no special precautions are needed, because the amount of radioactivity involved is minimal.

PATIENT TEACHING

Explain the purpose of the test and the procedure. Give the patient a receptacle for collecting urine, and emphasize the importance of collecting *all* urine for the 24-hour period following administration of the radioactive oral vitamin B_{12}. Reassure the patient that she is not "radioactive" and does not present any risk to others. If the patient is a nursing mother, verify any temporary restrictions on breast-feeding with the nuclear medicine department, and instruct the patient accordingly.

S ERUM STUDIES

NONSPECIFIC STUDIES

A number of blood tests can indicate a pathologic condition of the gastrointestinal tract or one elsewhere in the body; thus they are nonspecific diagnostic indicators. For example, a low hemoglobin and hematocrit may reflect gastrointestinal bleeding or bleeding elsewhere in the body. Similarly, an elevated white blood cell count (WBC) indicates infection but does not identify the source of the infection. Alterations in electrolyte balance and acid-base balance are commonly seen in a patient with abnormal losses from the gastrointestinal tract but may also be caused by a renal disorder, liver dysfunction, respiratory disease, or metabolic derangements. Table 3-1 displays normal values for commonly used nonspecific serum studies.

SPECIFIC STUDIES

Some blood tests provide more specific information about organ function. For example, liver function commonly is evaluated by a number of serum studies known collectively as liver function studies; the specific tests, normal values, and the significance of abnormal results are shown in Table 3-2 on p. 68. Pancreatic inflammation is reflected by rising levels of specific enzymes found in both serum and urine (Table 3-3, p. 69). Malnutrition may be evidenced by abnormally low serum protein levels and by a low total lymphocyte count (Table 3-4, p. 70), although these values are also seen in other diseases, such as liver disease and neutropenia.

TUMOR MARKERS

The carcinoembryonic antigen (CEA) is a glycoprotein found in the cell membranes of many tissues, including some malignant tumors of the gastrointestinal system (e.g., colorectal tumors). Elevated CEA levels are not specific for gastrointestinal cancer, because the elevation could also be caused by malignancies in other organ systems and by benign diseases. In addition, not all colorectal tumors secrete CEA; a significant number of patients with known colorectal cancer have normal CEA levels. For these reasons CEA is not valuable as a screening procedure for gastrointestinal malignancy. However, CEA is valuable for monitoring a patient for response to treatment and for recurrent disease; the patient with a gastrointestinal malignancy and elevated CEA before treatment whose CEA returns to normal after treatment has a good prognosis. The patient whose CEA remains elevated has a poor prognosis, and the patient whose CEA drops after treatment and then rises should be evaluated closely for recurrence. Normal CEA levels in nonsmoking adults are less than 2.5 ng/ml.

Table 3-1

COMMON NONSPECIFIC SERUM STUDIES

Test name	Normal values
Complete blood count with differential count (CBC and Diff)	
Red blood cell count (RBC)	Men: 4.7-6.1 million/mm^3 Women: 4.2-5.4 million/mm^3 Low values indicate anemia resulting from blood loss, hemolysis, dietary deficiency, drug ingestion, bone marrow failure, or chronic illness; high values may indicate compensation for high altitudes, chronic anoxia, or polycythemia vera.
Hemoglobin (Hb) concentration	Men: 14-18 g/dl Women: 12-16 g/dl Low and high values tend to be caused by the same processes that cause low or high values for RBC; dehydration causes an artificially high value.
Hematocrit (Hct)	Men: 42%-52% Women: 37%-47% Low and high values tend to be caused by the same processes that cause low or high RBC and Hb values.
Mean corpuscular volume (MCV)	Adults: 80-95/μm^3 High values may be seen in megaloblastic anemias (e.g., vitamin B$_{12}$ deficiency); low values may be seen with iron-deficiency anemia or thalassemia.
Mean corpuscular hemoglobin (MCH)	Adults: 27-31 pg Low and high values tend to be caused by the same processes that cause low or high values for MCV.
Mean corpuscular hemoglobin concentration (MCHC)	Adults: 32-36 g/dl Low values indicate hemoglobin deficiency and are seen in iron-deficiency anemia and thalassemia.
White blood cell count (WBC)	Adults: 5,000-10,000/mm^3
Differential	Neutrophils: 55%-70% Lymphocytes: 20%-40% Monocytes: 2%-8% Eosinophils: 1%-4% Basophils: 0.5%-1%

Continued.

Table 3-1

COMMON NONSPECIFIC SERUM STUDIES—cont'd

Test name	Normal values
	Elevated WBC commonly indicates infection or leukemia; decreased WBC may indicate bone marrow failure, overwhelming infection, dietary deficiency, or autoimmune disease; elevated neutrophil count may be seen in acute suppurative infection; decreased neutrophil count may be seen with overwhelming bacterial infection (especially in the elderly) or dietary deficiency; elevated lymphocyte count may be seen with chronic bacterial infection or viral infection; decreased lymphocyte count may be seen with sepsis; elevated eosinophil count may be seen with parasitic infestation, allergic reactions, or autoimmune diseases; a "shift to the left" means there is an increased percentage of neutrophils and immature leukocytes, which occurs with infection.
Platelet count	150,000-400,000/mm^3
	Reduced levels of platelets may result from decreased platelet production, increased sequestration (as is seen in hypersplenism), increased platelet destruction or consumption (e.g., disseminated intravascular coagulation), or loss of platelets through hemorrhage.
	Elevated levels may be seen with severe hemorrhage, polycythemia vera, postsplenectomy syndromes, and some malignant disorders.
Serum electrolytes	
Sodium (Na)	136-145 mEq/L
	Elevated levels may be seen with excessive sweating, extensive burns, osmotic diuresis, and excessive sodium intake or reduced sodium excretion; reduced levels may be seen with inadequate sodium intake, increased sodium losses (e.g., vomiting, nasogastric suction, diarrhea), renal disease, or third-space losses of sodium).
Potassium (K)	3.5-5 mEq/L
	Elevated levels may be seen with excessive intake or reduced excretion of potassium (e.g., renal failure), crushing injuries causing release of intracellular potassium, or with metabolic acidosis; reduced levels may be seen with inadequate intake or excessive losses (e.g., diarrhea, vomiting, use of diuretics, hyperaldosteronism) or as a result of metabolic alkalosis or administration of glucose, insulin, or calcium (which causes a shift of potassium from the bloodstream into cells).
Chloride (Cl)	90-110 mEq/L
	Changes in chloride concentration usually parallel changes in sodium concentration.
Carbon dioxide (CO_2)	23-30 mEq/L
	Elevated levels are seen with acidosis; reduced levels are seen with alkalosis.
Blood gas studies (arterial)	
pH	7.35-7.45
	High levels indicate alkalosis; low levels reflect acidosis.
Partial pressure of carbon dioxide (P_{CO_2})	35-45 mm Hg
	High levels indicate carbon dioxide retention due to respiratory depression or pulmonary disease (respiratory acidosis); low levels reflect excessive loss of carbon dioxide through hyperventilation (e.g., respiratory alkalosis due to overventilation or emotional trauma; may also be seen as compensatory response in metabolic acidosis).
Bicarbonate (HCO_3^-)	22-26 mEq/L
	Low levels indicate metabolic acidosis due to excessive acid production, resulting in depletion of HCO_3^- (e.g., diabetic acidosis); failure to eliminate H^+ ions, resulting in depletion of HCO_3^- (e.g., renal failure); or excessive loss of HCO_3^- (e.g., intestinal losses through diarrhea or fistula drainage); low levels may also be seen with insulin overdose, insulinoma, hypothyroidism, hypopituitarism, Addison's disease, and extensive liver disease.
	High levels indicate metabolic alkalosis resulting from bicarbonate overdose or excessive gastric losses; may also be seen as a compensatory response in a patient with prolonged respiratory acidosis, pancreatic disorders (e.g., adenoma, pancreatitis), corticosteroid therapy, diuretics, Cushing's disease, and hyperthyroidism.

Table 3-1

COMMON NONSPECIFIC SERUM STUDIES—cont'd

Test name	Normal values
Serum osmolality	275-300 mOsm/kg Elevated levels are seen with hyperglycemia, hypernatremia, dehydration, diabetes insipidus, and ketosis; low levels may result from fluid overload or inappropriate secretion of antidiuretic hormone (ADH).
Carcinoembryonic antigen (CEA)	<2 ng/ml Elevated levels may be seen in cancer of the colon, lung, pancreas, stomach, breast, head and neck, and prostate.
Cholesterol	150-250 mg/dl*
Vitamin and mineral levels (serum)	
Ascorbic acid	0.2-2 mg/dl Low levels may result from inadequate intake, compromised absorption, or excessive losses.
Folate	5-20 μg/ml Elevated levels may be seen with pernicious anemia; low levels may be seen during pregnancy or in patients with folic acid anemia, hemolytic anemia, malnutrition, malabsorption, malignancy, liver disease, sprue, or celiac disease.
Iron	60-190 μg/dl Low levels may indicate anemia due to inadequate iron intake, inadequate iron absorption, increased iron requirements, or blood loss; low levels may also be seen in patients with chronic illness (e.g., cancer, infections, cirrhosis). High levels may be caused by increased intake or absorption of iron (e.g., hemochromatosis).
Magnesium	1.2-1.9 mEq/L Low levels may be seen with a chronically deficient diet or severe malabsorption; high levels may be seen with renal failure.
Calcium	9-10.5 ng/dl Persistent high levels (three separate tests with elevated levels) may be seen with bone metastases, parathyroid hormone–producing tumors (e.g., lung or renal carcinoma), vitamin D intoxication, sarcoidosis, hyperparathyroidism, or excessive ingestion of calcium-containing antacids or concentrated milk; low levels may be seen with hypoparathyroidism, renal failure, or rickets.
Vitamin A	15-60 μg/dl High levels may be seen with excessive ingestion and absorption; low levels may be seen with inadequate intake or conditions causing fat malabsorption.
Vitamin B$_{12}$	160-950 pg/ml Low levels may be seen with pernicious anemia (inadequate production of intrinsic factor), malabsorption syndrome, liver disease, sprue, ileal resection, or hypothyroidism.
Zinc	0.66-1.1 μg/ml Low levels may be seen with chronic dietary deficiency, malabsorption, or excessive losses.

*There are discrepancies between reported normals; levels under 180 are desirable, but higher levels are common in the United States. Elevated levels are seen in cardiovascular disease, atherosclerosis, obstructive jaundice, and uncontrolled diabetes; reduced levels occur with fat malabsorption, liver disease, and hyperthyroidism.

Table 3-2

LIVER FUNCTION STUDIES

Test name	Normal values
Serum enzymes	
Alkaline phosphatase	13-39 U/ml
	Elevated levels are seen with biliary obstruction and cholestatic hepatitis.
Aspartate aminotrans-ferase (AST; previously SGOT)	5-40 U/ml
	Elevated levels are seen with hepatocellular injury.
Alanine aminotrans-ferase (ALT; previously SGPT)	5-35 U/ml
	Elevated levels are seen with liver dysfunction; the ratio of AST/ALT usually is more than 1 in alcoholic cirrhosis and liver congestion and less than 1 in acute hepatitis, viral hepatitis, and infectious mononucleosis.
Lactic dehydrogenase (LDH)	200-500 U/ml
	Elevated levels are seen with hepatitis and untreated pernicious anemia, as well as in a number of other conditions (e.g., acute myocardial infarction, renal disease, muscle disease, or malignant tumors).
5'-Nucleotidase	2-11 U/ml
	Elevated levels may be an early indication of metastasis to the liver.
Leucine aminopeptidase (LAP)	Men: 80-200 U/ml
	Women: 75-185 U/ml
	Elevated levels may be seen with liver metastasis and choledocholithiasis.
Gamma-glutamyltranspeptidase (GGTP)	Men: 8-38 U/L
	Women <45 yr: 5-27 U/L
	Elevated levels are seen in 75% of chronic alcoholics.
Bilirubin metabolism	
Serum bilirubin	
Indirect (unconjugated)	<0.8 mg/dl
	Elevated levels seen with hemolysis (lysis of RBCs).
Direct (conjugated)	0.2-0.4 mg/dl
	Elevated levels seen with hepatocellular injury or obstruction.
Total	<1 mg/dl
	Elevated levels may be seen with biliary obstruction.
Urine bilirubin	0
	Bilirubin in the urine may be seen with hepatic disease or biliary obstruction; only conjugated bilirubin spills into the urine, because unconjugated bilirubin is bound to albumin in the serum and thus cannot pass the glomerular membrane.
Urine urobilinogen	0-4 mg/24 h
	Increased levels are seen with hemolytic processes, shunting of portal blood flow, or increased intestinal bacteria.
Fecal urobilinogen	40-280 mg/24 h
	Reduced levels cause clay-colored stools and are seen in biliary obstruction.
Ammonia	Adult: 15-110 μg/dl
	Elevated levels may be seen with liver dysfunction, hepatic failure, or congestive heart failure.

Table 3-2

LIVER FUNCTION STUDIES—cont'd

Test name	Normal values
Serum proteins	
Albumin	3.5-5.5 g/dl
	Reduced levels are seen with hepatocellular injury.
Globulin	2.5-3.5 g/dl
	Increased levels are seen with hepatitis.
Total	6-7 g/dl
	Decreased levels may be seen with hepatocellular injury.
Albumin/globulin (A/G) ratio	1.5/1-2.5/1
	Ratio may be reversed with chronic hepatitis or other chronic liver disease.
Transferrin	250-300 μg/dl
	Reduced levels may be seen with liver damage; increased levels may be seen with iron deficiency.
Blood clotting functions	
Prothrombin time (PT)	11.5-14 sec *or* 90%-100% of control
	Increased levels may be seen with chronic liver disease (e.g., cirrhosis) or vitamin K deficiency.
	25-40 sec
Partial thromboplastin time (PTT)	Increased levels may be seen with severe liver disease or heparin therapy.

Table 3-3

TESTS OF PANCREATIC FUNCTION

Test name	Normal values
Serum amylase	60-180 Somogyi units/ml
	Elevated levels are seen with pancreatic inflammation.
Serum lipase	1.5 Somogyi units/ml
	Elevated levels may indicate pancreatic inflammation.
Urine amylase	35-260 Somogyi units/h
	Elevated levels are seen with pancreatic inflammation.
Secretin test	Volume 1.8 ml/kg/h
	HCO_3^- concentration >80 mEq/L
	HCO_3^- output >10 mEq/L/30 sec
	Reduced volumes are seen with pancreatic disease.

Table 3-4

LABORATORY INDICES OF NUTRITIONAL STATUS

Test name	Normal values
Albumin (serum)	3.5-5.5 mg/dl Decreased levels are seen in protein malnutrition and with hepatocellular injury.
Transferrin (serum)	250-300 mg/dl Decreased levels are seen in protein malnutrition; transferrin levels may be used to monitor a patient's response to nutritional support therapy, because transferrin's half-life is 8 to 10 days, whereas albumin's half-life is 19 to 20 days. (This means that transferrin levels reflect changes in the patient's visceral protein status much faster than do albumin levels.)
Prealbumin (serum)	15-32 mg/dl Decreased levels are seen in protein malnutrition; because the half-life of prealbumin is 2 to 3 days, these values reflect changes in the patient's visceral protein status even faster than transferrin levels.
Total lymphocyte count (serum)	$>150,000/mm^3$ Decreased levels may be seen in protein malnutrition; however, many other conditions affect the total lymphocyte count (e.g., infection or conditions affecting WBC production).
24-h urine for urea nitrogen (UUN)	Reflects renal excretion of nitrogen; used to determine nitrogen balance, which should be positive. Formula: $$\frac{\text{24-h Nitrogen intake (g of protein)}}{6.25} - (24\ h\ UUN + 4) = Balance$$

Inflammatory Disorders of the Gastrointestinal System

For a picture of gingivostomatitis, see Color Plate 1,
p. x.

Inflammatory disorders affecting the gastrointestinal system are very common and range in severity from a mild viral gastroenteritis to potentially fatal conditions such as hepatitis B and peritonitis. Most inflammatory disorders have an identifiable cause; common causes include bacterial, viral, and fungal infections; cytotoxic agents such as chemotherapeutic drugs or radiation therapy; and antigens that prompt an allergenic response. However, the gastrointestinal system is also subject to primary inflammatory disorders with no proven cause, such as chronic ulcerative colitis and Crohn's disease.

Inflammatory disorders can affect any structure of the gastrointestinal system; the symptoms produced depend on the specific structures involved. The principles of treatment are: eliminate the cause, when possible; rest the involved structure; and control the symptoms. Primary inflammatory disorders are managed with anti-inflammatory drugs and symptom control. Surgical intervention may be required to control infection (e.g., when perforation of an acutely inflamed structure is imminent or has occurred), to control bleeding, or to close fistulous tracts caused by the inflammation. Nursing management for patients with inflammatory gastrointestinal disorders includes attention to nutritional support, fluid and electrolyte balance, symptom control, and prevention of complications. Patient education and counseling are of prime importance, especially for patients coping with chronic inflammatory conditions or altered gastrointestinal structure or function, such as an ostomy.

Stomatitis

Stomatitis is a condition characterized by ulcers on the gums or the oral mucous membranes or both. The term "stomatitis" is also used to describe inflammation and ulceration of an intestinal stoma.

EPIDEMIOLOGY

Stomatitis is a common condition with a number of causes: mechanical trauma, oral irritants, viruses, fungi, nutritional deficits, and cytotoxic therapy (e.g., chemotherapy or radiation therapy). The severity ranges from a single lesion to several very painful lesions that affect nutrient intake.

Mechanical trauma can be caused by orthodontic appliances or poorly fitting dentures. The most common form of viral stomatitis is herpetic stomatitis. Primary infection usually occurs in childhood and is characterized by numerous vesicles that progress to ulcers, gingivitis, lymphadenopathy, fever, and mouth pain. After the initial infection, some individuals develop recurrent infections during times of stress or illness. These recurrent infections, known as herpes labialis, are characterized by ulcers around the lips at the mucocutaneous junction. Fungal stomatitis is also known as oral candidiasis and usually is seen in patients with fungal overgrowth stemming from antibiotic therapy, diabetes, or malnutrition. It is characterized by white plaques on the oral mucous membranes, gums, and tongue. Angular stomatitis refers to inflammatory changes caused by iron deficiency; these lesions appear at the corners of the mouth and range from erythema to ulcers and crusted fissures. Stomatitis caused by cytotoxic agents such as chemotherapy usually involves numerous, very painful ulcers on the oral mucous membranes, gums, tongue, and throat; ulcers may also be seen on intestinal stomas.

Besides the varieties of stomatitis with known causes, there is a type known as aphthous stomatitis. This condition is characterized by small, yellow, painful ulcers of unclear etiology. This type of stomatitis is seen most often in adolescents and young adults and affects women slightly more often than men.

PATHOPHYSIOLOGY

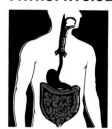

Prodromal symptoms may occur, including a burning or "prickling" sensation of the lips or mucous membranes. Initially the lesions appear as vesicles, which progress to open ulcers. These ulcers are very painful and may interfere with oral intake, especially when several lesions are involved. The open lesions also predispose to infection, especially in immunocompromised patients. In severely leukopenic patients, pathogenic invasion of the open ulcers can lead to septicemia.

The two types of stomatitis that do not progress from vesicles to ulcers are angular stomatitis, which in-

volves drying and cracking of the corners of the mouth, and fungal stomatitis, in which a patchy membrane forms over the mucosal surfaces.

To resolve the stomatitis, the cause must be eliminated. Aphthous stomatitis, which has no identified cause, usually resolves spontaneously within 1 to 2 weeks.

COMPLICATIONS
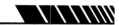

Altered nutritional status resulting from inadequate intake
Infection

DIAGNOSTIC STUDIES AND FINDINGS

Diagnostic test	Findings
Exudate culture (viral/fungal)	May be positive for fungi or viruses
Complete blood count (CBC)	May see reduced hemoglobin (Hb), hematocrit (Hct), mean corpuscular volume (MCV), mean corpuscular hemoglobin (MCH), and mean corpuscular hemoglobin concentration (MCHC) in patients with iron-deficiency stomatitis; may see reduced WBC in immunosuppressed patients

---

MEDICAL MANAGEMENT

GENERAL MANAGEMENT

Oral hygiene to reduce the risk of secondary infection; nutritional supplements as needed to maintain nutritional status; comfort measures (oral rinses and lubrication of lips).

DRUG THERAPY

Antiviral medications (e.g., acyclovir) for herpetic stomatitis; antifungal medications (e.g., nystatin) for fungal stomatitis; iron supplements (e.g., $FeSO_4$) for iron-deficiency stomatitis; topical anesthetics (e.g., viscous lidocaine) as needed for pain.

1 ASSESS

ASSESSMENT	OBSERVATIONS
Lips and oral cavity	May see vesicles or ulcers around lips or on oral mucous membranes; may see patchy white areas on oral mucous membranes; may see reddened areas or fissures around corners of mouth
Pain	May complain of burning or stinging mouth pain or extreme soreness in mouth
Nutritional status	May report recent weight loss; may refuse oral foods and fluids because of pain
Intestinal stoma (if applicable)	May see vesicles, ulcers, or patchy white membrane on surface of stoma

2 DIAGNOSE

NURSING DIAGNOSIS	SUBJECTIVE FINDINGS	OBJECTIVE FINDINGS
Altered oral mucous membranes related to inflammatory process	May complain of sore mouth; may report previous episodes of similar ulcers	Vesicles or ulcers on lips or oral mucous membranes or both; redness or fissures in corners of mouth; white patches on oral mucous membranes
Pain related to inflammation	Complains of mouth being sore; may describe pain as burning, stinging, or aching	Facial expressions of pain when performing oral care or eating (especially if eating spicy or textured foods); limits speech; limits food and fluid intake
Altered nutrition: less than body requirements related to difficulty eating and drinking	Describes inability to eat and drink; may report recent weight loss; may report altered taste	Consumes inadequate amounts of food and fluids; weight is below 90% of usual weight
Impaired tissue integrity (patient with intestinal stomatitis) related to inflammatory process	Describes lesions on stoma; may report bleeding when stoma is cleaned	Vesicles, ulcers, or white patches on intestinal stoma; stoma appears friable and bleeds easily

3 PLAN

Patient goals

1. The patient's oral mucous membranes will be intact.
2. The patient will be free of mouth pain.
3. The patient will maintain adequate nutrient and fluid intake.
4. The patient will have intact stomal mucosa (if applicable).

→ > >

4 IMPLEMENT

NURSING DIAGNOSIS	NURSING INTERVENTIONS	RATIONALE
Altered oral mucous membranes related to inflammatory process	Administer medications as ordered (e.g., antiviral or antifungal medications or iron supplements).	Stomatitis may be caused by viruses or fungi, and appropriate medications will eliminate them; stomatitis caused by iron deficiency is corrected by iron therapy.
	Help patient perform gentle, thorough oral hygiene after each meal and at bedtime (i.e., brushing teeth with soft-bristled toothbrush, using oral rinses).	Oral hygiene reduces the risk of secondary infection and prevents accumulation of plaque, which provides a medium for bacterial proliferation and further irritates the gums; gentle techniques must be used to prevent additional damage or bleeding.
Pain related to inflammation	Assess patient for mouth pain, and administer analgesics (e.g., viscous lidocaine) as needed, especially before meals.	Analgesics reduce pain and discomfort.
	Encourage patient to eat bland, nonirritating foods.	Spicy and "rough" foods may aggravate mouth pain.
	Apply pectin-based oral dressings (e.g., Orahesive) or oral pastes (e.g., Orabase) to lesions as ordered.	Pectin-based oral dressings and pastes provide a protective layer over the lesions and thus reduce pain.
	Provide soothing oral rinses as needed.	Oral rinses remove irritating debris and help promote comfort.
	Keep lips lubricated.	Lubrication prevents drying, which can cause cracking and aggravate pain.
Altered nutrition: less than body requirements related to difficulty eating and drinking	Compare patient's current weight to usual weight and ideal weight (for height and sex).	Recent weight loss or inadequate weight for height (below 90% of ideal body weight) indicates inadequate nutrient intake.
	Assess and document food and fluid intake.	Inadequate intake (less than 75% of prescribed diet, less than 1,500 ml fluid) requires adjustment in the plan for nutritional and fluid support.
	Encourage intake of bland, high-protein, high-calorie foods and at least 1,500 ml of fluid a day.	Bland foods cause less mouth pain; high-protein, high-calorie foods support the healing process and immune system functioning; adequate fluid intake prevents further drying of the mucous membranes.
	Consult the dietitian about patient with inadequate intake or patient whose weight is below 90% of usual weight.	The dietitian can do an in-depth nutritional assessment and can recommend appropriate measures for nutritional support.
Impaired tissue integrity (patient with intestinal stomatitis) related to inflammatory process	Clean stoma and peristomal skin gently.	Aggressive cleansing of damaged mucosal surface can cause increased trauma, bleeding, and possibly bacterial invasion.

NURSING INTERVENTIONS	RATIONALE
If stoma is very friable or bleeding, instill mineral oil into pouch.	Mineral oil lubricates the surface of the pouch and reduces friction between the pouch and the stoma.
If the patient is undergoing radiation therapy, tell the radiation oncologist about the stomatitis.	Severe stomatitis may necessitate a temporary interruption in radiation therapy to allow the mucosal surface to regenerate.

5 EVALUATE

PATIENT OUTCOME	DATA INDICATING THAT OUTCOME IS REACHED
Patient's oral mucous membranes are intact.	Inspection reveals no lesions in oral cavity.
Patient has no mouth pain.	Patient states that her mouth is no longer painful; she does not limit her speech or oral intake.
Patient maintains an adequate nutrient and fluid intake.	Patient consistently consumes 75% or more of her prescribed diet and ingests at least 1,500 ml of fluid daily.
Patient's stomal mucosa is intact.	Inspection reveals no stoma lesions; patient states that stomal bleeding has stopped.

PATIENT TEACHING

1. Explain the probable causes of stomatitis.
2. Explain the importance of oral hygiene in preventing infection and maintaining comfort.
3. If medications have been prescribed for the patient, explain the purpose and the dosage schedule. If the patient uses oral dressings or pastes, instruct her or her caregiver in the correct application and frequency of use.
4. Explain the importance of nutrient and fluid intake, and teach the patient measures for relieving pain (e.g., soothing rinses, oral anesthetics).
5. If the patient has herpetic stomatitis, explain the potential for infectious spread (e.g., to eyes), and stress the importance of handwashing; warn the patient to avoid touching the lesions.
6. If the patient has intestinal stomatitis, explain the importance of *very gentle* stoma care to prevent trauma.

Esophagitis

Esophagitis is an inflammation of the esophagus (Figure 4-1).

EPIDEMIOLOGY

Esophagitis may be caused by specific pathogens such as herpes simplex or *Candida* organisms, by ingested irritants, or by gastroesophageal reflux. Gastroesophageal reflux is the most common cause.

A number of interacting factors can contribute to gastroesophageal reflux: persistently low lower esophageal sphincter (LES) pressure; transient relaxation of the lower esophageal sphincter that causes a sudden drop in LES pressure; or an increase in intraabdominal pressure that "overrides" LES pressures. Studies have shown that gastroesophageal reflux occurs in asymptomatic individuals as well as in patients with reflux esophagitis; episodes of reflux are particularly common for a 2-hour period after eating. Normally reflux does not produce symptoms, because two mechanisms limit contact between gastric contents and the esophageal mucosa: esophageal peristalsis, which normally "clears" the esophagus of any refluxed material within 1 to 3 minutes, and saliva, which neutralizes the refluxed gastric contents.

Symptoms of esophagitis develop when there is prolonged or frequent contact between gastric contents and the esophageal mucosa, or when gastric contents are very acidic or contain bile salts or pancreatic enzymes. Studies show that patients with symptomatic esophagitis have more frequent episodes of transient LES relaxation, and lower LES resting pressures; frequent episodes of LES relaxation increase the frequency of reflux, and lower LES resting pressures are more easily "overridden" by increased intraabdominal pressures, resulting in reflux. Lower resting pressures may also permit spontaneous reflux of gastric contents.

Symptomatic gastroesophageal reflux is common during pregnancy, and studies have demonstrated lower LES pressures throughout pregnancy, apparently as a result of hormonal changes. Sphincter pressures return to normal after delivery, and symptoms subside.

Factors contributing to symptomatic gastroesophageal reflux include conditions that cause delayed gastric emptying, increased intraabdominal pressure, and impaired LES function. Gastric emptying is delayed by pyloric edema or strictures, which may result from peptic ulcer disease; intraabdominal pressures are affected by body position, body weight, and activities such as coughing. Impaired LES function frequently has been linked to sliding hiatal hernia; however, studies show that hiatal hernia does not necessarily lead to reflux.

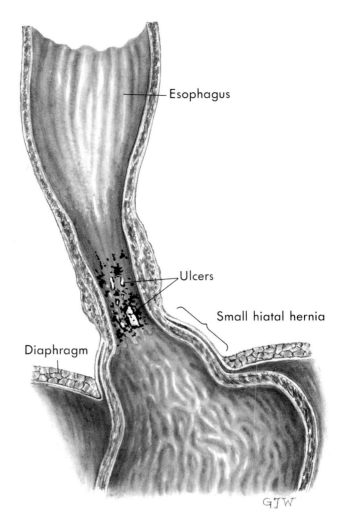

FIGURE 4-1
Esophagitis with esophageal ulcerations.

Some individuals with hiatal hernias have normal resting LES pressures and no symptomatic reflux; thus hiatal hernia is more appropriately considered an associated rather than a causative factor. Other factors associated with lower LES pressures are smoking, excessive alcohol consumption, some foods (e.g., fats, chocolate, orange juice, tomatoes), and side-lying or sitting positions.

PATHOPHYSIOLOGY

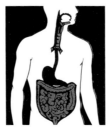

Pathologic changes usually can be seen with endoscopy; they include mucosal erythema, friability, superficial linear ulcers, and exudate formation. Infiltration of the esophageal mucosa with polymorphonuclear leukocytes may be seen on biopsy. Long-standing or recurrent inflammation may result in stricture formation and stenosis; superficial erosions are particularly likely to be associated with submucosal fibrosis and concentric thickening of the esophageal wall, which is the basis for stricture formation. Deeper ulcers may cause full-thickness damage but less concentric scarring.

The "heartburn" pain and dysphagia associated with symptomatic gastroesophageal reflux may be due to the irritating effect of gastric contents on sensory nerve endings in the esophageal mucosa, or they may be caused by esophageal muscle spasm that occurs in response to contact with gastric acid. Most probably the pain and difficulty swallowing stem from a combination of these two factors.

COMPLICATIONS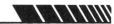

Esophageal stenosis

DIAGNOSTIC STUDIES AND FINDINGS

Diagnostic test	Findings
Esophageal endoscopy with mucosal biopsy	May show edema and superficial or deep erosions; may show stricture; biopsy may show mucosal infiltration with polymorphonuclear leukocytes
Barium swallow	Reflux may be demonstrated with severe disease; may reveal associated conditions (e.g., hiatal hernia, abnormal contours of esophageal lumen)
Esophageal manometry	LES pressures < 8 mm Hg commonly seen with gastroesophageal reflux
Acid perfusion (Bernstein test)	Abnormal in 85%-90% of patients with esophagitis; chest pain occurs within a few minutes of acid perfusion of esophagus. *Note:* There may be a delayed positive response (pain occurs 10-20 min after perfusion of acid) in patients with chest pain of unknown cause
Esophageal acidity test (pH monitoring)	Below normal with gastroesophageal reflux

MEDICAL MANAGEMENT

GENERAL MANAGEMENT

Measures to reduce intraabdominal pressure: Weight control; avoiding constrictive garments (e.g., girdles, tight belts); control of conditions such as chronic cough or constipation.

Measures to increase LES pressure: Dietary modifications (e.g., avoiding fats, chocolate, orange juice, and tomatoes); cessation of cigarette smoking; limiting alcohol intake.

Measures to promote gastric emptying and reduce reflux: Elevating the head of the bed 8 to 12 inches; avoiding eating for 4 hours before going to bed.

SURGERY

Surgery occasionally may be required to reduce the lumen of the lower esophagus or to treat complications such as stricture formation.

DRUG THERAPY

Antacids (e.g., Maalox): 30 ml 1 h and 3 h after meals to reduce gastric acidity.

H$_2$-receptor antagonists (cimetidine or ranitidine): To reduce production of gastric acid.

Cholinergic drugs (e.g., metoclopramide [Reglan]): To increase LES tone and promote gastric emptying.

1 ASSESS

ASSESSMENT	OBSERVATIONS
Pain	May report discomfort when swallowing acidic foods or fluids or alcohol; may report regurgitation or "heartburn" within 1-2 h after eating, when lying down, or with activities that cause increased intraabdominal pressure (e.g., coughing or straining at stool)

2 DIAGNOSE

NURSING DIAGNOSIS	SUBJECTIVE FINDINGS	OBJECTIVE FINDINGS
Impaired tissue integrity related to esophageal inflammation	May report regurgitation within 1-2 h after eating; reports discomfort with swallowing, particularly alcohol and acidic substances; describes substernal pain ("heartburn") after meals or with activities that increase intraabdominal pressure (e.g., coughing, straining at stool)	May limit intake of food and fluids; avoids recumbent position
Pain related to esophageal inflammation	Describes "heartburn"-type pain and may describe discomfort with swallowing	Facial expressions reflect discomfort when swallowing; may limit food and fluid intake

3 PLAN

Patient goals

1. The patient will regain normal esophageal tissue integrity.

2. The patient will have no "heartburn" pain or pain on swallowing.

4 IMPLEMENT

NURSING DIAGNOSIS	NURSING INTERVENTIONS	RATIONALE
Impaired tissue integrity related to esophageal inflammation	Elevate head of bed 8-12 in.	Elevating the head of the bed improves gastric emptying and reduces reflux.
	Teach patient to forgo food and fluids for 4 h before bedtime.	This reduces reflux by ensuring that the stomach is empty before the semirecumbent position is assumed.
	Encourage patient to eliminate cigarette smoking and to limit alcohol intake.	Cigarette smoking and large amounts of alcohol lower LES pressures, thus promoting reflux.
	Administer H_2-receptor antagonists (e.g., cimetidine) and antacids as ordered.	H_2-receptor antagonists reduce secretion of gastric acid, antacids help neutralize gastric acids; raising the pH of gastric secretions reduces esophageal damage if reflux occurs.

NURSING DIAGNOSIS	NURSING INTERVENTIONS	RATIONALE
	Administer cholinergic drugs (e.g., metoclopramide) as ordered.	Cholinergic drugs increase LES tone and promote gastric emptying, thus reducing reflux.
	Teach patient to avoid fats, chocolate, orange juice, and tomatoes.	These foods have been shown to lower LES pressure, thus promoting reflux.
	Prevent constipation by providing adequate fluid and fiber intake; monitor bowel movements.	Straining at stool increases intraabdominal pressure, which promotes reflux.
	Collaborate with physician and patient to establish management program for chronic cough.	Coughing increases intraabdominal pressure, which promotes reflux.
	Teach patient to avoid constrictive garments such as girdles or tight belts.	Constrictive garments may increase intraabdominal pressure, which increases reflux.
Pain related to esophageal inflammation	Administer antacids and H$_2$-receptor antagonists as ordered.	These medications reduce gastric acidity, thus reducing esophageal pain when reflux occurs.
	Provide a soft, bland, low-fat diet.	Acidic and highly textured foods may cause pain and esophageal spasm; fats reduce LES pressure, which may increase reflux.
	Instruct patient to avoid recumbent and side-lying positions.	These positions increase reflux.

5 EVALUATE

PATIENT OUTCOME	DATA INDICATING THAT OUTCOME IS REACHED
Patient has regained normal esophageal tissue integrity.	Patient tolerates regular diet without "heartburn" or discomfort.
Patient has no "heartburn" pain or pain on swallowing.	Patient states that "heartburn" pain and pain on swallowing are no longer present; he does not limit food or fluid intake.

PATIENT TEACHING

1. Explain that esophagitis is caused by reflux of gastric contents into the esophagus, and that treatment is directed toward eliminating reflux.
2. If the patient is pregnant, explain to her that "heartburn" is common during pregnancy because lower esophageal sphincter pressure is reduced; explain that this condition resolves spontaneously after delivery.
3. Explain that obesity, straining at stool, and chronic cough contribute to reflux by increasing intraabdominal pressure; discuss measures to control weight, prevent constipation, and control chronic cough.
4. Teach the patient measures to reduce reflux: eliminate smoking; avoid large amounts of alcohol; avoid fats, orange juice, tomatoes, and chocolate; forgo food and fluids for 4 hours before bedtime; elevate

→ > >

the head of the bed 8 to 12 inches; and avoid constrictive garments such as girdles and tight belts.

5. Teach the patient the importance of taking antacids and antisecretory medications (e.g., cimetidine) on schedule to reduce gastric acidity; emphasize that antacids should **not** be taken at the same time as antisecretory drugs, and that at least 1 hour should elapse between taking the antacid and taking the antisecretory drug.

Gastritis

Gastritis is any generalized inflammation of the gastric mucosa. Gastritis can be either acute or chronic.

ACUTE GASTRITIS

Acute gastritis is a temporary inflammation that can be caused by a number of factors: alcohol, aspirin, antiinflammatory drugs, corticosteroids, metabolic disorders (e.g., uremia), major physiologic stressors (e.g., burns or trauma), reflux of bile salts, or intense emotional reactions. Agents that cause acute gastritis appear to do so by damaging the mucosal barrier, allowing "back-diffusion" of hydrogen ions into the epithelial cells of the gastric mucosa. This damages the epithelial cells such that erosion, ulceration, and bleeding may result. Mechanisms of damage to the mucosal barrier are thought to include reduction of gastric blood flow, reduction of gastric mucus production, disruption of the tight junctions between the epithelial cells of the gastric mucosa, or inhibition of prostaglandins, which are thought to play a "cytoprotective" role for the gastric mucosal cells. Disruption of the tight junctions between the epithelial cells of the gastric mucosa is believed to be one of the most important factors in damaging the mucosal barrier, whereas reduced mucus production seems to be less significant. Certain drugs are thought to damage the mucosal barrier by interfering with the synthesis of prostaglandins.

"Stress ulceration" is the term commonly used for acute gastritis caused by major physiologic stress; this category includes both Cushing's ulcers and ischemic ulcers. Cushing's ulcer is an acute gastritis resulting from major intracranial processes; it is characterized by hypersecretion of gastric acid, probably in response to extreme vagal stimulation. Ischemic ulcer is an acute gastritis induced by reduction in gastric blood flow, which may occur after major burns, trauma, or sepsis. (Ulcers that occur after major burns are also called Curling's ulcers.) Stress ulceration rarely results in per-

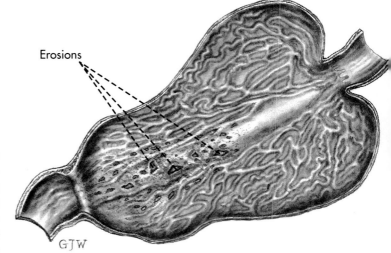

Erosions

GJW

FIGURE 4-2
Erosive gastritis (disruption of "tight cellular junctions" with back diffusion of H$^+$).

foration; bleeding is the major clinical manifestation, and it usually occurs 2 to 10 days after the stress event.

CHRONIC GASTRITIS

Chronic gastritis is a progressive condition that occurs primarily in the elderly. It can be further classified as type A (fundal) gastritis or type B (antral) gastritis. Chronic fundal gastritis (type A), also known as atrophic gastritis, is the most severe type; it involves marked degeneration of the mucosa in both the body and the fundus of the stomach, with subsequent changes in gastric function. The causes of atrophic gastritis are not known. One suggested cause is bile reflux; bile can disrupt the mucosal barrier, permitting back-diffusion of hydrogen ions with subsequent degeneration of the glandular layer of the stomach. Another theory is that the disorder is the result of an autoimmune process; evidence for this theory includes the presence of antibodies to parietal cells and intrinsic factor in the serum of many patients (60%) with atrophic gastritis, and the association between atrophic gastritis and other autoimmune conditions such as thyroid disease, diabetes mellitus, and adrenal insufficiency. Atrophic gastritis frequently is associated with pernicious anemia and is also associated with an increased incidence of gastric malignancies. Atrophic gastritis is more common in women than in men and occurs more frequently in families with a history of pernicious anemia.

Type B (antral) gastritis is much more common and less severe than fundal gastritis. Antral gastritis is limited to the antral area of the stomach and is characterized by mucosal inflammation; however, unlike fundal gastritis, it rarely causes mucosal atrophy or loss of gastric function. Parietal cell antibodies are not seen, and there is no association with pernicious anemia or gastric carcinoma. Antibodies to gastrin-producing cells are found in the serum of approximately 10% of patients with antral gastritis. The causes of this type of gastritis have not been clearly defined, but chronic reflux of bile is thought to contribute by frequently disrupting the mucosal barrier. Another possible cause is *Campylobacter pylori,* an organism frequently associated with antral gastritis and duodenal ulcer. Although a definite causal relationship has yet to be established, studies have demonstrated enhanced healing and reduced recurrence in patients with antral gastritis or duodenal ulcer who are known to have *C. pylori* and who are treated with appropriate antibiotics.

PATHOPHYSIOLOGY

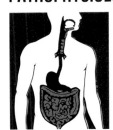

Acute gastritis involves a break in the mucosal barrier with subsequent back-diffusion of hydrogen ions (Figure 4-2); the hydrogen ions cause a number of adverse reactions, including the release of histamine. Histamine stimulates increased hydrogen-ion secretion by the parietal cells, increased capillary permeability, and edema; a vicious cycle is thus established. The acute inflammation causes superficial erosions and submucosal hemorrhages, and superficial, discrete ulcerations may occur also. Bleeding and even hemorrhage may result.

Chronic fundal gastritis (type A) is characterized by thinning of the gastric mucosa, atrophy of the muscle layer, and replacement of the gastric glands with glandular structures that produce mucus. Gastric function is markedly reduced; loss of chief cells and parietal cells results in reduced secretion of pepsinogen, hydrochloric acid, and intrinsic factor (IF). Serum gastrin may be elevated, because the chronically low levels of hydrochloric acid serve as a persistent stimulus for gastrin production. Pernicious anemia frequently develops, because intrinsic factor is insufficient to provide for transport and absorption of vitamin B_{12}.

Chronic antral gastritis is characterized by chronic inflammation of the antral region of the stomach, but atrophic changes are rare.

The symptoms associated with chronic gastritis frequently are vague; they include anorexia, fullness, nausea and vomiting, and epigastric pain. Low levels of acid production may foster bacterial overgrowth in the stomach and proximal small bowel and in some cases can result in absorptive disorders and steatorrhea. Gastric bleeding also may occur, and it sometimes is the only clinical manifestation of chronic gastritis. Atrophic gastritis resulting in pernicious anemia may produce symptoms such as glossitis, stomatitis, cheilosis, and peripheral neuropathy. However, liver stores of vitamin B_{12} usually delay the development of pernicious anemia for several years after the loss of intrinsic factor production.

COMPLICATIONS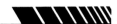

Bleeding/hemorrhage
Pernicious anemia (atrophic gastritis only)
Gastric carcinoma (increased risk with atrophic gastritis)

DIAGNOSTIC STUDIES AND FINDINGS

For a picture of erosive gastritis, see Color Plate 3, p. x.

Diagnostic test	Findings
Acute gastritis	
Nasogastric aspiration	May contain frank blood or may be positive for occult blood
Endoscopy (diagnostic procedure of choice)	Erosions, superficial ulcerations, and diffuse slow bleeding are commonly seen
Barium study	May show ulcerations, but very superficial lesions usually are not detectable
Angiography	May be used to identify the specific bleeding site in actively bleeding gastritis

Continued.

Diagnostic test	Findings
Chronic gastritis	
Endoscopy	May show chronic inflammation and gastric atrophy
Biopsy	Loss of normal gastric glands; atrophy of muscle layers; degeneration of mucosal structures; also done to rule out gastric carcinoma, which is associated with atrophic gastritis; silver stain of biopsy specimen can be used to identify *C. pylori*, which may be present in antral (type B) gastritis
Serum gastrin	Elevated in type A (fundal) gastritis; normal or low in type B (antral) gastritis
Serum antibodies to parietal cells and intrinsic factor (IF)	Presence suggests atrophic gastritis (type A)
Serum vitamin B_{12} levels	Low levels indicate pernicious anemia, which is associated with type A (atrophic) gastritis
Schilling test	Low levels indicate pernicious anemia, which is associated with type A gastritis

MEDICAL MANAGEMENT

GENERAL MANAGEMENT—ACUTE GASTRITIS

Elimination of gastric irritants (alcohol, aspirin, corticosteroids, antiinflammatory agents); nothing by mouth (NPO) status until acute bleeding and vomiting have resolved; nasogastric (N/G) tube with suction for gastric decompression and monitoring during acute bleeding episodes; iced saline (or tap water) lavage to control bleeding; intravenous (IV) fluids to maintain plasma volume (blood given as indicated during acute bleeding episodes to replace RBCs); soft, bland diet as tolerated once bleeding and vomiting have resolved; counseling for patient with significant emotional stress.

SURGERY

Laser coagulation of bleeding points: (may be performed in conjunction with endoscopy).

Partial or total gastrectomy: if medical management is ineffective in controlling the bleeding (the specific procedure is determined by the location of the bleeding).

Vagotomy and pyloroplasty: Vagotomy reduces the stimulus for acid production; pyloroplasty may be performed in conjunction with vagotomy because vagotomy reduces gastric motility, and enlarging the pylorus helps prevent pyloric obstruction.

DRUG THERAPY

Antacids (e.g., Maalox): 30 ml q 1-3 h to maintain gastric pH above 4.0 (studies have shown that stress ulcerations can be prevented by keeping the gastric pH above 3.5).

H_2-receptor antagonists (e.g., cimetidine, 300 mg IV or IM q 6 h or 300 mg PO qid; ranitidine, 50 mg IV or IM q 6 h or 300 mg PO daily): To reduce secretion of gastric acid.

Vasopressin (IV or by angiographic catheter): To induce vasoconstriction and reduce bleeding. **Note:** Vasoconstriction also compromises blood flow to gastric mucosa, which may contribute to inflammation.

GENERAL MANAGEMENT—CHRONIC GASTRITIS

Surveillance for development of pernicious anemia or gastric cancer (routine endoscopy and monitoring of serum vitamin B_{12} levels).

DRUG THERAPY

Antibiotics for patients with *C. pylori* infection; antacids (e.g., Maalox) to control epigastric distress; antiemetics (e.g., promethazine [Phenergan]) to control nausea; vitamin and mineral supplements (e.g., ascorbic acid to facilitate iron absorption); vitamin B_{12} injections for patients with pernicious anemia.

1 ASSESS

ASSESSMENT	OBSERVATIONS
Acute gastritis	
Medical history and medications	May report chronic use of aspirin, corticosteroids, antiinflammatory agents, or alcohol; may report recent major emotional stress; may have chronic renal failure or major physiologic stressors (e.g., intracranial process, major burn, trauma)
Epigastric distress	May report epigastric pain or vague epigastric or abdominal distress; abdominal palpation may reveal epigastric tenderness or guarding
Signs of bleeding	May report bloody emesis or tarry stools; may have hematemesis, melena, tachycardia, and hypotension
Chronic gastritis	
Medical and family history (type A)	May have history of thyroid disease, diabetes mellitus, adrenal insufficiency, or pernicious anemia; may report family history of pernicious anemia
Epigastric distress	May report anorexia, gastric fullness, nausea, vomiting, epigastric distress
Evidence of bleeding	Vomiting may occur and may reveal frank or occult blood
Evidence of pernicious anemia (type A)	May have glossitis, stomatitis, or cheilosis; may report numbness, tingling, or burning in fingers and toes

2 DIAGNOSE

NURSING DIAGNOSIS	SUBJECTIVE FINDINGS	OBJECTIVE FINDINGS
Impaired tissue integrity related to gastric inflammation	Reports epigastric pain or vague epigastric or abdominal distress; may report anorexia, nausea, vomiting, or gastric fullness; pain may be relieved by food (acute) or by antacid (acute or chronic)	Vomiting (emesis may test positive for occult or frank blood); epigastric or abdominal tenderness on palpation; stools may test positive for frank or occult blood
Altered renal, cerebral, cardiopulmonary, gastrointestinal, and peripheral tissue perfusion related to bleeding	Reports dizziness or faintness when standing; complains of shortness of breath, feelings of anxiety	Bleeding may be evidenced by hematemesis or melena; hypovolemia is evidenced by tachycardia, tachypnea, hypotension (initially orthostatic), diaphoresis, cool extremities, oliguria
Pain related to gastric inflammation	Reports epigastric pain or tenderness	Facial expressions indicate pain; may "hold" abdomen with hands; abdominal guarding may be noted on palpation
Sensory/perceptual alterations (tactile) related to pernicious anemia (atrophic gastritis only)	Reports numbness, burning, or tingling in fingers and toes	May have lesions caused by painless trauma; may have diminished sensation of touch

→ > >

3 PLAN

Patient goals

1. The patient will regain normal integrity of the gastric mucosa.
2. The patient will maintain adequate perfusion of the renal, cerebral, cardiopulmonary, gastrointestinal, and peripheral tissues.
3. The patient will have no epigastric pain or distress.
4. The patient with atrophic gastritis will have normal sensory tactile perception.

4 IMPLEMENT

NURSING DIAGNOSIS	NURSING INTERVENTIONS	RATIONALE
Impaired tissue integrity related to gastric inflammation	Administer H_2-receptor antagonists (e.g., cimetidine) and antacids (e.g., Maalox) as ordered.	H_2-receptor antagonists reduce gastric acid secretion, and antacids help neutralize gastric acids; raising the pH of gastric secretions reduces mucosal damage from those secretions.
	Collaborate with physician to minimize use of aspirin, corticosteroids, and antiinflammatory drugs.	These medications are known to damage the gastric mucosal barrier, thus contributing to gastritis.
	Instruct patient to avoid ingesting alcohol and caffeine.	Alcohol is a major cause of gastritis; it can damage the mucosal barrier. Caffeine may increase gastric acidity and delay healing.
	Administer antibiotics as ordered for the patient with chronic antral gastritis who has *C. pylori* infection.	Elimination of the *C. pylori* is associated with better healing and reduced recurrence.
Altered renal, cerebral, cardiopulmonary, gastrointestinal, and peripheral tissue perfusion related to bleeding	Monitor stools, emesis, and N/G aspirate (if applicable) for frank or occult blood; measure volumes of bloody stools, emesis, or aspirate.	Bleeding is a complication of gastritis and results in hematemesis or melena; measuring stool and emesis volume helps quantify blood loss.
	Monitor vital signs for evidence of hypovolemia: tachycardia, tachypnea, hypotension.	Hypovolemia is reflected by changes in blood pressure; compensatory responses to hypovolemia produce tachycardia and tachypnea.
	During bleeding episodes, keep the patient NPO and place an N/G tube as ordered (or assist with placement).	Placement of an N/G tube permits monitoring of gastric aspirate and provides access for gastric lavage; N/G intubation and NPO status provide gastric decompression and reduce vomiting.
	Carry out iced saline or tap water lavage as ordered.	Iced saline promotes mucosal vasoconstriction, which helps stop the bleeding. Some clinicians prefer tap water, because it breaks up blood clots more readily and because lowering the body temperature with iced saline can inhibit platelet function and prolong bleeding.

NURSING DIAGNOSIS	NURSING INTERVENTIONS	RATIONALE
	Administer IV fluids and blood replacement as ordered; observe for transfusion reactions if blood is given.	IV fluids are administered to maintain plasma volume; blood may be required for replacement of RBCs and platelets during massive bleeding episodes.
	Prepare patient for endoscopy and laser coagulation if bleeding does not respond to conservative management. Administer vasopressin IV as ordered (or prepare patient for arteriography and intraarterial administration of vasopressin as ordered).	Endoscopy and laser coagulation are commonly used to control bleeding. Vasopressin significantly reduces mesenteric blood flow and also reduces secretion of gastric acid; thus helping to control bleeding.
	If bleeding continues, prepare patient for surgery.	Emergency surgery (e.g., partial or total gastrectomy) may be required if massive bleeding fails to respond to lesser measures.
Pain related to gastric inflammation	Administer antacids and H_2-receptor antagonists as ordered.	These medications reduce gastric acidity and thus reduce irritation of sensory receptors in the damaged gastric mucosa.
	When oral food and fluids are permitted, provide a soft, bland diet with frequent small feedings.	Acidic and highly textured foods may cause pain; large meals may cause epigastric distress.
Sensory/perceptual alterations (tactile) related to pernicious anemia (atrophic gastritis only)	Monitor patient with atrophic gastritis for signs and symptoms of pernicious anemia (or monitor serum vitamin B_{12} levels).	Atrophic gastritis is commonly associated with pernicious anemia because of inadequate secretion of IF.
	Administer vitamin B_{12} as ordered.	Lifelong parenteral administration of vitamin B_{12} is required for patients who lack IF and thus cannot absorb ingested vitamin B_{12}.

5 EVALUATE

PATIENT OUTCOME	DATA INDICATING THAT OUTCOME IS REACHED
Patient has regained normal integrity of gastric mucosa.	Patient tolerates regular diet without epigastric distress (pain, nausea, or sense of fullness).
Patient maintains adequate perfusion of renal, cerebral, cardiopulmonary, gastrointestinal, and peripheral tissues.	Stools and N/G aspirate (if applicable) are negative for blood; vital signs are normal; urine output is normal.
Patient has no epigastric pain or distress.	Patient states that she no longer feels epigastric pain and distress.

→ > >

PATIENT OUTCOME	DATA INDICATING THAT OUTCOME IS REACHED
Patient with atrophic gastritis has normal sensory tactile perception.	Patient demonstrates normal sensory awareness of touch and states that she has no numbness, tingling, or burning.

PATIENT TEACHING

1. Explain the relationship between gastritis and the following: substances known to damage the mucosal barrier (e.g., aspirin, corticosteroids, antiinflammatory agents, alcohol), severe emotional stress, and acute physical stress.
2. Teach the patient the importance of taking antacids and antisecretory drugs (e.g., cimetidine) on schedule to reduce gastric acidity; instruct the patient to wait at least 1 hour after taking antacids before taking antisecretory medications.
3. Teach patient to adjust dietary intake according to tolerance: initially spicy foods and caffeine are likely to cause discomfort and should be omitted; small, frequent feedings help neutralize gastric acidity.
4. Teach the patient to recognize signs of bleeding (e.g., tarry stools) and to report evidence of bleeding to her physician promptly.
5. If the patient is suffering from severe emotional stress, discuss the value of counseling and offer to refer her to a counseling center.
6. If the patient has atrophic (fundal) gastritis, teach her the importance of routine medical follow-up to detect and treat the associated conditions of pernicious anemia and gastric carcinoma. Teach her the signs and symptoms of pernicicous anemia, and emphasize the importance of reporting these symptoms promptly.

Peptic Ulcer Disease

Peptic ulcer disease is an umbrella term that refers to ulcerations in the mucosal lining of the lower esophagus, stomach, or proximal small intestine. The two most common types of peptic ulcers are duodenal ulcers and gastric ulcers.

Ulcers may be acute or chronic and shallow or deep. They are differentiated from the erosions characteristic of gastritis by the depth of penetration; erosions involve the superficial mucosa but do not penetrate the muscularis mucosae, whereas ulcers extend through the muscularis mucosae to involve the submucosal layer and possibly even the muscular layer of the involved organ.

EPIDEMIOLOGY

Duodenal Ulcers

Duodenal ulcers (Figure 4-3) are about four times more common than gastric ulcers. They occur most often between 40 and 60 years of age and are three times as

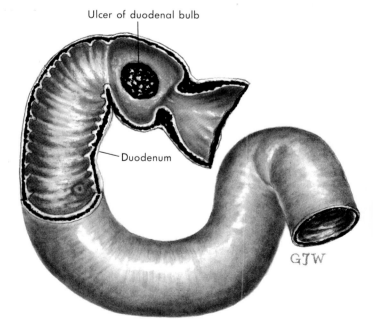

FIGURE 4-3
Duodenal peptic ulcer.

common in men as in women. Although it is commonly believed that duodenal ulcers occur more often in executives under high pressure, they actually are more common among unskilled laborers and in lower-income families with less education.

The primary cause of duodenal ulcers appears to be increased levels of gastric acid. These increased levels can be caused by a number of different pathologic processes. Factors that are believed to contribute to the state of hyperacidity are outlined in the box. Another factor that may contribute to the development of a duodenal ulcer is rapid gastric emptying, which may overwhelm the buffering effect provided by pancreatic secretions.

There is some evidence that genetic factors may play a role in the development of duodenal ulcers; for example, it has been documented that people with type O blood have a higher incidence of duodenal ulcers than people with other blood types. Also, considerable data support the link between long-standing anxiety or emotional tension and ulcer development. It is thought that chronic emotional stress predisposes to ulcer development by reducing mucosal resistance or increasing acid production (or both), and that usually a precipitating event exacerbates these processes and causes the ulcer to develop. Other factors thought to contribute to development of duodenal ulcers include cigarette smoking, caffeine, alcohol, and certain drugs (e.g., corticosteroids, aspirin, and antiinflammatory agents). Diseases associated with development of duodenal ulcers include chronic lung disease, cirrhosis, chronic pancreatitis, and Zollinger-Ellison syndrome. Zollinger-Ellison syndrome involves pancreatic islet cell tumors without hyperinsulinism; it is characterized by massive hypersecretion of gastric acid. More than half of these tumors are malignant.

Gastric Ulcers

Gastric ulcers (Figure 4-4) are much less common than duodenal ulcers. They usually occur in people between 45 and 70 years of age and are about equally common in men and women. Unlike duodenal ulcers, gastric ulcers do not involve increased production of gastric acid; acid production in these patients is normal or decreased. Gastric ulcers are commonly associated with chronic gastritis, which is characterized by thinning of the gastric mucosa. Gastric ulcers are thought to develop as a result of changes in the mucosal barrier that make the mucosa more permeable to hydrogen ions and thus more susceptible to damage. These changes are probably induced by reflux of bile and by ulcerogenic drugs. It is thought that chronic reflux of bile may occur as a result of inadequate pyloric sphincter function; studies have shown that the pylorus in these patients fails to re-

FACTORS CONTRIBUTING TO GASTRIC HYPERACIDITY

- Increased production of hydrochloric acid (HCl) by parietal cells
- Increased number of parietal cells producing hydrochloric acid
- Increased sensitivity of parietal cells to secretory stimuli
- Prolonged production of acid by parietal cells in response to stimuli
- Increase in vagal stimulation (which increases gastric secretion)
- Increased levels of serum gastrin (which stimulate parietal cells to produce HCl)
- Loss of ability to "turn off" gastrin secretion and acid production

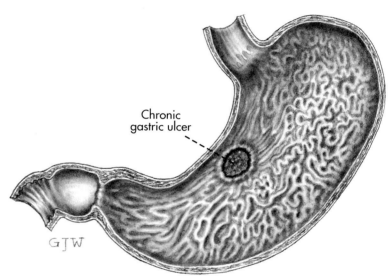

Chronic gastric ulcer

FIGURE 4-4
Gastric peptic ulcer.

spond to acid chyme in the duodenum with increased tone. As a result, duodenal contents can reflux into the stomach. Duodenal contents commonly contain bile, which is thought to damage the gastric mucosal barrier. The drugs considered ulcerogenic are corticosteroids, aspirin, and antiinflammatory agents; these drugs damage the mucosal barrier through the mechanisms already discussed in the section on gastritis. Smoking does not seem to play a causative role in the development of gastric ulcers, but it does retard healing of these ulcers.

PATHOPHYSIOLOGY

Duodenal Ulcers

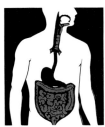

Duodenal ulcers usually are found in the 2 cm just distal to the pylorus and usually are less than 1 cm in diameter. They may occur on either the anterior or posterior wall. Posterior wall ulcers tend to be larger and are more likely to cause massive bleeding (because of the proximity of the pancreatoduodenal artery), whereas anterior wall ulcers are more likely to perforate.

Ulceration occurs when the increased acidity overwhelms the gastric mucosal barrier, resulting in back-diffusion of hydrogen ions into the gastric epithelial cells. The hydrogen ions damage the cells and prompt the release of histamine, which triggers an inflammatory response and further stimulates production of acid. The inflammatory response increases capillary permeability, which causes mucosal edema. Pain occurs as a result of acid gastric contents bathing the surface of the ulcer; the acid may stimulate nerve fibers directly or may cause muscle spasms that cause pain. (The pain occurs when the stomach is empty and usually is relieved by food or antacids, leading to the pain-food-relief pattern commonly reported.) The pain usually is localized to the epigastric area. Pain that radiates through to the back usually indicates posterior penetration of the ulcer. Other symptoms that may occur with a duodenal ulcer include vomiting, which is uncommon, and mild diarrhea. Some patients with a duodenal ulcer have no symptoms.

Duodenal ulcer disease tends to be intermittent, with ulcers sometimes healing spontaneously. Recurrences are most common during the spring and fall. Remission of the pain is associated with healing of the ulcer.

Gastric Ulcers

Gastric ulcers typically are found in the antral area of the stomach. These ulcers tend to be chronic, as opposed to the intermittent nature of duodenal ulcers. Benign gastric ulcers are round or oval and have a punched-out appearance and a smooth base. About 8% of gastric ulcers are malignant; these ulcers usually have an irregular, necrotic base.

Gastric ulcers develop when acid penetrates a damaged gastric mucosal barrier. Penetration of the barrier permits back-diffusion of hydrogen ions into the epithelial cells, which initiates release of histamine. Histamine stimulates the production of acid and increases capillary permeability; this results in leakage of proteins and fluid, which causes edema of the stomach wall. The pain associated with gastric ulcers usually is located to the left of the midepigastric area. The pain is not necessarily relieved by eating and may even occur immediately after eating or a short time later. Other symptoms sometimes produced by gastric ulcers include a sense of fullness, nausea, vomiting, and weight loss, which may be profound.

COMPLICATIONS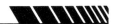

Bleeding or hemorrhage
Perforation
Penetration into surrounding structures
Obstruction
Intractability

Complications from peptic ulcer disease include bleeding, perforation, penetration, obstruction, and intractability. *Bleeding* results from damage to mucosal blood vessels and may produce hematemesis or melena (60 ml of blood can produce a tarry stool). Minor bleeding may go undetected, and over time it can cause iron-deficiency anemia. Massive bleeding occurs in 15% to 20% of patients with peptic ulcer disease and is more comon with chronic ulcers; 90% of patients who suffer an episode of massive bleeding have had ulcer symptoms for over a year.

Perforation is not common but occurs more frequently with duodenal ulcers than with gastric ulcers. Perforation usually occurs with a chronic ulcer and is the most common cause of death from peptic ulcer disease.

Penetration refers to a perforation that is sealed off; penetration occurs only with chronic ulcers and may result in fistulas to other organs or in acute pancreatitis (if the penetration involves the pancreas).

Obstruction occurs in about 5% of patients with peptic ulcer disease; it may result from severe edema or from stenosis of the pylorus. Patients may be functionally obstructed even when the lumen is open because of spasticity and atony affecting the stomach and duodenum.

Peptic ulcer disease is considered intractable when ulcers recur while the patient is being treated or soon after treatment has been discontinued.

Intractability most commonly results from complications of peptic ulcer disease or from a persistent pathologic condition, such as a hypersecretory syndrome. Surgery is not recommended for intractable disease until the cause of the recurrent ulcerations has been determined and all medical options have been exhausted.

DIAGNOSTIC STUDIES AND FINDINGS

Diagnostic test	Findings
Upper gastrointestinal (GI) study (barium study)	May show anatomic deformity created by ulcer crater (in stomach or duodenum); may show delayed gastric emptying (if partial obstruction caused by edema or scarring is present)
Endoscopy (esophagogastroduodenoscopy)	Ulcer visualized; location and stage of healing determined
Biopsy	Reveals or rules out gastric cancer or malignant gastric ulcer
Gastric analysis	May show hyperacidity (duodenal ulcer); normal or reduced acidity (gastric ulcer); may show blood in gastric secretions
Serum gastrin levels	May be elevated
Hemoglobin (Hb) and hematocrit (Hct)	May be reduced if ulcer is complicated by bleeding
Stool for occult blood	Positive results indicate bleeding
Abdominal x-rays (flat plate and upright of abdomen)	Free air under diaphragm indicates perforation
Serum amylase	Elevated if penetration into pancreas causes acute pancreatitis
Serum albumin and transferrin	May be decreased with weight loss and malnutrition

MEDICAL MANAGEMENT

GENERAL MANAGEMENT

Elimination of causative and contributing factors (aspirin, corticosteroids, antiinflammatory agents, alcohol) and of factors known to inhibit healing (e.g., smoking).

During episodes of active bleeding: NPO status; N/G intubation and suction; iced saline or plain water lavage; IV administration of fluids; blood replacement. Soft diet with small, frequent feedings once bleeding has stopped and oral food and fluids are permitted; counseling for patient with severe emotional stress.

SURGERY

The goals of surgical intervention are to reduce the stimuli for acid secretion, reduce the number of acid-secreting cells in the stomach, eliminate bleeding, correct obstruction, or close perforations. Procedures include laser coagulation of bleeders by means of esophagogastroduodenoscopy; partial gastrectomy with anastomosis of the gastric stump to the duodenum (Billroth I procedure) or the jejunum (Billroth II procedure) to eliminate bleeding sites, reduce the number of acid-secreting cells in the stomach, or resect areas of perforation or stenosis; vagotomy to reduce the stimuli for acid production.

DRUG THERAPY

The primary focus in medical management is to treat the patient with medications that reduce acid secretion, neutralize gastric acid, or enhance mucosal resistance. Treatment with these agents induces healing in 60% to 75% of duodenal ulcers after 4 weeks and 80% to 90% of duodenal ulcers after 12 weeks.

Histamine H_2-receptor antagonists (e.g., cimetidine, 300 mg IV or IM q 6 h or 300 mg PO qid; ranitidine, 50 mg IV or IM q 6 h or 300 mg PO daily): To reduce secretion of gastric acid.

Anticholinergic drugs (e.g., Pro-Banthine, 15 mg before meals and 30 mg at bedtime PO): To reduce acid secretion.

Antacids (e.g., Maalox, 30 ml 1 and 3 h after meals): To neutralize gastric acid, relieve ulcer pain, and inactivate pepsin.

Continued.

MEDICAL MANAGEMENT—cont'd

Omeprazole: To inhibit production of gastric acid.

Cytoprotective drugs (e.g., sucralfate, 1 g PO qid): To form a protective coating over the surface of the ulcer, protecting it from gastric secretions.

Antiemetics (e.g., promethazine): To control nausea and vomiting.

Antiulcer agents (e.g., misoprostol, 100-200 μg qid for duration of treatment with antiinflammatory agents): To reduce production of gastric acid and protect mucosa.

Vasopressin (IV or by intraarterial injection): To cause mesenteric vasoconstriction and thus reduce bleeding. **Note:** Reduction of blood flow to stomach or duodenal wall may induce further inflammation and actually prolong bleeding.

1 ASSESS

ASSESSMENT	OBSERVATIONS
Ingestion of ulcero-genic substances, including over-the-counter (OTC) and prescription drugs	May report excessive or chronic use of drugs known to be barrier breakers (e.g., aspirin or aspirin-containing compounds, corticosteroids, antiinflammatory agents); ingestion of large amounts of caffeine and alcohol; cigarette smoking
History of medical and psychologic conditions associated with peptic ulcer disease	May report chronic lung disease, cirrhosis, chronic pancreatitis, Zollinger-Ellison syndrome, chronic gastritis, previous ulcers; also may report long-standing anxiety and recent stressful events
Pain patterns and location	*Duodenal ulcer:* may report epigastric pain relieved by food or antacids. *Gastric ulcer:* may report pain to left of midepigastrium that is not necessarily relieved by food or antacids and may be worse after large meals. *Perforating ulcer:* may report epigastric pain radiating to back
Evidence of bleeding	Melena or hematemesis may be seen or reported; chronic blood loss may be evidenced by fatigue, pallor, activity intolerance
Signs of obstruction	May report anorexia, gastric fullness, early satiety, nausea and vomiting
Current and usual weight	*Chronic gastric ulcer:* may report profound weight loss. *Duodenal ulcer:* may report weight gain

2 DIAGNOSE

NURSING DIAGNOSIS	SUBJECTIVE FINDINGS	OBJECTIVE FINDINGS
Impaired tissue integrity related to gastric or duodenal ulcer	Reports epigastric pain relieved by food or antacids (duodenal ulcer), *or* pain located to left of midepigastrium that may not be relieved by food or antacids and may be worsened by large meals (gastric ulcer); may report hematemesis or melena; may report additional signs of gastric or duodenal inflammation: anorexia, nausea, vomiting, sense of fullness; may complain of epigastric or abdominal tenderness on palpation	Vomiting; emesis may test positive for frank or occult blood; stools may test positive for frank or occult blood
Altered renal, cerebral, cardiopulmonary, gastrointestinal, and peripheral tissue perfusion related to bleeding or to septic shock caused by perforation	Reports dizziness or faintness when standing, shortness of breath, feelings of anxiety	Bleeding may be evidenced by hematemesis or melena; hypovolemia may be evidenced by tachycardia, tachypnea, hypotension (initially postural hypotension), diaphoresis, cool extremities, and oliguria
Pain related to gastric inflammation	Reports pain in epigastric area or to left of midepigastric area or radiating from epigastric area to back	Facial expressions indicate pain; may "hold" abdomen with hands; knees may be drawn up; abdominal guarding may be noted on palpation
Altered nutrition: less than body requirements related to anorexia, nausea, and vomiting	Reports inability to eat usual amounts; reports recent weight loss, loss of appetite, nausea and vomiting	Weight is below 90% of usual weight; intake record indicates inadequate protein and calorie intake, *or* patient vomits after eating (or both)

3 PLAN

Patient goals

1. The patient will regain normal integrity of gastric and duodenal mucosa.
2. The patient will maintain adequate perfusion of renal, cerebral, cardiopulmonary, gastrointestinal, and peripheral tissues.
3. The patient will have no abdominal pain or epigastric distress.
4. The patient will maintain adequate weight and ingest adequate food and fluids daily.

4 IMPLEMENT

NURSING DIAGNOSIS	NURSING INTERVENTIONS	RATIONALE
Impaired tissue integrity related to gastric or duodenal ulcer	Administer H_2-receptor antagonists (e.g., cimetidine), omeprazole, anticholinergic drugs, ulcer-coating agents, and antacids as ordered.	H_2-receptor antagonists, omeprazole, and anticholinergic drugs reduce gastric acid secretion, and antacids help neutralize gastric acid; reducing gastric acidity prevents further mucosal damage and promotes healing of ulcers; agents that coat the ulcer's surface protect the lesion from further irritation by gastric acid and thus promote healing.
	Collaborate with physicians to minimize the use of aspirin, corticosteroids, and antiinflammatory agents.	These medications are known to damage the gastric mucosal barrier, thus contributing to ulcer development.
	Instruct patient to avoid alcohol and caffeine ingestion and cigarette smoking.	Alcohol may further damage the mucosal barrier; caffeine may increase gastric acidity; cigarette smoking has been shown to inhibit healing of ulcers and may contribute to development of duodenal ulcers.
Altered renal, cerebral, cardiopulmonary, gastrointestinal, and peripheral tissue perfusion related to bleeding or to septic shock caused by perforation	Monitor stools, emesis, and N/G aspirate for frank or occult blood; measure volumes of bloody stools and emesis or N/G aspirate.	Bleeding is the most common complication of peptic ulcer disease and is evidenced by melena or hematemesis; measuring stool and emesis or aspirate volumes helps to quantify blood loss.
	Monitor vital signs, central venous pressure (CVP) readings, Swan-Ganz catheter pressure readings, and urinary output for evidence of hypovolemia: i.e., falling blood pressure, tachycardia, tachypnea, falling CVP and Swan-Ganz readings, and reduced urinary output.	Hypovolemia is reflected by falling blood pressure, CVP, and Swan-Ganz readings, and reduced urinary output; compensatory responses to hypovolemia produce tachycardia and tachypnea.
	Keep patient NPO and place N/G tube as ordered (or assist with placement) during episodes of bleeding.	Placement of an N/G tube permits monitoring of gastric aspirate and provides access for gastric lavage; N/G intubation and NPO status maintain gastric decompression and reduce vomiting.
	Carry out iced saline, iced water, or plain water lavage as ordered.	Iced saline or iced water lavage promotes vasoconstriction, which helps stop the bleeding; some clinicians prefer plain water lavage, because it breaks up clots more readily and because lowering the body temperature with iced lavage can inhibit platelet function and prolong bleeding.
	Administer IV fluids and blood replacement as ordered; observe for transfusion reactions if blood is given.	IV fluids are administered to maintain plasma volume; blood may be required for replacement of RBCs and platelets during episodes of massive bleeding.

NURSING DIAGNOSIS	NURSING INTERVENTIONS	RATIONALE
	Prepare patient for endoscopy and laser coagulation.	Endoscopy with laser coagulation is commonly used to control bleeding.
	Administer vasopressin IV as ordered (or prepare patient for arteriography and intraarterial administration of vasopressin as ordered).	Vasopressin significantly reduces mesenteric blood flow and also reduces secretion of gastric acid, thus helping to control bleeding; however, vasopressin can also cause mucosal ischemia, so its use is controversial.
	If bleeding continues (or for patients with perforation): prepare patient for surgery.	Emergency surgery (e.g., partial gastrectomy) may be required when massive bleeding fails to respond to lesser measures or for management of perforation.
Pain related to gastric inflammation	Monitor patient for pain of increasing intensity, pain that radiates to the back, or pain associated with abdominal rigidity or rebound tenderness.	These types of pain indicate complications such as perforation.
	Administer antacids, coating agents, and H_2-receptor antagonists as ordered.	These medications reduce gastric acidity and protect the ulcer's surface, thus reducing irritation of sensory receptors in the exposed base of the ulcer.
	When oral food and fluids are permitted, provide a soft, bland diet with frequent small feedings.	Acidic and highly textured foods may cause pain; frequent small feedings help to neutralize gastric acid and to prevent epigastric distress.
Altered nutrition: less than body requirements related to anorexia, nausea, and vomiting	Consult the dietitian for nutritional assessment and recommendations for patient with any of the following: recent weight loss, weight below 90% of usual weight, inadequate food and fluid intake (less than 75% of prescribed diet, less than 1,500 ml of fluid daily), or frequent vomiting.	These patients are at significant risk for nutritional deficits; thorough assessment is required to establish an appropriate plan for nutritional support.
	Administer antiemetics and antacids as ordered and needed.	Antiemetics and antacids reduce nausea and epigastric distress and may improve dietary intake and tolerance.
	Provide high-calorie, high-protein diet with frequent small feedings.	Frequent small feedings help neutralize gastric acid and are better tolerated than large meals; patients with nutritional compromise require increased amounts of protein and calories.
	Monitor nutritional status: intake, weight, laboratory parameters (e.g., serum albumin, serum transferrin).	Continual evaluation is required to determine adequacy of nutritional support plan.

→ > >

5   EVALUATE

PATIENT OUTCOME	DATA INDICATING THAT OUTCOME IS REACHED
Patient has regained normal integrity of gastric and duodenal mucosa.	Patient tolerates regular diet without epigastric distress (pain, nausea, sense of fullness).
Patient maintains adequate perfusion of renal, cerebral, cardiopulmonary, gastrointestinal, and peripheral tissues.	Stools and N/G aspirate (if applicable) test negative for blood; patient is free of pain; vital signs are within normal limits.
Patient has no abdominal pain or epigastric distress.	Patient states that epigastric pain and distress are no longer present.
Patient maintains adequate weight and ingests adequate food and fluids daily.	Patient's weight is 90% or more of usual weight; patient tolerates food and fluids without distress and routinely ingests at least 75% of prescribed diet and 1,500 ml of fluid daily.

PATIENT TEACHING

1. Explain how development of a peptic ulcer is linked to ingestion of ulcerogenic medications and substances and to long-standing or severe emotional stress.
2. Teach the patient the importance of taking antacids and antisecretory medications (e.g., cimetidine) on schedule to reduce gastric acidity; instruct the patient to wait at least 1 hour after taking antacid before taking antisecretory medications, because antacids can inhibit the absorption of antisecretory medications.
3. Teach the patient the importance of taking antisecretory medications for the prescribed period of time to promote healing of the ulcer or ulcers.
4. Explain to the patient the need to eliminate cigarette smoking to promote healing of ulcers.
5. Teach the patient to adjust dietary intake according to her tolerance: spicy foods and caffeine may cause discomfort and initially should be avoided; frequent feedings help neutralize gastric acidity.
6. Teach the patient to recognize the signs of bleeding or perforation (e.g., tarry stools, sudden increase in pain) that should be reported to the physician promptly.
7. If the patient is coping with severe or long-standing emotional stress, discuss the value of counseling and offer to refer her to a counseling center.
8. Explain that peptic ulcer disease tends to recur and that preventive measures need to be incorporated on a long-term basis.

Gastroenteritis

Gastroenteritis is a general term for an inflammation of the stomach and intestinal tract (Figure 4-5). It commonly is caused by viral or bacterial infections and is characterized by varying degrees of anorexia, nausea, vomiting, cramping pain, and diarrhea.

EPIDEMIOLOGY

A number of specific illnesses fall under the heading of gastroenteritis. The most common are the bacterial infections that cause "traveler's diarrhea" and the viral infections that frequently cause epidemic outbreaks of "GI flu." Most forms of infectious gastroenteritis are transmitted through contaminated food and water or by direct or indirect fecal-oral transmission from an infected person.

Resistance to gastroenteritis normally is provided by several components at work in a healthy gastrointestinal tract; a change in these components leaves an individual more susceptible to pathogenic invasion. The resistance factors are the normal bacterial flora of the intestinal tract, the marked acidity of the stomach, and the normal motility of the gastrointestinal (GI) tract. The normal bacterial flora protect the intestinal tract by competing with pathogens for mucosal attachment sites or by producing volatile organic acids. Conditions or treatments that alter the normal bacterial flora (e.g., antibiotics and malnutrition) increase the individual's risk of pathogenic invasion. The normal gastric acidity is important in eliminating ingested pathogens; most bacteria cannot survive a gastric pH of 3.0 or less. Individuals at increased risk for bacterial gastroenteritis as a result of loss of normal gastric acidity include patients with atrophic gastritis, patients who are taking antacids or antisecretory drugs such as H_2-receptor antagonists, and patients who have had gastric surgery. Normal gastrointestinal motility provides protection by purging the intestinal tract of pathogens; individuals with reduced motility are at greater risk for pathogenic proliferation that results in disease. Besides these factors, age and physical condition affect resistance; children, the elderly, and debilitated individuals are at greater risk than healthy adults.

Bacterial gastroenteritis ("traveler's diarrhea") is more likely to occur in individuals traveling from "low-risk" (highly industrialized) countries to "high-risk" (developing) countries. For example, an individual traveling from the United States to Mexico is more likely to be affected than an individual traveling from Mexico to the United States.

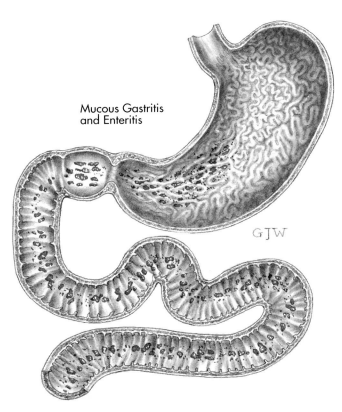

Mucous Gastritis and Enteritis

GJW

FIGURE 4-5
Gastroenteritis.

PATHOPHYSIOLOGY

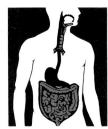

Viral and bacterial gastroenteritis is different from food poisoning in that the viruses or bacteria invade and multiply within the gastrointestinal tract, whereas food poisoning is caused by ingestion of food contaminated with bacteria that have already multiplied within the food. Pathogens that cause gastroenteritis do so by one of the following mechanisms: (1) secretion of an enterotoxin that causes severe inflammation and secretory diarrhea (e.g., enterotoxigenic *Escherichia coli*); (2) invasion of

Table 4-1

BACTERIAL AND VIRAL GASTROENTERITIS

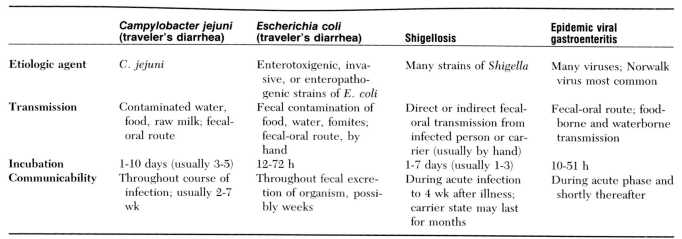

	Campylobacter jejuni (traveler's diarrhea)	*Escherichia coli* (traveler's diarrhea)	Shigellosis	Epidemic viral gastroenteritis
Etiologic agent	*C. jejuni*	Enterotoxigenic, invasive, or enteropathogenic strains of *E. coli*	Many strains of *Shigella*	Many viruses; Norwalk virus most common
Transmission	Contaminated water, food, raw milk; fecal-oral route	Fecal contamination of food, water, fomites; fecal-oral route, by hand	Direct or indirect fecal-oral transmission from infected person or carrier (usually by hand)	Fecal-oral route; foodborne and waterborne transmission
Incubation	1-10 days (usually 3-5)	12-72 h	1-7 days (usually 1-3)	10-51 h
Communicability	Throughout course of infection; usually 2-7 wk	Throughout fecal excretion of organism, possibly weeks	During acute infection to 4 wk after illness; carrier state may last for months	During acute phase and shortly thereafter

the intestinal wall, with resultant cellular destruction, necrosis, and possible ulceration (e.g., *Shigella* and *Campylobacter* organisms); or (3) mucosal attachment, with resultant destruction of absorptive cells in the intestinal villi (e.g., rotavirus). Pathologic conditions resulting from the above processes include reduced absorption of fluids and electrolytes and increased intestinal motility, with resultant diarrhea and the potential for fluid and electrolyte imbalance. Pathogens that secrete enterotoxins cause excessive secretion of fluids and electrolytes into the intestinal lumen, resulting in large-volume diarrhea and the probability of severe fluid-electrolyte imbalance. (Examples of this type of gastroenteritis include cholera and enterotoxigenic *E. coli.*)

The incubation period for viral and bacterial gastroenteritis ranges from 12 hours to 10 days, depending on the specific organism involved. The onset of illness usually is marked by nausea, vomiting, abdominal cramping, and fever; diarrhea may accompany the onset of illness or may begin the following day. Viral gastroenteritis tends to be self-limiting, usually lasting for 24 to 48 hours. Bacterial gastroenteritis frequently lasts for as long as 5 to 10 days and may require antibiotics for eradication. Table 4-1 provides a comparative overview of the most common types of viral and bacterial gastroenteritis.

COMPLICATIONS

Fluid and electrolyte imbalance (possibly severe)
Ulcerative colitis (*Campylobacter jejuni*)
Febrile convulsions (*Campylobacter jejuni*)

WHO FORMULA FOR REHYDRATION SOLUTION

5 tsp glucose or 10 tsp sucrose
¾ tsp salt
½ tsp baking soda
¼ tsp KCl
1 liter drinking water

DOSAGE: 250 to 500 ml/hour for adults; 125 to 250 ml/hour for children over age 2.

WHO provides this formula in anhydrous packages (Oralyte).

DIAGNOSTIC STUDIES AND FINDINGS

Diagnostic test	Findings
Stool analysis and culture	*C. jejuni:* tests positive for leukocytes, erythrocytes, *C. jejuni* organisms; *E. coli:* tests positive for enterotoxigenic or invasive strains of *E. coli; Shigella:* tests positive for pus and *Shigella* organisms; *epidemic viral gastroenteritis:* virus seen on immune electron microscopy or radioimmunoassay of feces; *rotavirus:* electron microscopy or immunologic examination of feces or rectal swab positive for rotavirus (1 million per gram of feces)
Serology	Fourfold increase in antibody titer (*C. jejuni, E. coli,* rotavirus, epidemic viral gastroenteritis)
Electrolytes	Fluid-electrolyte imbalance

MEDICAL MANAGEMENT

The primary goals in medical management are to maintain the fluid-electrolyte balance and to control symptoms. Antibiotics may be prescribed to treat bacterial gastroenteritis and sometimes are prescribed for prophylaxis of bacterial gastroenteritis ("traveler's diarrhea").

GENERAL MANAGEMENT

Oral rehydration solutions (balanced, buffered, isotonic mixture of glucose and electrolytes): See box for WHO (World Health Organization) formula and formula for home-made solution; IV fluid and electrolyte replacement (more rapid replacement is indicated if patient is hypovolemic).

DRUG THERAPY

Antidiarrheal agents: Drugs that reduce intestinal motility (e.g., loperamide and diphenoxylate) are **contraindicated** in bacterial gastroenteritis but may be used for viral gastroenteritis.

Diphenoxylate (Lomotil): 5 mg PO qid.

Loperamide (Imodium): 4 mg initial dose, then 2 mg after each loose stool, not to exceed 16 mg a day.

Bismuth subsalicylate (Pepto-Bismol) may be prescribed for viral or bacterial gastroenteritis: 30 ml (or 2 tablets) q 30-60 min, not to exceed 8 doses for more than 2 days.

Antibiotics (for *Shigella* and *E. coli* organisms): Trimethoprim-sulfamethoxazole (Septra, Bactrim), 1 tablet (80 mg trimethoprim and 400 mg sulfamethoxazole) q 12 h for 5 days.

Antibiotics for prophylaxis: Trimethoprim-sulfamethoxazole, 1 tablet q 12 h or doxycycline (Vibramycin), 100 mg daily for 2 wk before travel to high-risk area.

Note: Prophylaxis is controversial because of the development of resistant organisms; prophylaxis usually is recommended primarily for high-risk individuals.

1 ASSESS

ASSESSMENT	OBSERVATIONS
Recent history	May report travel outside of country to developing country or exposure to individual with similar illness
Food and fluid intake	May report: anorexia, nausea, vomiting; change in usual dietary intake because of illness
Bowel movements	May report: cramping pain with diarrheal stools; as many as 20 to 30 stools per day; blood or mucus in stools or foul odor to stools
Urine output	May report reduced urine output and increased urine concentration (due to fluid loss)
Skin turgor	May be reduced (due to fluid volume deficit)

ASSESSMENT	OBSERVATIONS
Vital signs (blood pressure lying and sitting or standing)	May see orthostatic hypotension, hypotension, tachycardia, and tachypnea due to severe fluid volume deficit; fever is common (low grade with viral gastroenteritis, higher with bacterial type)
Level of consciousness and orientation	May see lethargy or confusion with severe fluid-electrolyte disturbances

2 DIAGNOSE

NURSING DIAGNOSIS	SUBJECTIVE FINDINGS	OBJECTIVE FINDINGS
Diarrhea related to intestinal inflammation	Reports increased number and frequency of stools; may report cramping, blood and mucus in stool, foul odor to stool	Frequent loose stools; mucus and blood may be seen in stool
Fluid volume deficit related to diarrhea, vomiting, or both	Reports dry mouth, thirst; may report: reduced urine output and increased urine concentration; dizziness or weakness; weight loss	Reduced skin turgor; increased urine concentration and decreased urine output; postural hypotension, tachycardia, tachypnea; altered mental status (lethargy, confusion); dry mucous membranes
Hyperthermia related to intestinal infection and dehydration	May report flushing, chills	Fever; flushed skin
Altered nutrition: less than body requirements related to anorexia, nausea, and vomiting	Reports reduced food and fluid intake; may report anorexia, nausea, and cramping	Vomiting; diarrhea; eats and drinks minimal amounts; weight loss

3 PLAN

Patient goals

1. The patient's diarrhea will resolve, and normal bowel function will be reestablished.
2. The patient will demonstrate normal fluid balance.
3. The patient's temperature will remain within normal limits.
4. The patient will resume intake of adequate amounts of food and fluids.

4 IMPLEMENT

NURSING DIAGNOSIS	NURSING INTERVENTIONS	RATIONALE
Diarrhea related to intestinal inflammation	Assess all stools for volume, consistency, odor, and abnormal constituents.	Stool characteristics provide clues to cause of gastroenteritis.

NURSING DIAGNOSIS	NURSING INTERVENTIONS	RATIONALE
	Administer antidiarrheal medications as ordered. **Note:** Agents that slow intestinal motility (e.g., loperamide, diphenoxylate) are **contraindicated** in bacterial gastroenteritis.	Antidiarrheal medications reduce intestinal secretion and may reduce intestinal motility, thus reducing diarrhea; agents that reduce motility should not be given with bacterial gastroenteritis because motility helps purge the bowel of offending organisms.
	Obtain stool cultures as ordered (check with laboratory about optimal collection and transport procedures).	Stool cultures provide identification of the causative organism, which directs treatment.
	Administer antibiotics as ordered.	Antibiotics may be ordered for treatment of bacterial gastroenteritis.
	Gently cleanse perianal area after each stool, and apply moisture-barrier ointments or films; use enteric precautions in caring for patient.	Gentle cleansing and use of protective skin products prevent skin breakdown; enteric precautions prevent transmission of disease.
Fluid volume deficit related to diarrhea, vomiting, or both	Keep accurate records of intake and fluid loss (urine output, emesis, liquid stools).	Accurate records provide the basis for accurate fluid replacement.
	Monitor indicators of intravascular volume depletion (B/P, pulse, skin turgor urine output).	Monitoring permits prompt recognition of hypovolemia and early intervention.
	Administer IV fluids and electrolytes as ordered.	Intravenous fluid and electrolytes restore plasma volume and correct fluid volume deficits.
	Provide oral fluid intake as soon as tolerated; encourage fluids that are isotonic and contain a balanced mixture of glucose and electrolytes, and discourage fluids containing caffeine.	Oral fluid replacement is begun as soon as possible; fluids that are isotonic and balanced are more readily absorbed. Caffeine may increase diarrhea, because it can increase intracellular levels of cyclic adenosine monophosphate (cAMP).
Hyperthermia related to intestinal infection and dehydration	Monitor patient's temperature, and administer antipyretics as ordered.	Monitoring permits prompt recognition of fever and timely intervention.
Altered nutrition: less than body requirements related to anorexia, nausea, and vomiting	Administer antiemetics as ordered.	Antiemetics reduce nausea and vomiting, thus improving oral intake and tolerance.
	Encourage small amounts of balanced glucose-electrolyte solutions until nausea resolves; then administer oral fluids in volumes equivalent to output.	Balanced glucose and electrolyte solutions usually are well tolerated during episodes of gastroenteritis.
	Monitor oral intake and tolerance, and body weight.	Measuring oral intake and body weight provides data on nutrient intake and nutritional status.

→ > >

5   EVALUATE

PATIENT OUTCOME	DATA INDICATING THAT OUTCOME IS REACHED
Patient's diarrhea has resolved, and normal bowel function has been reestablished.	Patient reports normal stool frequency and consistency.
Patient demonstrates normal fluid balance.	Oral fluid intake balances fluid output (urine and stool); mucous membranes are moist; urine is straw colored; skin turgor is normal; patient is alert and oriented; B/P is normal.
Patient's temperature remains within normal limits.	Temperature is normal.
Patient has resumed intake of adequate amounts of food and fluids.	Oral fluid intake balances urine output; patient states that anorexia and nausea have resolved and resumes normal dietary intake.

PATIENT TEACHING

1. Explain the infectious nature of the illness, and stress the importance of infection control measures: thorough handwashing after using the toilet and forgoing food preparation and handling until the illness has resolved. Explain that people with *Shigella* infections are not allowed to handle food or to provide child care until two successive fecal samples or rectal swabs show no *Shigella* organisms.
2. Teach outpatients to recognize the signs and symptoms of fluid volume deficit: dry mucous membranes, dizziness or weakness, decreased urine output and increased urine concentration, and lethargy or mental confusion. Explain the importance of promptly reporting these signs and symptoms to the physician.
3. Explain the guidelines for fluid replacement: drinking small volumes of clear, caffeine-free fluids containing glucose and electrolytes until nausea has resolved; then fluid replacement in volumes equal to losses.
4. Explain guidelines for medication administration:
   - If patient has bacterial gastroenteritis, instruct him to take antidiarrheal agents **only** if prescribed by physician; explain that some antidiarrheal agents, such as Imodium, may actually prolong the illness.
   - If antidiarrheal agents are prescribed, explain the guidelines for taking them.
   - If antibiotic agents are ordered, explain the importance of completing the full course.
5. Instruct the patient in measures that reduce the risk of acquiring "traveler's diarrhea" when traveling in high-risk countries:
   - Avoid drinks served with ice cubes, which may be contaminated by foodhandlers
   - Avoid foods served in cafeterias or purchased from street vendors
   - Avoid raw vegetables, raw meat, raw fish and shellfish, and food that has not been refrigerated or has been left out for several hours
   - Food that is served "piping hot" usually is safe, as is tap water.

   Tell the individual that if mild to moderate diarrhea does occur, the safest over-the-counter medication is Pepto-Bismol (bismuth subsalicylate); severe diarrhea or diarrhea with fever requires medical attention.

Appendicitis

Appendicitis is an inflammation of the vermiform appendix (Figure 4-6). It can be further classified as simple, gangrenous, or perforated. Simple appendicitis is an inflammation of an intact appendix; gangrenous appendicitis is an inflamed appendix that involves focal or extensive necrosis with microscopic perforations; perforated appendicitis is a gross disruption of the wall of the appendix.

EPIDEMIOLOGY

Appendicitis is the most common reason for emergency abdominal surgery. The incidence rate is 1 to 2 per 1,000, with young adults between 20 and 30 years of age the most commonly affected. However, appendicitis can affect any age group, including the elderly, in whom the diagnosis may be obscured because the symptoms frequently are vague and abdominal tenderness may be mild.

The causes of appendicitis vary, but all involve occlusion of the lumen of the appendix. In children and young adults, systemic infections (especially respiratory infections) may cause hyperplasia of the abundant lymphoid tissue in the appendix; this hyperplastic response may occlude the appendiceal lumen and initiate the development of appendicitis. Other causes include obstruction of the lumen by hardened stool (fecaliths), seeds, or tumors.

PATHOPHYSIOLOGY

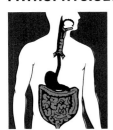

Occlusion of the appendiceal lumen prevents the normal mucosal secretions from draining. As the secretions accumulate, the intraluminal pressure increases, impairing mucosal blood flow and causing hypoxia. The mucosal ischemia may progress to ulceration, which provides an entry point for bacterial invasion. Bacterial invasion triggers an acute inflammatory response, with increased mucosal edema; the edema causes further obstruction of the lumen and further impairs blood flow. Because the appendiceal artery is an end artery branching from the ileocolic artery, it is particularly susceptible to occlusion from increased intraluminal pressure. Occlusion usually results in necrosis and perforation of the appendix.

Initial symptoms of appendicitis include vague epigastric, periumbilical, or generalized abdominal pain that gradually increases in intensity; the pain probably is due to appendiceal distention caused by edema or

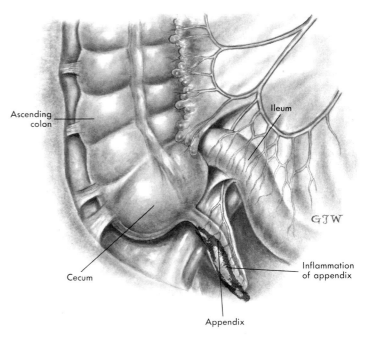

FIGURE 4-6
Acute appendicitis.

colic caused by appendiceal obstruction. The pain eventually localizes in the right lower quadrant, probably because of inflammation involving the peritoneal surfaces of adjacent loops of bowel. (The pain may subside before localizing.) Other symptoms include anorexia, nausea, and vomiting; low-grade fever is also common. Physical examination reveals tenderness to palpation (especially over McBurney's point), rebound tenderness, and involuntary guarding.

Appendicitis does not always exhibit these typical signs and symptoms; varying clinical pictures may result if the patient is older or pregnant or if the appendix is in an atypical position.

COMPLICATIONS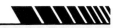

    Perforation
    Abscess formation
    Peritonitis

DIAGNOSTIC STUDIES AND FINDINGS

Diagnostic test	Findings
White blood cell count (**WBC**)	Elevated (10,000-16,000/mm^3), with shift to the left (75% neutrophils)
Abdominal x-ray	May show fecalith in right lower quadrant or localized ileus; used to differentiate appendicitis from perforated ulcer (free air under diaphragm indicates perforation)
Urinalysis	No or few leukocytes and RBCs; used to differentiate appendicitis from urinary tract disease

MEDICAL MANAGEMENT

GENERAL MANAGEMENT

NPO status; IV fluids and electrolytes; preparation for surgery (informed consent; preoperative teaching).

SURGERY

Appendectomy

DRUG THERAPY

Antibiotic prophylaxis may be given (metronidazole or cefamandole as a single dose before surgery); antibiotics may be continued after surgery if perforation with peritoneal contamination is present at time of surgery; analgesics may be given after diagnosis has been established.

1   ASSESS

ASSESSMENT	OBSERVATIONS
Pain location and pattern	May report initial onset of pain several hours previously, involving entire abdomen or epigastric/periumbilical area; may report later localization of pain to right lower quadrant; may report interval of reduced pain before localization Reports increased pain with walking or coughing Can point to localized point midway between iliac crest and umbilicus (McBurney's point) as site of pain May report atypical pain pattern: less intense pain that is poorly localized and not exacerbated by activity (retrocecal or retroileal appendix); severe pain that is localized on the left with tenderness on rectal examination and urge to urinate or defecate, but no abdominal tenderness (pelvic appendix); vague symptoms (elderly patient); altered location (pregnancy)
Associated gastrointestinal symptoms	May report anorexia; may have vomiting; may report diarrhea or constipation and failure to expel flatus

ASSESSMENT	OBSERVATIONS
Abdominal examination	May exhibit rebound tenderness and muscle rigidity on palpation or percussion
Rectal examination	May be normal or may cause tenderness (with atypical appendix location)
Vital signs	May have low-grade fever and shallow, rapid respirations
Anxiety	May express fear, anxiety, and concern about medical procedures and surgery

2 DIAGNOSE

NURSING DIAGNOSIS	SUBJECTIVE FINDINGS	OBJECTIVE FINDINGS
Pain related to inflammation of appendix	Describes abdominal pain that is initially vague but becomes progressively more intense and localized to right lower quadrant (McBurney's point); states that pain is exacerbated by movement (may have atypical pain pattern if appendix is in different position, or if patient is elderly or pregnant)	Shallow, rapid respirations; knees may be drawn up; facial expression indicates pain; may limit movement and may "guard" abdomen
High risk for infection related to perforation	Reports sudden relief of pain followed by increasing generalized abdominal pain	Fever >38.8° C (102° F); tachycardia; abdominal distention; increased abdominal rigidity and guarding
Anxiety related to medical procedures and surgery	Reports feeling "anxious, worried, scared"; reports lack of knowledge about surgery	Increased alertness; tachycardia; restlessness; frequent requests for reassurance; focus is on self; overexcited behavior

3 PLAN

Patient goals

1. The patient's pain will be relieved.
2. The patient will have no infection.

3. The patient's anxiety will be controlled.

4 IMPLEMENT

NURSING DIAGNOSIS	NURSING INTERVENTIONS	RATIONALE
Pain related to inflammation of appendix	Assess patient's pain (location, severity, and exacerbating factors).	Pattern and location of pain provide important etiologic clues.
	Help patient find a comfortable position (usually semi-Fowler's); limit activity.	Pain is exacerbated by movement such as walking or coughing; knees-up position helps reduce traction on abdominal organs and reduces pain.

➔ ❯ ❯

NURSING DIAGNOSIS	NURSING INTERVENTIONS	RATIONALE
	Administer analgesics as ordered after diagnosis has been established.	Analgesics may be withheld so that an accurate assessment can be made; once the diagnosis has been determined, analgesics are indicated for pain relief.
High risk for infection related to perforation	Monitor patient for signs of perforation or peritonitis: sudden relief of pain followed by increasingly intense, generalized abdominal pain; increasing abdominal distention, rigidity, and guarding; fever; tachycardia; tachypnea.	Continual assessment promotes prompt recognition and early intervention; perforation requires immediate surgical intervention.
	Prepare patient for surgery.	Prompt surgical removal of an inflamed appendix prevents complications such as perforation and peritonitis; prompt removal of a perforated appendix and removal of purulent material from the abdominal cavity reduce the risk of peritonitis.
	Administer antibiotics as ordered.	Antibiotics are indicated for surgical prophylaxis or to eradicate intraabdominal infection.
Anxiety related to medical procedures and surgery	Explain all procedures (e.g., venipuncture); provide preoperative teaching, with amount of detail determined by patient's and family's desire for information and level of comprehension.	Fear of the unknown is a significant contributor to anxiety; explanations reduce the "unknown" factor and increase trust in caregivers.
	Monitor the patient's and family's anxiety level; identify specific concerns and address them.	Anxiety and fear increase pain and reduce an individual's ability to cope; identifying increasing anxiety and specific concerns permits prompt intervention.
	Provide support to patient and family; permit family to remain with patient before surgery.	Illness and surgery are traumatic events affecting both patient and family; separation from one's support system increases anxiety.
	Provide comfort measures; limit painful procedures (e.g., abdominal examinations) as much as possible.	Pain increases anxiety; comfort measures reduce pain and increase trust in caregivers.

5 EVALUATE

PATIENT OUTCOME	DATA INDICATING THAT OUTCOME IS REACHED
Patient's pain has been relieved.	Patient does not require analgesics; he states that abdominal pain is gone (may exhibit mild incisional tenderness).
Patient has no infection.	Temperature is normal; abdominal examination reveals no distention, rigidity, or guarding. (Patient may have mild incisional tenderness, but incision shows no signs of infection, i.e., purulence, induration, or erythema.)

PATIENT OUTCOME	DATA INDICATING THAT OUTCOME IS REACHED
Patient's anxiety has been eased.	Patient rests quietly; he states his relief from feelings of fear and dread; he asks appropriate questions and cooperates with caregivers.

PATIENT TEACHING

1. Explain preoperative care and rationales (e.g., purpose of venipuncture, intravenous fluids, nothing by mouth status).
2. Explain the surgical procedure for appendectomy and its rationale.
3. Explain postoperative care, including gradual dietary advancement, gradual increase in activity, and measures for controlling pain.

For a picture of Crohn's disease, see Color Plate 5, p. x.

Crohn's Disease

Crohn's disease is a chronic inflammatory disease that can affect any area of the alimentary canal from the mouth to the anus. Crohn's disease is one type of inflammatory bowel disease (IBD), a general category that includes ulcerative colitis, Crohn's disease, and indeterminate IBD (a term used to describe inflammatory bowel disease that cannot be clearly diagnosed as either Crohn's disease or ulcerative colitis because it has features of both). Table 4-2 compares features of Crohn's disease and ulcerative colitis.

Other names for Crohn's disease are ileitis, regional enteritis, ileocolitis, granulomatous colitis, and transmural colitis.

EPIDEMIOLOGY

Crohn's disease was first described, by Crohn and associates, in 1932. It is now recognized as a fairly common problem of the gastrointestinal tract, with a prevalence currently estimated at 20 to 70 cases per 100,000 population. Crohn's disease can affect any ethnic group, but it is most common among Western whites of European Anglo-Saxon descent and is three to five times more common among European or North American Jews than among non-Jews. Onset of the disease most often occurs during adolescence or young adulthood; the most common age at onset is 15 to 30. There is some familial tendency toward development of Crohn's disease; siblings have an increased risk of about 30%. Crohn's disease affects men and women about equally.

Much research has been devoted to determining the cause of Crohn's disease; to date, the answer remains elusive. Research has focused primarily on the possible role of infectious agents and immunologic disturbances; other factors that may play a causative role are dietary agents and psychosomatic factors.

A number of viral and bacterial organisms have been studied in relation to Crohn's disease, but none has been shown to act as a causative agent, and at this time Crohn's disease is not considered an infectious process. However, recent research has implicated a previously unstudied mycobacterium that was isolated from surgical specimens obtained from patients with Crohn's disease. When these organisms were fed to baby goats, the kids developed Crohn's disease and the mycobacterium was found in their lymph nodes. Research in this area is continuing.

The second major theory of causation is immunologic disturbances. This seems to be logical in view of the fact that Crohn's disease involves recurrent inflammation, formation of granulomatous lesions, systemic manifestations, and a positive response to corticosteroids. Crohn's disease initially was theorized to be an autoimmune process, because these patients were

Table 4-2

COMPARISON OF CROHN'S DISEASE AND ULCERATIVE COLITIS

	Crohn's disease	Ulcerative colitis
Bowel segments involved	May involve any segment of bowel; terminal ileum and ascending colon most commonly involved; skip lesions common	Involves colon and rectum only; begins in rectum and proceeds proximally; no skip lesions
Extent of involvement	Transmural	Mucosal
Clinical features	Abdominal pain; low-volume, non-bloody diarrhea; fever	Rectal bleeding, diarrhea
X-ray/endoscopic findings	"Rake" ulcers, cobblestoning, thickening of bowel wall, strictures	Friable, edematous mucosa; pseudopolyps; shortening of colon
Complications	Fistulas, abscesses, anorectal disease, short bowel syndrome (if multiple resections are required)	Hemorrhage, toxic megacolon with perforation, increased risk of colorectal cancer

found to have autoantibodies that were thought to attack intestinal epithelium. However, studies have shown that the autoantibodies are nonspecific and that the level of autoantibodies does not correlate with the severity of Crohn's disease; in addition, cellular damage from the autoantibodies has not been demonstrated. Another theory is that Crohn's disease results from lymphocyte-mediated reactions. This theory is based on the fact that lymphocytes from patients with Crohn's disease have been shown to be cytotoxic for intestinal epithelial cells. However, further studies indicated that the presence of sensitized lymphocytes is nonspecific and that the cytotoxicity to intestinal epithelium disappears within 10 days after the diseased bowel has been resected. These findings seem to suggest that altered immune responses may be the result rather than the cause of Crohn's disease. A third immunologic disturbance theory is altered host resistance. A number of studies report reduced lymphocyte counts and diminished response to mitogens, and some studies suggest impaired neutrophil function. However, it is unknown whether these changes represent an etiologic factor or a response to the disease process. A hypersensitivity response mediated by IgE has been suggested, and large numbers of degranulating mast cells have been found in the intestinal wall of patients with Crohn's disease; however, elevated levels of IgE have not been demonstrated. It is clear that Crohn's disease is associated with immunologic disturbances; at this time it is not known whether these changes represent cause or effect.

Additional theories of causation include dietary factors and psychosomatic illness. Dietary factors have been implicated because the disease is much more common in Western cultures. Specific agents suggested as etiologic factors include chemical food additives, highly refined carbohydrates, the food stabilizer carrageenan, heavy metals such as mercury, breakfast cereals, and low-fiber diets. At this time there is no evidence to support an etiologic role for dietary factors.

There also is no evidence to support emotional factors as a cause. Although stress has been associated with exacerbations of the disease, it has not been shown to cause the disease and the disease has not been found to occur more frequently in people with emotional problems. Much has been written about the "IBD personality"; however, it is likely that the emotional problems associated with Crohn's disease are a result of the chronic illness and the debilitating symptoms rather than a causative factor.

PATHOPHYSIOLOGY

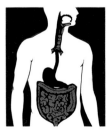

Crohn's disease involves transmural inflammation of the bowel wall. It tends to be recurrent and can affect any segment of the alimentary canal. About 90% of patients with Crohn's disease have involvement of the terminal ileum, which is the segment most commonly affected. In some patients, the disease is limited to the small intestine; however, in most patients the disease involves both the small bowel and the colon (ileocolitis). Other segments may be involved as well, such as the stomach or duodenum. Perianal disease is common and can occur even in patients who have no colon involvement. Perianal disease is characterized by abscesses, fissures, fistulas, and ulcerations of the perineal skin. In addition to the bowel disease, there are systemic manifestations associated with Crohn's disease.

Microscopically, Crohn's disease involves transmural, granulomatous inflammation; the entire bowel wall is edematous and infiltrated with inflammatory cells. "Skip" lesions are common, with normal bowel seen between diseased segments. The regional lymph nodes are always involved.

Aphthous ulcers are probably the earliest pathologic finding. These ulcers begin as microabscesses in lymphoid follicles and develop into superficial ulcers surrounded by normal or mildly edematous mucosa. As the disease advances, the ulcers become more invasive, forming fissures that may extend into the submucosal layer; these are known as "rake ulcers." The ulcers run both longitudinally and transversely and tend to coalesce; the combination of deep ulcers and edematous mucosa creates the classic "cobblestoned" appearance of the mucosa. With advanced disease, these fissures can penetrate the bowel wall to create fistulas or abscesses.

Changes in the submucosal layer include lymphocyte infiltration and lymphedema; these changes may extend into the muscular and serosal layers, resulting in thickening of the bowel wall. As the disease progresses, the bowel wall becomes fibrotic and stenotic, with narrowing of the lumen. Granulomas are found in the bowel wall of most patients, and in some patients granulomas are found in the enlarged mesenteric lymph nodes.

The serosa frequently is inflamed and exudative, with engorged vessels and lymphatics. This serosal inflammation predisposes to fistula formation, because the inflamed loops of bowel tend to stick to each other, to uninvolved loops of bowel, to adjacent organs, or to the abdominal wall; the deep fissures then erode through the bowel wall to create fistulas. The mesentery adjacent to the diseased bowel becomes inflamed and edematous, with enlarged lymph nodes. The mesenteric fat may extend onto the serosal surface and may even wrap around the bowel wall, a phenomenon referred to as "fat wrapping." The mesentery may also become shortened, resulting in fixation of the bowel.

Because early clinical manifestations of Crohn's disease are vague and episodic, the disease may go unrecognized for several years. Initial symptoms include general malaise, anorexia, fever, mild abdominal discomfort, and diarrhea. Children and adolescents may also experience growth retardation or failure to mature sexually. As the disease progresses, the symptoms become more severe. The most consistent symptoms are abdominal pain and diarrhea. Abdominal pain resulting from partial obstruction is intermittent and crampy, whereas pain associated with an acute exacerbation of the disease is more persistent and frequently associated with abdominal tenderness and the formation of ab-

scesses or fistulas. The diarrhea may be severe during exacerbations of the disease and usually is characterized by frequent small-volume, nonbloody stools without mucus or pus. The diarrhea may be caused by partial obstruction; impaired absorption of bile salts, resulting in colonic irritability; colonic disease; a fistula between the small bowel and the sigmoid colon; or, in some patients, lactose intolerance. Other clinical manifestations include anorexia, weight loss, and fever. Rectal bleeding may occur but is not as common as with ulcerative colitis.

Advanced disease may be associated with obstruction, abscess formation, and fistula development. As the disease progresses, the bowel may become strictured, resulting in obstructive symptoms: colicky abdominal pain, obstipation, abdominal distention, nausea, and vomiting. Abscess formation may result from perforations that are walled off by adjacent loops of bowel or by the mesentery. Signs and symptoms of abscess formation include fever, leukocytosis, pain, a tender abdominal mass, and guarding. Abscesses extending into the retroperitoneum can result in ureteral entrapment and hydronephrosis or a psoas muscle abscess, which produces hip flexion and a limp. Fistulas develop as a result of serosal inflammation and may or may not produce signs and symptoms, depending on the organs involved. Fistulas between loops of bowel rarely produce significant symptoms, whereas fistulas between the bowel and the skin, bladder, or vagina can cause significant morbidity.

Perianal disease is common with Crohn's disease and may be the most distressing aspect of the disorder for the patient. Perianal disease may precede the development of intestinal disease, may occur concurrently with Crohn's colitis, or may occur in Crohn's disease limited to the small bowel. Perianal lesions commonly include edematous skin tags and wide, painless fissures. There may be several fissures with undermined edges and subcutaneous communication. Anal canal ulcers may occur, causing pain on defecation and rectal examination. Stenosis of the anal canal may occur with long-standing disease but does not usually cause problems with bowel movements. Perianal abscesses are common and may occur in association with fissures or fistulas or as a result of infection of the anal glands. These abscesses may be simple or may involve the anal sphincters. Abscesses usually require drainage to relieve pain and to prevent spontaneous rupture with possible fistula formation. Fistulas in ano are less common than fissures in Crohn's disease. They may occur spontaneously or secondary either to an abscess extending from the anal canal or rectum to the perineum or to a deep rectal ulcer penetrating the vaginal wall. The fistula may drain stool and pus intermittently.

Nutritional deficits are common in Crohn's disease.

The severity of the deficiency depends on the severity of the disease, the segment of bowel involved, and the type of treatment. Reduced absorption of multiple nutrients is associated with involvement or resection of the jejunum and ileum; deficits may involve carbohydrates, amino acids, fats, water-soluble and fat-soluble vitamins, and folate. Involvement or resection of the distal ileum may result in anemia and fat intolerance secondary to malabsorption of vitamin B_{12} and bile salts. Lactase deficiency may occur with small bowel disease. Stricture formation may result in partial obstruction, which causes bacterial overgrowth in the lumen of the bowel; bacterial overgrowth impairs absorption of carbohydrates, fats, and vitamin B_{12}. (Bacterial overgrowth may also occur after resection of the ileocecal valve or surgical creation of a blind loop of bowel.) Folate deficiency is common and results from a number of factors: reduced intake, reduced absorption (resulting from jejunal and ileal involvement or resection, or administration of sulfasalazine), and possible increased requirements stemming from a catabolic state and chronic blood loss. Low zinc levels have also been reported in patients with Crohn's disease. The chronic inflammation of Crohn's disease may increase the need for protein and calories, and this increased need may widen the gap between needed nutrients and ingested nutrients, creating a chronic state of malnutrition.

Extraintestinal manifestations occur in addition to the bowel disease. Common systemic manifestations include joint problems (arthritis, sacroiliitis, and ankylosing spondylitis), skin lesions (erythema nodosum and pyoderma gangrenosum), ocular disorders (uveitis and conjunctivitis), and aphthous ulcers of the mouth. Extraintestinal manifestations are more common in Crohn's disease involving the colon than in Crohn's disease limited to the small bowel, and they often respond to treatment of the underlying disease. The arthritis associated with Crohn's disease usually involves one large joint in the lower limb and resolves spontaneously without residual damage to the joint; some patients have migrating arthralgias or polyarthritis. Arthritis most often occurs when the Crohn's disease is active and rarely precedes the onset of intestinal disease. Ankylosing spondylitis occurs 20 to 30 times more frequently in patients with Crohn's disease than in the general population; it does not necessarily reflect the activity of the intestinal disease and may even precede it by several years. Sacroiliitis frequently is asymptomatic. Skin lesions tend to recur during exacerbations of the disease and subside when the disease has been brought into remission. Erythema nodosum occurs more frequently with Crohn's disease involving the colon; pyoderma gangrenosum is uncommon with Crohn's disease. Ocular disorders are more likely to occur with Crohn's colitis than with Crohn's disease limited to the small intestine. Uveitis is the most serious of these disorders, requiring prompt intervention to preserve sight. Aphthous oral ulcers may precede or accompany an exacerbation of the disease; granulomatous lesions also have been reported in the mouth.

Other systemic disorders associated with Crohn's disease include gallstones, kidney stones, osteoporosis, liver disorders, vascular problems, and psychiatric disorders. The increased incidence of gallstones is limited to patients with small bowel disease and probably results from reduced absorption of bile salts, which alters the ratio of bile salts to cholesterol and thus promotes cholesterol precipitation. Kidney stones result from changes in intestinal absorption and are of two types: uric acid stones and oxalate stones. Uric acid stones may form in patients with small bowel disease; the reduced absorption of water and increased loss of bicarbonate (HCO_3^-) result in concentrated urine with low pH and high levels of uric acid. Oxalate stones form in patients with extensive ileal dysfunction (or resection) and an intact colon. The basis for oxalate stone formation is unclear. One theory is as follows: (1) dietary oxalates usually are bound to calcium in the bowel and excreted through the stool; (2) with steatorrhea (which results from ileal dysfunction and loss of bile salts), the fats trap the calcium so that it is not available to bind with the oxalates; (3) the oxalates are absorbed and may then precipitate in the urine. Osteoporosis, if present, may be worsened by steroid therapy. Liver disease may occur and may be mild or may involve pericholangitis. Depression affects many patients with Crohn's disease and frequently precedes the onset of disease. There is some increased risk of cancer; however, the risk is not as great as for the patient with ulcerative colitis.

The course of the disease varies. Many individuals have long periods of remission between exacerbations, whereas others have a more fulminant disease pattern. Studies have shown that most patients live fairly normal lives despite the relentless and recurrent nature of the disease.

Medical intervention is the primary approach to management of Crohn's disease; surgical intervention is reserved for complication management or intractable disease. Statistically, most patients will require surgical intervention at some point.

COMPLICATIONS

Fistulas
Abscess formation
Intestinal obstruction
Perianal disease (fissures, fistulas, abscesses)
Malnutrition
Growth retardation

DIAGNOSTIC STUDIES AND FINDINGS

Diagnostic test	Findings
Complete blood count (CBC)	Decreased Hb and Hct; decreased RBCs; increased or decreased MCV and MCH; decreased MCHC; elevated WBCs
Vitamin B$_{12}$ levels	May be reduced with distal ileitis or distal ileal resection
Total protein and albumin	May be decreased with advanced disease and malnutrition
Liver function studies	May be altered in patient with liver disease
Folic acid (folate)	May be reduced
Flat plate of abdomen	May show dilated loops of bowel with obstruction
Barium studies (barium enema, upper GI)	Aphthous ulcers; rake ulcers; longitudinal and transverse fissures ("cobblestoning" of mucosa); skip lesions; stenosis; stricture; areas of diffuse narrowing; asymmetric disease; pseudodiverticula; sinus tracts; fistula formation
Endoscopy	Aphthous ulcers; discrete ulcers; fissures; "cobblestoning" of the mucosa; skip areas; asymmetric disease; rectal sparing; fistulas
Biopsy	May show granulomas; diagnoses or rules out malignancy
Computed tomography (CT) scan	May show mesenteric abnormalities; thickening of bowel wall; abscess and fistula formation
Stool for guaiac	May be positive
Hydrogen breath test	May show lactose intolerance

MEDICAL MANAGEMENT

GENERAL MANAGEMENT

Nutritional Support

Regular balanced diet as tolerated during periods of remission. **Note:** Lactose restriction is indicated only if patient is demonstrated to have lactose intolerance. No specific dietary restrictions during remission; emphasis is on adequate caloric and protein intake and maintaining ideal body weight.

Restricted-residue diets may be indicated for patient with stenotic lesions causing partial obstruction.

Oral intake as tolerated during periods of exacerbation. Chemically defined diets may be given orally or by feeding tube to supplement oral intake.

Continuous enteral administration of elemental formulas may be beneficial during exacerbations (may induce remission) and may promote closure of enteric fistulas (as long as feedings do not increase fistula output).

Specific supplements as indicated for correction of specific deficits: Folic acid, vitamin B$_{12}$, minerals (calcium, magnesium, zinc, iron), and electrolytes (e.g., potassium). Total parenteral nutrition (TPN) for preoperative preparation and postoperative support of malnourished patients, treatment of short bowel syndrome, management of growth retardation, and to avert or delay surgery in patients with intractable disease who are poor surgical risks. **Note:** Remissions obtained with TPN usually are of short duration. Bowel rest (NPO with IV fluid and nutritional support) may be required during acute exacerbations.

General support measures

Emotional support to patient and family (e.g., referral to patient support groups, general supportive counseling, referral for counseling).

Continued.

MEDICAL MANAGEMENT—cont'd

SURGERY

Resection of diseased segment of bowel with reanastomosis for severe segmental disease or complications involving specific segments (e.g., small bowel resection, ileocolic resection, colon resection).

Subtotal colectomy with Hartmann's pouch and temporary end ileostomy or ileorectal anastomosis (for severe colonic disease with rectal sparing).

Temporary ileostomy or colostomy to provide bowel rest for distal bowel or as adjunct to procedures involving resection and reanastomosis when risk of anastomotic leakage is thought to be significant.

Total proctocolectomy with end ileostomy for severe disease involving the colon and rectum.

Stricturoplasty for relief of obstruction caused by strictures.

Bypass procedure for patient who is a poor risk for resection.

DRUG THERAPY

Sulfasalazine (Azulfidine): 3-4 g daily in divided doses; maintenance dose 1.5-2 g daily in divided doses. **Note:** Effective only for colonic disease; not active in small intestine.

Mesalamine (Rowasa enema or suppository): Enema administered daily; suppository administered bid. **Note:** A delayed-release oral form of mesalamine is awaiting FDA approval; because mesalamine is active only in the colon, it is effective only for Crohn's colitis.

Prednisone: 50-80 mg daily during exacerbations (PO or IV); 5-15 mg daily for maintenance with gradual tapering and withdrawal of drug once remission has been achieved. **Note:** Drug may be given qod to reduce side effects, especially growth retardation.

Mercaptopurine (6-MP): Initial dose, 1.5 mg/kg daily with dose titrated according to patient's response and effects on WBC and platelet counts; frequently allows reduction in steroid dosage or withdrawal from steroids without relapse.

Metronidazole (Flagyl): 15-20 mg/kg daily in divided doses; primarily indicated for patient with colonic disease, specifically fistula formation or perianal disease; long-term use may cause peripheral neuropathy.

Antidiarrheal agents: Diphenoxylate (Lomotil); loperamide (Imodium); codeine; tincture of opium; psyllium derivatives (for bulking action); cholestyramine (Questran) for diarrhea related to malabsorption of bile salts; aluminum hydroxide.

1 ASSESS

ASSESSMENT	OBSERVATIONS
Bowel function	May report diarrhea, diarrhea alternating with constipation, bloating and cramping after meals, anorexia, nausea, or vomiting, blood in stool, fecal urgency (rectal involvement)
Nutritional and hydration status	May report weight loss; weight may be less than 85%-90% of ideal body weight; may have signs of nutritional depletion (dry skin, sparse hair that comes out easily, dull eyes, listlessness, fatigue, joint edema); may have signs of fluid volume deficit (dry mucous membranes, oliguria, orthostatic hypotension)

ASSESSMENT	OBSERVATIONS
Vital signs	Fever may be present with exacerbations or abscess formation
Perianal tissue	May see perianal denudation with chronic or acute diarrhea; may see fissures or fistulous tracts with perianal disease; may see skin tags; may see induration, erythema, tenderness with perirectal abscess
Evidence of fistula formation	May see fistulous tracts exiting on abdominal surface; patient may report passage of gas or stool per urethra or vagina
Extraintestinal manifestations	May see inflammation of conjunctiva, or patient may report blurred vision; may see edematous, inflamed joint, and patient may report joint pain or soreness and stiffness in back; may see skin lesions, such as erythema nodosum lesions on legs
Emotional status/ coping skills	May report feeling stressed, depressed, unable to cope

2 DIAGNOSE

NURSING DIAGNOSIS	SUBJECTIVE FINDINGS	OBJECTIVE FINDINGS
Diarrhea related to intestinal inflammation	Reports frequent stools; states, "I know every bathroom in town"; reports alterations in life-style related to diarrhea; reports frequent use of antidiarrheal medications	Loose, frequent stools (more than three per day); perianal skin irritation
Nutrition, altered: less than body requirements related to anorexia and diarrhea	Reports reduced intake of food and fluids and weight loss	Weight is below 85%-90% of ideal body weight; dry skin; sparse, pluckable hair; joint edema; fissures at corners of mouth; apathy; fatigue
Impaired adjustment related to chronic illness	Verbalizes nonacceptance of diagnosis and altered health status; statements reflect compromised self-esteem; noncompliance with care plan; reports persistent feelings of anger or depression about illness with no change in feelings over time	Excessive dependency on family members or health team; unable to set realistic goals or to plan for future; lack of adequate support
Coping, ineffective family: compromised related to chronic illness in family member	Statements of patient and family reflect increased family conflict; patient complains that family members do not provide needed assistance and support; family members express difficulty handling their feelings and patient's care and support needs	"Hovering," overly protective behavior; lack of supportive behavior on part of family members; care provided by family members is inadequate
High risk for fluid volume deficit related to diarrhea or fistula output	Reports severe diarrhea or large-volume fistula output; reports feelings of dizziness and faintness; complains of dry mouth and thirst, weakness, fatigue	Output exceeds intake; oliguria; increased urine concentration; dry mucous membranes; reduced skin turgor; postural hypotension; lethargy

→ > >

NURSING DIAGNOSIS	SUBJECTIVE FINDINGS	OBJECTIVE FINDINGS
Impaired skin integrity related to diarrhea or fistula drainage	Reports skin pain around anus or fistula opening	Denudation of perineum or perifistular skin
Altered sexuality patterns related to chronic illness and ineffective coping	Patient or partner or both describe compromised sexual relationship	None

3 PLAN

Patient goals

1. The patient's diarrhea will be controlled.
2. The patient will attain and maintain ideal body weight.
3. The patient will demonstrate appropriate adjustment to the illness.
4. The family will demonstrate effective coping skills.
5. The patient will maintain adequate fluid and electrolyte balance.
6. The patient's skin will be intact.
7. The patient and partner will achieve a satisfactory sexual relationship.

4 IMPLEMENT

NURSING DIAGNOSIS	NURSING INTERVENTIONS	RATIONALE
Diarrhea related to intestinal inflammation	Monitor stools for volume, consistency, and characteristics (e.g., occult blood, steatorrhea).	Goal of therapy is to establish near-normal pattern of defecation; antidiarrheal drugs must be titrated according to patient's response; occult blood indicates active disease and the potential for anemia; steatorrhea indicates ileal dysfunction.
	Administer antiinflammatory medications as ordered (e.g., sulfasalazine, prednisone).	Control of the underlying inflammatory process reduces diarrhea.
	Administer antidiarrheal drugs as ordered: psyllium derivatives for watery stools; diphenoxylate, loperamide, codeine, and tincture of opium for frequent stools; cholestyramine for diarrhea resulting from malabsorption of bile salts.	Psyllium derivatives act as a bulking agent; diphenoxylate, loperamide, codeine, and tincture of opium reduce peristalsis and thus reduce cramping and diarrhea; cholestyramine binds bile salts.
	Assess patient for fecal urgency associated with low-volume diarrhea; notify physician if present.	Fecal urgency indicates rectal inflammation and may indicate a need for local antiinflammatory drugs (enema or suppository).
Nutrition, altered: less than body requirements related to anorexia and diarrhea	Monitor patient's weight and nutrient intake and laboratory indicators of malnutrition (e.g., reduced albumin or transferrin).	Prompt recognition of nutritional deficits permits early intervention; correction of nutritional deficits helps prevent complications and may improve condition of bowel wall.

NURSING DIAGNOSIS	NURSING INTERVENTIONS	RATIONALE
	Work with patient and dietitian to provide high-calorie, high-protein diet based on patient's preferences and tolerance.	Maintaining body weight and positive nitrogen balance reduces morbidity and improves health status.
	Provide nutritional supplements as ordered and indicated (e.g., high-calorie, high-protein beverages, and iron, folic acid, or magnesium supplements).	Nutritional supplements can improve protein and calorie intake and can replace specific nutrients.
	If patient has inadequate intake or signs of malnutrition, obtain order for nutritional support.	Patients with acute exacerbations or short bowel syndrome may require continuous elemental enteral feedings or TPN.
Impaired adjustment related to chronic illness	Provide information on the disease according to patient's readiness for teaching.	Information about the disease reduces the "fear of the unknown."
	Provide supportive counseling.	Supportive counseling helps patient explore his feelings and identify major concerns; confronting these issues is the first step in adjustment.
	Refer patient to local support group (e.g., Crohn's and Colitis Foundation of America).	Sharing concerns and experiences reduces patient's sense of isolation and expands his support system.
	Offer professional counseling as an option.	Professional counseling helps patient deal with the numerous issues associated with a chronic illness.
Coping, ineffective family: compromised related to chronic illness in family member	Provide information about the disease to family members according to their readiness for information.	Information reduces the "fear of the unknown" and may increase the ability to cope.
	Talk with family members separately about their feelings, concerns, and frustrations.	Family members must adapt to the changes in the patient's health; they must have an opportunity to express their feelings and confront their personal issues.
	Encourage family members to share their feelings and concerns with each other and with patient.	Open communication reduces resentment and misunderstanding and improves ability to cope with frustrations.
	If patient cannot carry out usual family roles, help him and family renegotiate tasks so that patient contributes as much as possible.	Renegotiating tasks maintains patient's feelings of worth and reduces other members' overload and resentment.
	Suggest family counseling as an effective management approach.	Counseling supports each member in dealing with the illness and their feelings in an effective manner.
	Encourage patient and family to share recreational and pleasurable activities when possible.	Shared activities reduce stress and promote closeness, which improves the ability to cope.
	Acknowledge negative feelings as normal and "OK."	Acknowledging normality of negative feelings reduces guilt and enhances coping.

NURSING DIAGNOSIS	NURSING INTERVENTIONS	RATIONALE
High risk for fluid volume deficit related to diarrhea or fistula output	Monitor patient's intake and output, and watch for signs of hypovolemia (dry mucous membranes, oliguria, orthostatic hypotension, reduced skin turgor).	Prompt recognition permits early correction of fluid volume deficits.
	Provide fluid replacement as ordered and tolerated (PO or IV).	Maintaining fluid volume is essential for maintaining tissue perfusion.
Impaired skin integrity related to diarrhea or fistula drainage	For patient with diarrhea or perianal fistulas: (1) Cleanse skin gently with tap water, mineral oil, or gentle cleanser; (2) protect skin with skin sealants or moisture barrier ointment; if skin is denuded, apply pectin-based powder before applying sealant or ointment.	Liquid stool and fistula drainage can erode the skin; prevention involves avoiding trauma and using moisture barrier products.
	For patient with enterocutaneous fistula: (1) Use ostomy or wound pouches to contain drainage; (2) protect perifistular skin with pectin-based paste; if skin is denuded, apply pectin powder before applying paste.	Small bowel output contains proteolytic enzymes that can rapidly erode the skin; pectin barrier products are resistant to small bowel output.
Altered sexuality patterns related to chronic illness and ineffective coping	Assess patient's and partner's concerns about sexual relationship.	Assessment data provide basis for intervention.
	Provide accurate information about the disease and sexuality.	Accurate information dispels myths.
	Provide specific suggestions as indicated (e.g., alternatives to intercourse for patient with severe perianal disease).	Specific suggestions validate importance of sexual concerns and provide new options for management.

5 EVALUATE

PATIENT OUTCOME	DATA INDICATING THAT OUTCOME IS REACHED
Patient's diarrhea has been controlled.	Patient states that he has fewer than four or five stools per day; he states that diarrhea is no longer limiting his life-style.
Patient has achieved and maintains ideal body weight.	Patient's weight is within 10% of his ideal body weight.
Patient demonstrates appropriate adjustment to illness.	Patient can discuss disease realistically and is open about his feelings; he makes appropriate plans for the future.
Family demonstrates effective coping skills.	Patient and family discuss disease and its impact openly and honestly; they discuss their feelings, negotiate tasks appropriately, and engage in pleasurable activities when possible.

PATIENT OUTCOME	DATA INDICATING THAT OUTCOME IS REACHED
Patient maintains an adequate fluid-electrolyte balance.	Skin turgor is normal: urine volume and dilution are normal; B/P is normal in all positions (no orthostatic hypotension); laboratory values for electrolytes are normal.
Patient's skin is intact.	There is no erythema or denudation.
Patient and partner have attained a satisfactory sexual relationship.	Patient's and partner's statements indicate satisfaction with sexual relationship.

PATIENT TEACHING

1. Explain that the cause of Crohn's disease is not known; stress that it is *not* a psychosomatic disease or a result of dietary indiscretion.
2. Explain that the disease is chronic and recurrent, but emphasize the probability of long periods of remission.
3. Explain the importance of a healthy diet; explain that dietary restrictions are based on individual tolerance, and teach the patient to monitor his response to various foods. Encourage the patient to eat a variety of healthful, enjoyable foods within his limits of tolerance.
4. Explain that high levels of stress may cause exacerbations, and help the patient plan effective ways of dealing with stress (e.g., routine exercise or relaxation therapy).
5. Emphasize the importance of both routine medical follow-up and prompt reporting of any symptoms of an exacerbation, such as abdominal pain, fever, increased diarrhea, malaise, anorexia.
6. Provide instruction about all prescribed medications: purpose, dose, side effects, and signs or symptoms to report to physician. If the patient is taking steroids, emphasize the importance of gradually tapering the drug before it is discontinued. If the patient is taking metronidazole, emphasize the importance of avoiding alcohol because of the Antabuse-like reaction, and teach the patient to report any signs of peripheral neuropathy promptly.
7. Teach the patient the signs and symptoms of complications that should be reported **immediately**: flatus or stool from the urethra or vagina; increasing abdominal distention associated with cramping pain; and increasing abdominal tenderness associated with fever.
8. Provide information on support services and counseling centers in area (e.g., Crohn's and Colitis Foundation of America).

Ulcerative Colitis

> For a picture of ulcerative colitis, see Color Plate 6, p. X.

Ulcerative colitis is a chronic inflammatory condition affecting the mucosa of the colon and rectum.

Ulcerative colitis is one type of inflammatory bowel disease (IBD), a general category that includes Crohn's disease, ulcerative colitis, and indeterminate IBD (inflammatory bowel disease that cannot be clearly identified as either ulcerative colitis or Crohn's disease because it has features of both). Table 4-2 compares Crohn's disease and colitis.

EPIDEMIOLOGY

The annual incidence of ulcerative colitis in the United States is about six to eight cases per 100,000 people. The groups commonly affected are the same as those affected by Crohn's disease; European and American Jews are affected more commonly than non-Jews or

Jews living in Israel, and whites are affected more commonly than nonwhites. There is some familial tendency, and some families have an increased incidence of both Crohn's disease and ulcerative colitis. The incidence of disease onset peaks in the third and fifth decades of life, and men and women are affected equally.

As with Crohn's disease, the cause of ulcerative colitis remains unknown. The theories of causation parallel those already discussed under Crohn's disease and include viral or bacterial organisms, psychosomatic origins, and immunologic disorders. No virus, bacterium, or fungus has been consistently identified as a cause, and at this time ulcerative colitis is not thought to be infectious in origin. The psychosomatic theory of causation is based partly on animal studies that revealed colonic ulceration after intense parasympathetic stimulation. However, the studies done in humans have failed to consistently demonstrate a pathologic personality pattern, and psychosomatic factors currently are thought to play more of an exacerbating role than a causative one. Immunologic abnormalities definitely are present in ulcerative colitis. The abnormalities parallel those discussed under Crohn's disease and can be summarized as follows: (1) anticolon antibodies have been found in the plasma of patients with ulcerative colitis, but they are not colon specific and their significance is not known; (2) lymphocytes obtained from patients with ulcerative colitis have been found to damage colonic epithelial cells in culture media; (3) a factor that inhibits migration of macrophages has been found in the serum of patients with ulcerative colitis; and (4) ulcerative colitis frequently is associated with other diseases thought to be caused by immunologic abnormalities. One aspect of immune function currently under investigation is the role of inflammatory mediators, the chemicals that regulate the immune response. A number of inflammatory mediators have been identified (e.g., arachidonic acid, prostaglandins, and leukotrienes), and it is known that drugs currently used to treat inflammatory bowel disease suppress some inflammatory mediators. It is hoped that further study will identify the specific mediators involved in IBD and that drugs to regulate these mediators can be developed.

PATHOPHYSIOLOGY

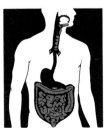

In its usual form ulcerative colitis primarily affects the mucosal layer of the colon. It begins in the rectum and proceeds proximally and may eventually involve the entire colon. The course of the disease commonly involves remissions and exacerbations, although a small percentage of patients have fulminant disease that involves the deeper layers of the bowel wall and that may progress

to toxic megacolon. In addition to the bowel disease, ulcerative colitis may produce systemic manifestations.

The pathologic changes that occur in ulcerative colitis begin with inflammation at the base of the crypts of Lieberkühn. This inflammatory process damages the epithelial cells in the crypts, resulting in leukocyte migration into the crypts and the formation of crypt abscesses. As the abscesses in an area coalesce, the inflammatory process spreads, causing frank epithelial necrosis; the result is ulceration and denudation of the mucosa. The mucosa surrounding the ulcerations may appear "heaped up," because the muscularis mucosae (the thin layer of smooth muscle that separates the mucosa and submucosa) tends to contract; these mucosal "humps," commonly called pseudopolyps, are one diagnostic finding in ulcerative colitis.

Mucosal repair proceeds concurrently with the inflammation. A thin layer of very vascular granulation tissue covers the ulcer's surface and serves as a base for epithelial migration. Hypertrophy of the muscularis mucosae may occur, and contraction of this hypertrophic muscle causes apparent spasm, stricture, loss of haustrations, and even shortening of the colon. However, these changes are all reversible, since true fibrosis does not occur.

Rectal bleeding (hematochezia) and diarrhea are the most prominent clinical manifestations of ulcerative colitis. The bleeding may be mild and intermittent or severe enough to cause circulatory collapse. The bleeding is the result of mucosal ulceration, vascular engorgement, and highly vascular granulation tissue. Two types of diarrhea may occur with ulcerative colitis. The first type is caused by severe rectal inflammation and is characterized by fecal urgency and frequent passage of small amounts of stool mixed with blood, pus, and mucus. High-volume, watery diarrhea may also occur. This is caused by destruction of the mucosal layer, resulting in loss of sodium and water absorption and reduced motility, which in turn results in loss of the normal "back-and-forth" contractions that promote fluid reabsorption. (The acute inflammation reduces motility.)

Ulcerative colitis ranges in severity from mild disease with intermittent bleeding, mild diarrhea, and no systemic manifestations to severe disease that may be either chronic or fulminant. Chronic severe disease is characterized by marked diarrhea, bleeding severe enough to cause anemia, abdominal cramping and tenderness, anorexia, and weight loss. Fever and leukocytosis may occur as well. Fulminant disease may occur with the initial bout of the disease or may occur in well-established disease; it is characterized by steadily worsening disease that fails to respond to intensive medical therapy.

The major complications associated with ulcerative colitis include massive bleeding, hypovolemia secondary to severe diarrhea, toxic megacolon, perforation, and an increased risk of adenocarcinoma of the colon. The pathophysiology underlying massive bleeding and severe diarrhea has already been described. Toxic megacolon is a rare complication, occurring in about 5% of patients with ulcerative colitis; however, it is a very serious complication, with a mortality rate averaging 25%. It appears to result from a spread of the mucosal inflammation to the submucosal, muscular, and possibly the serosal layers of the colon; the smooth muscle is paralyzed, which permits the colon to passively dilate, and the barrier function of the epithelium appears to be lost, permitting uptake of bacterial toxins and antigens. Factors contributing to the development of toxic megacolon are thought to include severe inflammation compounded by excessive use of opiates, narcotics, or anticholinergic drugs or by vigorous colonic preparation for surgery and diagnostic examinations. In many cases, however, there is no definable cause. Clinical manifestations of toxic megacolon include severe abdominal distention, abdominal pain and tenderness, and signs of toxicity: chills, fever, leukocytosis with a shift to the left, anorexia, nausea and vomiting, and bloody diarrhea. The goal in managing toxic megacolon is to prevent perforation and peritonitis, which carries a 25% to 40% mortality rate. Aggressive medical management is instituted, and the patient is closely monitored; immediate surgical intervention is indicated for signs of impending perforation or failure to respond to medical therapy.

Ulcerative colitis is also associated with an increased risk of colon cancer; patients at increased risk include those who have had the disease for 10 years or longer, and patients whose disease involves most or all of the colon. The severity of the disease does not seem to affect the risk; patients with mild disease are as likely to develop cancer as those with severe disease. Cancer associated with ulcerative colitis is commonly infiltrative in nature and may involve several sites; thus it is more difficult to detect with routine screening. In addition, the early signs of malignancy (painless bleeding) frequently are attributed to the ulcerative colitis. Careful, annual surveillance (e.g., double-contrast barium enemas or colonoscopy with several biopsies, or both) is indicated for patients considered at risk as a result of the duration and extent of their disease. However, even with careful surveillance, some lesions are missed, leading some practitioners to recommend prophylactic proctocolectomy for high-risk patients. This is a major decision for these patients, since proctocolectomy requires some type of fecal diversion (i.e., ileostomy, continent ileostomy, or ileoanal anastomosis with proximal reservoir). Such patients must be given current information about risk factors and treatment options and must be supported in making their own informed decisions.

In addition to the bowel disease, ulcerative colitis is associated with systemic manifestations, including skin lesions, eye lesions, arthritis, and liver disease. The skin lesions include erythema nodosum and pyoderma gangrenosum. Erythema nodosum is a dermatosis marked by tender, raised lesions on the arms and legs. Pyoderma gangrenosum, which occurs less frequently but can cause significant skin and tissue loss, is characterized by painful lesions with purulent drainage and results in dermal destruction. Exacerbation of skin lesions is commonly seen with flare-ups of the ulcerative colitis and usually subsides when the disease is brought under control; however, pyoderma gangrenosum may recur even after proctocolectomy and may require systemic steroids for management.

Eye lesions include iritis, uveitis, episcleritis, and conjunctivitis. Uveitis is the most common and is characterized by blurred vision, eye pain, and photophobia. Prompt consultation with an ophthalmologist is important to preserve sight.

Arthritis commonly involves migratory joint pain and edema that coincide with exacerbations of the disease and resolve when the disease is brought under control; no residual joint deformity occurs. Ankylosing spondylitis is another type of arthritis commonly seen with ulcerative colitis. It causes back pain and stiffness, may result in deformity, and tends to be progressive. Physical therapy and antiinflammatory drugs may be required for these patients.

The most serious of the extracolonic manifestations are those involving the liver; fortunately, these are uncommon, occurring in about 7% of patients with ulcerative colitis. Liver disease may be limited to mild abnormalities in liver function tests. However, more serious disease can occur as well, such as fatty liver, sclerosing cholangitis, chronic active hepatitis, and cancer of the bile duct. The liver disease does not always improve after the inflammatory bowel disease has been brought under control.

COMPLICATIONS

Massive bleeding
Toxic megacolon
Perforation
Adenocarcinoma of the colon
Extracolonic manifestations: skin lesions (erythema nodosum, pyoderma gangrenosum); eye lesions (uveitis, conjunctivitis, episcleritis); joint abnormalities (migratory arthritis, ankylosing spondylitis); and liver disease (fatty liver, sclerosing cholangitis, chronic hepatitis, bile duct cancer)

DIAGNOSTIC STUDIES AND FINDINGS

Diagnostic test	Findings
Stool (for blood)	Positive during active disease
Stool (for culture)	Negative (rules out bacterial source of disease)
Complete blood count (CBC)	Hb and Hct may be low (blood loss, anemia); MCV, MCH, MCHC may be low (anemia); RBCs may be low (blood loss, anemia); WBCs may be elevated (toxic megacolon)
Serum albumin	May be decreased with severe disease
Barium enema	Mucosal irregularities; ulcerations; loss of haustrations; colonic shortening; pseudopolyps (*Note:* A barium enema is contraindicated with acute disease; caution must be used in administering bowel preparation)
X-ray (flat plate) of abdomen	May show: shortening of colon and loss of haustrations; irregular mucosal surface (because of ulcerations and pseudopolyps); severe dilation of colon, especially transverse colon (toxic megacolon)
Endoscopy	Hyperemic, friable, intensely inflamed mucosa with exudate (early disease); deep mucosal ulcerations; coarse granular appearance of mucosa; pseudopolyps; shortening of colon; loss of haustrations (late disease) (*Note:* With acute disease, sigmoidoscopy is permitted but colonoscopy is contraindicated due to the risk of perforation)
Biopsy	Reveals inflammatory changes in mucosa; helps differentiate ulcerative colitis and Crohn's disease; also used in surveillance for colon cancer in long-standing disease involving entire colon
Liver studies	May be altered in patient with liver involvement

MEDICAL MANAGEMENT

GENERAL MANAGEMENT

Fluid replacement during exacerbations resulting in severe diarrhea:

Oral fluids as tolerated, IV fluids and electrolytes when oral fluids cannot be tolerated or when volume tolerated is inadequate to maintain fluid balance.

Blood replacement may be required for episodes of massive bleeding.

Nutritional support: No routine dietary restrictions; patient is encouraged to eat well-balanced diet and to base restrictions on foods she finds to be irritating; high-protein, high-calorie supplements may be required during severe exacerbations associated with reduced oral intake and hypoalbuminemia; parenteral nutrition occasionally is required for severe, unremitting disease that prevents oral intake (or for patient requiring nutritional repletion before surgery).

Bowel rest (NPO status and placement of N/G or small bowel tube for decompression) for patient with toxic megacolon.

Surveillance for colon cancer for patients with long-standing disease involving the entire colon.

Emotional support for patient and family.

MEDICAL MANAGEMENT—cont'd

SURGERY

Subtotal colectomy with ileostomy and Hartmann's pouch: or mucous fistula for severe disease with toxic megacolon and impending or actual perforation.

Total proctocolectomy with Brooke ileostomy: for severe disease or premalignant changes in colon (in patient who is not a candidate for or does not desire a continent procedure).

Total colectomy with subtotal proctectomy: (sphincter-sparing procedure); construction of ileal reservoir (e.g., J-pouch or S-pouch) and anastomosis of reservoir to anal canal. (Mucosal proctectomy may also be done with this procedure.) This procedure is indicated for severe disease or premalignant changes in colon in patient who is a candidate for and desires a continent procedure. **Note:** These procedures may be done in one, two, or three stages. The two-stage procedure is most common (stage 1: total colectomy, subtotal proctectomy, mucosal proctectomy, creation of reservoir, and anastomosis to anal canal, diverting loop ileostomy; stage 2: ileostomy takedown). The three-stage procedure is indicated for a very ill patient or one who is overweight and steroid dependent; the three-stage procedure permits weaning from steroids and weight loss (which provides increased mesenteric mobility and improves the potential for successful anastomosis of reservoir to anal canal). (Stage 1: diverting ileostomy, subtotal proctocolectomy, Hartmann's pouch or mucous fistula; stage 2: takedown of ileostomy, construction of reservoir, mucosal proctectomy, anastomosis of reservoir to anal canal, diverting loop ileostomy; stage 3: ileostomy takedown.)

Total proctocolectomy with continent ileostomy: (Kock pouch or continent ileal reservoir) for patient who has severe disease or premalignant changes in colon and is a candidate for and desires a continent ileal reservoir.

DRUG THERAPY

Sulfasalazine (Azulfidine): 3-4 g daily in divided doses during acute phase, then 1.5-2 g daily in divided doses for maintenance.

Hydrocortisone enema (Cortenema): Administered nightly for 21 days or until remission has been achieved (if no improvement is shown within 21 days, drug is discontinued). If drug is given for more than 21 days, dosage is tapered before discontinuing. **Note:** Primarily indicated for proctitis and left-sided colitis.

Hydrocortisone rectal foam (Cortifoam): 1 applicator 1-2 times daily for 2-3 wk, then qod.

Mesalamine (Rowasa) enema: Daily for 3-6 wk; suppository twice daily for 3-6 wk. Suppository is for treatment of proctitis only; enema is for treatment of proctosigmoiditis. (A delayed-release form of mesalamine is in the final stages of FDA approval.)

Olsalazine (Dipentum): Maximum dosage 3 g daily (this is a new drug to be used as an alternative to sulfasalazine for patients who cannot tolerate sulfasalazine).

Prednisolone: 100 mg daily IV for 10-14 days during acute phase of severe disease.

Prednisone: 60-100 mg daily PO for severe disease (taper slowly based on patient's response); 40-60 mg daily PO for moderate disease (taper slowly); qod regimen may be used to reduce adverse effects.

Antidiarrheal medications: Psyllium products (for bulking effect with watery diarrhea); diphenoxylate (Lomotil); loperamide (Imodium); codeine.

Note: Anticholinergic drugs, opiates, and narcotics (diphenoxylate, loperamide, and codeine) should be used with extreme caution in severe disease because of the risk of toxic megacolon.

Iron supplements may be administered to patient with chronic bleeding and iron-deficiency anemia.

Antibiotics (e.g., gentamycin, metronidazole, second- or third-generation cephalosporin) may be ordered for patient with toxic megacolon.

1 ASSESS

ASSESSMENT	OBSERVATIONS
Bowel function	May report mild diarrhea *or* fecal urgency with frequent passage of small amounts of stool, pus, and mucus *or* severe diarrhea with large volumes of watery stool; may report abdominal cramping and tenderness; may report anorexia or nausea; in toxic megacolon, hypoactive bowel sounds, severe abdominal distention and tenderness, infrequent bloody stools, or constant oozing of bloody stool may be seen
Bleeding	May report intermittent, chronic, or severe rectal bleeding; stool may test positive for occult blood; hematochezia may be present; may exhibit signs of anemia with chronic blood loss (fatigue, pallor, activity intolerance)
Vital signs	Fever may be present with severe disease or toxic megacolon; postural hypotension and tachycardia may be present with fluid volume deficit related to severe diarrhea; hypotension, tachycardia, and tachypnea may be present with massive bleeding
Perianal skin	May be erythematous and denuded in patient with chronic or severe diarrhea
Fluid-electrolyte balance	Decreased skin turgor, oliguria, increased concentration of urine, dizziness, weakness, and fatigue may be present with fluid volume deficit and electrolyte imbalance
Nutritional status	May report anorexia and weight loss; weight may be less than 85% to 90% of ideal body weight; may have signs of nutritional depletion (dry skin, joint edema, sparse hair that is easily pluckable, listlessness, fatigue)
Evidence of extracolonic manifestations	Conjunctivae may appear inflamed, or patient may complain of blurred vision or eye pain; may have joint pain and swelling affecting one or more large joints; may complain of back pain or stiffness; may have skin lesions (erythema nodosum or pyoderma gangrenosum); may have signs of liver disease (malaise, anorexia, jaundice, right upper quadrant tenderness)
Emotional status/coping skills	May report feeling "stressed," depressed, or unable to cope

2 DIAGNOSE

NURSING DIAGNOSIS	SUBJECTIVE FINDINGS	OBJECTIVE FINDINGS
Diarrhea related to chronic inflammation	Reports frequent stools; may report fecal urgency; states, "I know every bathroom in town"; reports alterations in life-style related to diarrhea; reports frequent use of antidiarrheal medications	Loose stools; frequent stools (more than three per day); perianal skin irritation
Altered renal, cerebral, cardiopulmonary, gastrointestinal, and peripheral tissue perfusion related to massive bleeding or to toxic megacolon or perforation	Reports severe bleeding or severe abdominal pain; complains of dizziness, anxiety, and shortness of breath	Massive or continuous rectal bleeding; severe abdominal distention and tenderness; hypotension, tachycardia, tachypnea, and diaphoresis; restlessness; fever; pallor

NURSING DIAGNOSIS	SUBJECTIVE FINDINGS	OBJECTIVE FINDINGS
Fluid volume deficit related to diarrhea	Reports severe diarrhea or a combination of diarrhea and anorexia/vomiting; reports feelings of dizziness and faintness; complains of dry mouth and thirst, weakness, fatigue	Output exceeds intake; oliguria; increased urine concentration; dry mucous membranes; reduced skin turgor; postural hypotension; lethargy
Nutrition, altered: less than body requirements related to anorexia	Reports reduced intake of food and fluids and weight loss	Weight below 85%-90% of ideal body weight; dry skin; sparse, pluckable hair; joint edema; fatigue
Impaired skin integrity related to diarrhea	Reports skin pain around anus	Denudation of perianal skin
Impaired adjustment related to diarrhea and chronic illness	Expresses rejection of diagnosis and altered health status; statements reflect compromised self-esteem; reports persistent feelings of anger or depression about illness with no change in feelings over time	Excessive dependency on family members or health team; unable to set realistic goals or to plan for future; lack of adequate support; noncompliance with care plan
Coping, ineffective family: compromised related to illness of family member.	Statements of patient and family reflect increased family conflict; patient complains that family members do not provide needed assistance and support; family members express difficulty handling their feelings and patient's support needs	Overly protective behavior toward patient; lack of supportive behavior by family members

3 PLAN

Patient goals

1. The patient's diarrhea will be controlled.
2. The patient will have normal tissue perfusion.
3. The patient will maintain an adequate fluid-electrolyte balance.
4. The patient will attain and maintain ideal body weight.
5. The patient's skin will be intact.
6. The patient will demonstrate appropriate adjustment to the illness.
7. The family will demonstrate effective coping skills.

4 IMPLEMENT

NURSING DIAGNOSIS	NURSING INTERVENTIONS	RATIONALE
Diarrhea related to chronic inflammation	Monitor stools for volume, consistency, and presence of blood.	Goal of therapy is to establish near-normal pattern of defecation; antidiarrheal drugs must be titrated according to patient's response. Severity of diarrhea and bleeding are indicators of disease activity.

→ > >

NURSING DIAGNOSIS	NURSING INTERVENTIONS	RATIONALE
	Administer antiinflammatory drugs as ordered (e.g., sulfasalazine, steroid enemas, prednisone)	Control of the underlying inflammation reduces diarrhea.
	Administer antidiarrheal drugs as ordered: psyllium derivatives for watery stools; diphenoxylate, loperamide, and codeine for frequent stools. *Note:* Do not administer diphenoxylate, loperamide, or codeine to patient with severe inflammation or signs of toxic megacolon.	Psyllium derivatives act as bulking agents; diphenoxylate, loperamide, and codeine reduce peristalsis and thus cramping and diarrhea; drugs that slow peristalsis are **contraindicated** in patient with severe inflammation and toxic megacolon.
	Assess patient for fecal urgency associated with low-volume diarrhea; if present, review medication profile for antiinflammatory enemas or suppositories. (If patient is not receiving antiinflammatory enemas or suppositories, notify physician of patient's symptoms.)	Fecal urgency indicates rectal inflammation and may indicate need for local antiinflammatory drugs (enema or suppository).
Altered renal, cerebral, cardiopulmonary, gastrointestinal, and peripheral tissue perfusion related to massive bleeding or to toxic megacolon or perforation	Measure bloody stools if possible; monitor patient for increasing abdominal distention and tenderness.	Measuring stool volume helps quantify blood loss; increasing distention and tenderness may indicate toxic megacolon and impending perforation; acute blood loss causes hypovolemic shock unless adequate replacement is provided; perforation may precipitate septic shock.
	Monitor vital signs and urinary output for evidence of circulatory compromise: hypotension, tachycardia, tachypnea, and reduced urinary output.	Circulatory compromise is reflected by changes in B/P and urinary output; compensatory responses to circulatory compromise produce tachycardia and tachypnea.
	For patient with toxic megacolon: keep patient NPO, and place N/G or small bowel tube as ordered (or assist with placement); irrigate tube as needed to maintain patency.	Decompression of proximal bowel reduces the risk of perforation, which can precipitate peritonitis and septic shock.
	Administer IV fluids and blood replacement as ordered; observe for transfusion reactions if blood is given.	IV fluids are administered to maintain plasma volume; blood replacement may be required for replacement of RBCs and platelets during episodes of massive bleeding.
	Administer antiinflammatory drugs as ordered.	Control of the underlying inflammation reduces bleeding and may help reverse toxic megacolon.
	If patient fails to improve with conservative therapy, prepare patient for surgery.	Emergency surgery may be required to control bleeding or to prevent or manage perforation.
Fluid volume deficit related to diarrhea	Monitor patient for intake and output and for signs of hypovolemia (e.g., dry mucous membranes, oliguria, orthostatic hypotension, reduced skin turgor).	Prompt recognition of fluid deficits permits early intervention.

NURSING DIAGNOSIS	NURSING INTERVENTIONS	RATIONALE
	Provide fluid replacement as ordered and tolerated (PO or IV).	Maintaining fluid volume is essential for adequate tissue perfusion.
Nutrition, altered: less than body requirements related to anorexia	Monitor patient's weight, nutrient intake, and laboratory indicators of malnutrition (e.g., reduced albumin levels).	Prompt recognition of nutritional deficits permits early intervention; correcting nutritional deficits helps prevent complications.
	Collaborate with patient and dietitian to provide high-calorie, high-protein diet based on patient's preferences and tolerance.	Maintaining body weight and positive nitrogen balance reduces morbidity and improves health status.
	Provide nutritional supplements as ordered and indicated (e.g., high-protein, high-calorie beverages; iron supplements). If patient has inadequate intake or signs of malnutrition, obtain order for nutritional support.	Nutritional supplements can improve protein and calorie intake and can replace specific nutrients.
Impaired skin integrity related to diarrhea	Cleanse perianal skin gently after each bowel movement with tap water, mineral oil, or gentle cleanser; protect the skin with skin sealant or moisture-barrier ointment; if skin is denuded, apply pectin-based powder before applying sealant or ointment.	Liquid stool can erode the skin; prevention involves avoidance of trauma and using moisture-barrier products.
Impaired adjustment related to diarrhea and chronic illness	Provide realistic information about the disease based on patient's readiness for teaching.	Information about the disease reduces "fear of the unknown" and increases ability to cope.
	Provide supportive counseling (encourage ventilation, and use reflective listening to promote self-awareness).	Supportive counseling helps patient explore her feelings and identify major concerns; exploring and confronting issues is the first task in the adjustment process.
	Refer patient to local support group (e.g., Crohn's and Colitis Foundation of America).	Sharing concerns and experiences reduces the patient's sense of isolation and expands her support system.
	Discuss with the patient the benefits of professional counseling.	Professional counseling helps patient to deal with the numerous issues associated with a chronic illness.
Coping, ineffective family: compromised related to chronic illness in family member.	Provide realistic information about the disease to family members according to their readiness for information.	Information reduces "fear of the unknown" and increases ability to cope.
	Provide opportunities for family members to discuss their feelings, concerns, and frustrations in private (away from the patient).	Family members must adapt to changes in patient's health status; they need an opportunity to ventilate their feelings and confront their personal issues.
	Encourage family members to share their feelings and concerns with each other and the patient.	Open communication reduces resentment and misunderstanding and improves ability to cope with frustrations.

→ ❭ ❭

NURSING DIAGNOSIS	NURSING INTERVENTIONS	RATIONALE
	If patient cannot carry out usual family roles, help patient and family renegotiate tasks so that patient contributes as much as possible.	Renegotiating tasks maintains patient's feelings of worth and reduces other members' overload and resentment.
	Suggest family counseling as an effective management approach.	Counseling supports each member in dealing with the illness and their feelings in an effective manner.
	Encourage patient and family to share recreational and pleasurable activities when possible.	Shared activities reduce stress and promote closeness, which improves ability to cope.
	Acknowledge negative feelings as normal and "OK."	Acknowledging the normality of negative feelings reduces guilt and enhances coping ability.

5 EVALUATE

PATIENT OUTCOME	DATA INDICATING THAT OUTCOME IS REACHED
Patient's diarrhea is under control.	Patient has fewer than four or five stools per day; she states that diarrhea is no longer limiting her life-style.
Patient has normal tissue perfusion.	Bleeding is controlled; abdominal distention and tenderness are gone; vital signs are normal; urine output is normal.
Patient maintains an adequate fluid-electrolyte balance.	Skin turgor is normal; urine volume and concentration are normal; B/P is normal in all positions (no orthostatic hypotension); laboratory values for electrolytes are normal.
Patient attains and maintains ideal body weight.	Patient's weight is 90% or more of her ideal body weight.
Patient's perianal skin is intact.	Perianal skin is intact and without erythema or denudation.
Patient demonstrates appropriate adjustment to illness.	Patient can discuss disease realistically, is open about her feelings, and makes appropriate plans for the future.
Family demonstrates effective coping skills.	Patient and family discuss disease and its impact openly and honestly; they discuss their feelings and negotiate tasks appropriately; they engage in pleasurable activities when possible.

PATIENT TEACHING

1. Explain that the cause of ulcerative colitis is not known; stress that it is *not* a psychosomatic disease.
2. Explain that the disease is chronic and recurrent; tell the patient that the disease usually can be controlled with drugs, with long periods of remission. Explain that the disease can be cured by surgery, although most patients never require surgery.
3. Explain the importance of a healthy diet; explain that dietary restrictions are based on individual experience, and teach the patient to monitor her response to various foods. Encourage her to eat a variety of healthful, enjoyable foods within her limits of tolerance.
4. Explain that high levels of stress may cause exacerbations, and help the patient plan effective ways of dealing with stress (e.g., routine exercise or relaxation therapy).
5. Emphasize the importance of routine medical follow-up and prompt reporting of any symptoms of an exacerbation (increased diarrhea and bleeding, anorexia, and abdominal cramping).
6. Teach the patient about all prescribed medications: their purpose, dosage, and side effects, and any signs or symptoms to report to the physician. If the patient is taking steroids, emphasize the importance of gradually tapering the dosage of the drug before it is discontinued.
7. Teach the patient the signs and symptoms of complications that should be reported *immediately:* increasing abdominal pain and distention, fever, massive bleeding, and blurred vision or eye pain.
8. Teach the patient about extracolonic manifestations that may occur: skin lesions, eye disorders, joint problems, and liver problems. Tell her to report any such signs or symptoms to the physician.
9. Provide the patient with information on local support services and counseling options (e.g., Crohn's and Colitis Foundation of America).

Pseudomembranous Enterocolitis

Pseudomembranous enterocolitis is an antibiotic-associated diarrhea characterized by inflammation and necrosis of the mucosal and submucosal layers of the bowel wall. It is called pseudomembranous enterocolitis, because the inflammation causes exudative plaques ("pseudomembranes") to form on the mucosal surface.

For a picture of pseudomembranous colitis, see Color Plate 4, p. x.

Pseudomembranous enterocolitis can involve both the small bowel and the colon (enterocolitis), but most commonly it is limited to the colon (pseudomembranous colitis).

EPIDEMIOLOGY

Pseudomembranous enterocolitis results from infection with *Clostridium difficile*, a gram-positive anaerobic bacillus. It is considered an antibiotic-related diarrhea because *C. difficile* is inhibited by the normal intestinal flora and flourishes only when the normal flora have been suppressed or eliminated by antibiotics. Two groups of people may acquire pseudomembranous enterocolitis: individuals who are carriers of *C. difficile* who are given antibiotics and noncarriers who are given antibiotics and then exposed to *C. difficile* through environmental contamination. Environmental contamination is particularly common in health care facilities; *C. difficile* has been isolated from the hands and stools of hospital staff and from furniture, toilets, bedding, and floors in the vicinity of patients infected with the organism. It is known that *C. difficile* forms hardy spores that are difficult to eradicate; these spores have been found to survive for weeks to months after an infected patient has been discharged. Environmental contamination is especially likely to occur when the patient is incontinent and fecal contamination of linens and floors occurs; in addition, one study reports probable spread by means of a bedside commode shared by patients in a semiprivate room.

The development of pseudomembranous enterocolitis is not related to the underlying illness, the antibiotic dose, or the route of administration. The type of antibiotic *may* be significant; drugs most frequently associated with pseudomembranous enterocolitis are ampicillin, clindamycin, and the cephalosporins. However, almost any antibiotic can alter the normal flora enough to permit *C. difficile* to proliferate; the exceptions are vancomycin and parenteral aminoglycosides such as gentamycin and tobramycin. The incidence of pseudomembranous enterocolitis seems to be higher among patients who are elderly or generally debilitated or who have had abdominal surgery.

The illness may develop during the course of antibiotic therapy or in the 6 weeks after the antibiotic regimen has been completed. The severity ranges from mild to fatal; death occurs in 10% to 20% of elderly or debilitated patients when the disease is not recognized and treated correctly.

PATHOPHYSIOLOGY

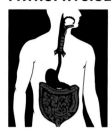

Proliferation of *C. difficile* results in production of two toxins that damage the epithelial cells of the intestinal mucosa and cause cell necrosis. The inflammation produces an inflammatory exudate (pseudomembranes) composed of fibrin, mucin, sloughed epithelial cells, and inflammatory cells. In mild disease focal damage to the mucosa occurs, with characteristic "summit" lesions;

more advanced disease involves damage to the mucosal glands and production of raised, yellow-white plaques (pseudomembranes). Severe disease causes extensive damage to the mucosa and a thick layer of inflammatory exudate, or pseudomembranes. Sloughing of the pseudomembranes reveals large areas of denuded mucosa.

The clinical picture varies, depending on the severity of the disease. Mild disease may be evidenced by two to five semisolid or liquid stools per day. More severe disease causes extensive mucosal damage, with severe diarrhea resulting from the impaired absorption of fluids and electrolytes. Patients may have up to 30 bowel movements a day and may also have abdominal tenderness, cramping, and fever. Severe mucosal necrosis may also cause loss of albumin. Occasionally the disease manifests as an "acute abdomen" syndrome that may result in toxic megacolon, colonic perforation, and peritonitis rather than diarrhea.

COMPLICATIONS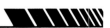

Fluid-electrolyte imbalance
Toxic megacolon
Perforation
Peritonitis

DIAGNOSTIC STUDIES AND FINDINGS

Diagnostic test	Findings
Complete blood count (CBC)	May show leukocytosis
Serum albumin	May be decreased
Serum electrolytes	May show abnormalities
Stool assay for *Clostridium difficile* toxin	Positive; cytopathic toxin is neutralized by clostridial antitoxin (*Note:* Negative results do not rule out disease)
X-ray (flat plate) of abdomen	May show edema and distention of colon; distorted haustral markings
Endoscopy (sigmoidoscopy or colonoscopy)	Erythematous, friable mucosa; distorted haustra; ulcerations; yellow-white plaques (pseudomembranes)

MEDICAL MANAGEMENT

GENERAL MANAGEMENT

Antibiotics are omitted if possible.

Monitoring of fluid-electrolyte balance: Intake and output, vital signs, and patient's weight are measured; patient is observed for signs of fluid-electrolyte imbalance.

Fluid-electrolyte replacement: Oral replacement if tolerated; IV fluid administration if oral fluids are not tolerated or if patient cannot maintain fluid balance with oral intake.

MEDICAL MANAGEMENT—cont'd

Safety measures for ambulatory patient: Patient assisted to bathroom as necessary; call bell kept within reach; bedside commode provided if needed.

Skin care: Gentle cleansing after each stool; protection of perianal skin.

Infection control measures: Private room if patient is incontinent or has poor personal hygiene; gowns for caregiver if soiling is likely; gloves for caregivers handling stool or giving perineal care; thorough handwashing by patient and caregivers; disposal of contaminated equipment or proper decontamination techniques (e.g., bag and label contaminated articles and send for decontamination; sterilize heavily contaminated objects such as endoscopes or bedpans with heat or sporicidal disinfectants).

SURGERY

Colectomy or diverting ileostomy for control of fulminant disease (not common)

DRUG THERAPY

Cholestyramine (Questran): 4 g 3-4 times daily, mixed with applesauce or noncarbonated beverage. **Note:** Primarily used for mild disease, it works by binding toxins in bowel lumen rather than eradicating organism; usually is *not* given in conjunction with vancomycin, because cholestyramine binds the vancomycin and renders it inactive.

Vancomycin: 125-500 mg 4 times daily for 10-14 days (drug of choice); metronidazole: 1.2-1.5 g daily for 7-14 days.

Note: Drugs that slow peristalsis (e.g., opiates, diphenoxylate, and loperamide) are *contraindicated,* since they promote retention of the *C. difficile* toxins, which may increase mucosal damage.

1 ASSESS

ASSESSMENT	OBSERVATIONS
Antibiotic intake	May be currently receiving antibiotics or may report antibiotic therapy within past 6 wk
Bowel function	May report diarrhea ranging from mild to severe; stools may test positive for blood; may report abdominal cramping and tenderness; may have episodic or frequent bowel incontinence; may report nausea and vomiting; may have reduced bowel sounds and abdominal distention
Fluid-electrolyte balance	May report dry mouth, thirst, dizziness and weakness when standing, reduced urine output; may have concentrated urine, decreased skin turgor, orthostatic hypotension, output that exceeds intake
Perianal skin integrity	May report perianal soreness and tenderness; may have erythema and denudation in perianal area
Vital signs	May have fever; may have orthostatic hypotension and tachycardia

→ › ›

ASSESSMENT	OBSERVATIONS
Mobility	May report difficulty getting to the bathroom; weakness and dizziness when walking
Hygiene practices	May demonstrate careful attention to handwashing and personal hygiene or may demonstrate carelessness in this area

2 DIAGNOSE

NURSING DIAGNOSIS	SUBJECTIVE FINDINGS	OBJECTIVE FINDINGS
Diarrhea related to bowel wall inflammation	Reports increased number and frequency of stools; describes stools as semisolid, liquid, or watery; may report blood or mucus in stool	Increased number and frequency of stools (more than two per day); stools are more fluid in consistency than usual (based on knowledge of patient's usual bowel function); blood or mucus or both in stool
Fluid volume deficit (II) related to diarrhea	Reports dry mouth, thirst, weakness, dizziness, reduced urinary output, increased concentration of urine (dark urine)	Dry mucous membranes; orthostatic hypotension; tachycardia; reduced skin turgor; oliguria; increased urine concentration; lethargy
High risk for trauma related to general debilitation and diarrhea	Reports weakness, dizziness, need to hurry to bathroom, unwillingness to use bedpan	Unsteady gait; orthostatic hypotension; altered mental status; frequent trips to bathroom
Impaired perianal skin integrity related to diarrhea	Reports perianal pain	Liquid stools; perianal erythema and denudation
Altered renal, cerebral, cardiopulmonary, gastrointestinal, and peripheral tissue perfusion related to toxic megacolon and impending perforation	Reports increasing abdominal pain, chills	Severe abdominal distention; fever and chills; hypotension and tachycardia

3 PLAN

Patient goals

1. The patient's diarrhea will be resolved.
2. The patient will maintain fluid and electrolyte balance.
3. The patient will remain free of injury.
4. The patient's perianal skin will be intact.
5. The patient will maintain normal tissue perfusion.

4 IMPLEMENT

NURSING DIAGNOSIS	NURSING INTERVENTIONS	RATIONALE
Diarrhea related to bowel wall inflammation	Monitor all patients receiving antibiotics for diarrhea.	Early recognition of pseudomembranous enterocolitis permits prompt treatment.
	For patient receiving antibiotics and developing diarrhea: send stool specimen for toxin assay (*Note:* Protect specimen from heat; refrigerate until specimen is delivered to laboratory).	Pseudomembranous enterocolitis must be differentiated from other diarrheal syndromes; the *C. difficile* toxin is heat labile.
	Administer medications as ordered (i.e., vancomycin, metronidazole, bacitracin, or cholestyramine). Do *not* administer cholestyramine in conjunction with vancomycin.	Vancomycin is the drug of choice for eliminating *C. difficile;* metronidazole and bacitracin have also been used; cholestyramine binds the toxin but also binds vancomycin, rendering it inactive.
	Do *not* administer antiperistaltic agents such as opiates, diphenoxylate, or loperamide.	Antiperistaltic agents delay elimination of the toxin, which may result in increased mucosal damage.
	Monitor number, volume, and consistency of stools.	Continuous assessment provides data on patient's response to therapy.
	Maintain enteric precautions (i.e., private room for patient who is incontinent or has poor personal hygiene; gloves for contact with stool; gowns if contamination is possible; disposal or decontamination of contaminated articles).	*C. difficile* is a spore-producing, opportunistic pathogen that can be spread through the environment as well as by the fecal-oral route.
Fluid volume deficit related to diarrhea	Monitor patient for intake and output, weight (daily), vital signs, and clinical signs of fluid volume deficit.	Output exceeding intake, weight loss, orthostatic hypotension, tachycardia, weakness, dizziness, dry mucous membranes, lethargy, reduced skin turgor, and thirst are all indicators of fluid volume deficit.
	Provide fluid replacement, oral (as tolerated) or IV (as ordered); if oral fluids are tolerated, encourage intake of fluids containing electrolytes (e.g., sports drinks, broth, tea, juice).	Replacement of fluid losses is essential for maintaining plasma volume and neuromuscular function.
	Administer antiemetics as ordered and needed.	Antiemetics reduce nausea and vomiting, thus reducing fluid loss and improving oral intake.
High risk for trauma related to general debilitation and diarrhea	Assess patient for orientation, weakness, and dizziness, and assess frequency and urgency of bowel movements.	Disorientation, weakness, and dizziness increase the risk of injury with independent ambulation; frequency and urgency related to defecation increase the risk of unassisted ambulation.

NURSING DIAGNOSIS	NURSING INTERVENTIONS	RATIONALE
	Initiate measures to reduce risk of falls: call bell at bedside, bedside commode,* bedpan at bedside.*	Providing for assisted ambulation or reducing the need for ambulation reduces the risk of injury.
Impaired perianal skin integrity related to diarrhea	Cleanse perianal skin gently after each bowel movement with tap water, mineral oil, or gentle cleanser; protect skin with skin sealants or moisture-barrier ointment; if skin is denuded, apply pectin-based powder before applying sealant or ointment.	Liquid stool can erode skin; prevention involves avoiding trauma and using moisture-barrier products.
	With an incontinent patient with severe diarrhea, consider using a fecal incontinence collector.	Pouching contains the stool and thus protects the skin.
Altered renal, cerebral, cardiopulmonary, gastrointestinal, and peripheral tissue perfusion related to toxic megacolon and impending perforation	Monitor patient for increasing abdominal distention and tenderness and fever.	Increasing distention and fever and tenderness may indicate toxic megacolon and impending perforation; perforation may precipitate septic shock.
	Monitor vital signs and urinary output for evidence of circulatory compromise: hypotension, tachycardia, tachypnea, and reduced urinary output.	Circulatory compromise is reflected by reduced B/P and urinary output; compensatory responses to circulatory compromise produce tachycardia and tachypnea.
	For patient with increasing distention: keep patient NPO and place N/G or small bowel tube as ordered (or assist with placement); irrigate tube as needed to maintain patency.	Decompression of the proximal bowel reduces the risk of perforation, which can precipitate peritonitis and septic shock.
	Administer IV fluids as ordered.	IV fluids are administered to maintain plasma volume.
	If patient fails to improve with conservative therapy, prepare patient for surgery.	Emergency surgery may be required to prevent or manage perforation.

5   EVALUATE

PATIENT OUTCOME	DATA INDICATING THAT OUTCOME IS REACHED
Patient's diarrhea is resolved.	Stool consistency is soft to formed; patient has no more than three stools per day.
Patient maintains fluid and electrolyte balance.	Intake and output are balanced; urine output is of normal volume and concentration; B/P and pulse rate are normal; patient has no dizziness, weakness, or dry mouth; skin turgor is normal.
Patient remains free of injury	There is no evidence of tissue trauma; patient states that no falls have occurred.

*Use of bedside commodes or bedpans increases the risk of environmental contamination.

PATIENT OUTCOME	DATA INDICATING THAT OUTCOME IS REACHED
Perianal skin is intact.	Perianal skin is intact and there is no erythema.
Patient maintains normal tissue perfusion.	Vital signs and urinary output are normal; abdomen is soft, nondistended, and nontender.

PATIENT TEACHING

1. Teach patients taking antibiotics to report diarrhea, especially if it is severe or if the stools contain mucus or blood.
2. Explain the infectious nature of the diarrhea, and teach the patient measures for controlling infection: prompt emptying and cleansing of bedpans or bedside commodes after use (notify staff of use); scrupulous perianal hygiene after each bowel movement; thorough handwashing after each bowel movement.
3. Explain the importance of accurate intake and output, and instruct the patient to save urine, emesis, and liquid stools for measurement.
4. Explain the importance of fluid replacement, and encourage the patient to drink fluids containing electrolytes (e.g., broth, sports drinks, juices, and tea).
5. For outpatients: Instruct the patient to avoid antidiarrheal agents unless approved by the physician; provide instruction on prescribed medications, including purpose, dosage, administration guidelines, and side effects to be reported. For patients taking cholestyramine, emphasize the importance of taking all other medications either 1 hour before or 4 hours after cholestyramine, and explain the potential for constipation and the importance of monitoring stools for consistency.
6. Teach the patient the signs and symptoms of fulminant disease that should be reported: increasing fever, abdominal distention, and abdominal tenderness.

Diverticulitis

Diverticulitis is an inflammation of one or more diverticula, which are saclike outpouchings of the colon wall caused by herniation of the mucosal and submucosal layers through weak points in the colonic musculature (Figure 4-7). Diverticulitis is the pathologic extreme in a spectrum of conditions known collectively as diverticular disease. The term "diverticular disease" includes prediverticular disease, diverticulosis, and diverticulitis.

EPIDEMIOLOGY

Diverticular disease is primarily a disease of Western cultures, which has led investigators to implicate the Western diet as a causative or contributing factor. It is also associated with increasing age; diverticula are uncommon in people under 35 years of age, but the incidence gradually increases, and autopsy studies reveal diverticula in two thirds of those 85 years of age or older.

Diverticula can develop in any or all segments of the colon, but the sigmoid is most likely to be involved, in both single-segment and multiple-segment disease. Diverticula are most likely to develop at the point where nutrient blood vessels penetrate the colon wall,

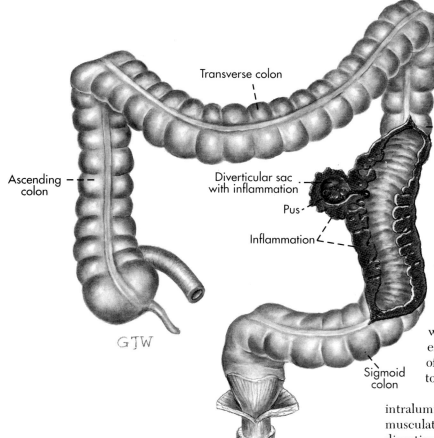

Ascending colon

Transverse colon

Descending colon

Diverticular sac with inflammation

Pus

Inflammation

Sigmoid colon

Anus

GTW

FIGURE 4-7
Diverticulosis (diverticulitis).

creating a "weak point" in the muscular coat. This proximity of the blood vessel to the diverticular sac explains why diverticular disease is the most common cause of bleeding from the lower gastrointestinal tract.

Diverticular disease seems to be progressive. The earliest stage is labeled prediverticular disease; although no diverticula are present, pathologic changes occur in the colonic musculature and intraluminal pressures that are consistent with diverticular disease. The second stage is diverticulosis, in which diverticula are present but there is no inflammation. Most individuals with diverticulosis are asymptomatic, and in fact diverticulosis frequently is diagnosed incidentally during diagnostic workups for unrelated symptoms or at autopsy. Diverticulitis occurs when perforation of the diverticular sac or sacs causes local inflammation (and possibly abscess formation) or even diffuse peritonitis.

The causes of diverticular disease are not clear, but current data indicate a complex interplay among factors producing excessive intraluminal pressures and factors contributing to weak points in the colonic musculature. Studies have demonstrated intraluminal pressures as high as 90 mm Hg in patients with diverticular disease; normal pressures, even with segmental contractions, do not usually exceed 10 mm Hg. These excessive pressures are thought to cause mucosal herniation in areas where the muscular coat is deficient.

Factors contributing to excessive intraluminal pressures are thought to include low-fiber diets, hypertrophy of the colonic musculature, and a colonic motility disorder characterized by excessive segmentation in response to stimuli such as eating. Low-fiber diets tend to produce small-caliber stools; small-caliber stools fail to distend the colon lumen and thus contribute to luminal narrowing. Narrowing of the lumen increases intraluminal pressure, as explained by Laplace's law: the pressure within a cylinder is inversely related to the radius of the cylinder. In addition, small-caliber stools are associated with reduced peristaltic activity (stemming from loss of colon distention), which results in prolonged transit times and excessive drying of the stools within the lumen of the colon; small, dry stools require more force to propel distally than do soft, bulky stools.

A second factor contributing to excessive intraluminal pressures is hypertrophy of the colonic musculature. Studies indicate that most patients with diverticular disease have thickening of the muscle layer in the area where the diverticula are located; this hypertrophy frequently precedes the development of diverticula. The thickening of the muscle layer causes further narrowing of the lumen, which in turn causes increased intraluminal pressures.

The third factor thought to contribute to excessive intraluminal pressures is a colonic motility disorder. Many patients with diverticular disease have been found to have shortening of the colon in addition to thickening of the muscle layer; this is thought to result from abnormal and prolonged contraction of the colonic muscles. In addition, patients with diverticular disease frequently respond to stimuli such as eating, morphine, and parasympathetic stimulation with excessive segmentation contractions. The end result of excessive segmentation and prolonged muscle contraction is increased intraluminal pressure. It is interesting to note that the pattern of excessive segmentation seen in some patients with diverticular disease is almost identical to that found in patients with irritable bowel syndrome; it has been hypothesized that in some cases irritable bowel syndrome may actually result in diverticular disease.

As explained earlier, diverticula occur in areas where the muscle coat of the bowel wall is deficient. The colon wall has congenital "weak points" where the nutrient blood vessels penetrate the muscle layer, and hypertrophy of the circular muscle layer may create additional deficiencies in the muscle layer. This is because the hypertrophied fibers may become concentrated in thick bands, resulting in areas that essentially are devoid of muscular support. These areas are subject to mucosal herniations with excessive intraluminal pressure.

Although muscular hypertrophy, excessive intraluminal pressures, and abnormal motility are common to many patients with diverticular disease, they cannot be demonstrated in *all* patients with the disorder. This fact underscores the incomplete understanding of the factors contributing to this complex spectrum of diseases.

PATHOPHYSIOLOGY

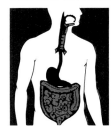

Prediverticular disease is characterized by hypertrophy of the colonic musculature, altered colonic motility, and increased intraluminal pressure; diverticula are not present. Most patients with prediverticular disease are asymptomatic, although some have symptoms that probably are caused by the underlying motility disorder, such as intermittent or chronic abdominal pain that may worsen after eating or before bowel movements and altered patterns of bowel elimination (i.e., constipation or diarrhea or both).

The development of diverticula heralds the progression from prediverticular disease to diverticulosis. The mucosal layer of the colon herniates through the defects in the muscular coat, resulting in flask-shaped sacs with thin walls composed mainly of mucosa and serosa. Because the openings of the sacs are narrow and difficult to see, the diverticula may be missed during endoscopic procedures. Because the diverticula push through the colon wall at points where the wall is penetrated by blood vessels, the diverticular sacs lie directly under or immediately adjacent to these blood vessels, and bleeding or even hemorrhage is a potential complication of diverticulosis. In many instances bleeding is the first indication of diverticulosis, because most patients are asymptomatic. Patients who do have symptoms complain of cramping abdominal pain, intermittent distention, and constipation or alternating bouts of constipation and diarrhea. These symptoms are thought to result from the underlying changes in colonic musculature and motility rather than from the diverticula themselves.

Diverticulitis is an inflammation of one or more diverticula. Whereas diverticulosis is common, diverticulitis is relatively uncommon. Diverticulitis results when one or more diverticula become acutely inflamed and perforate; the perforations may be small or large. The inflammation is thought to be caused by fecal plugs that become trapped in the diverticular sac, dehydrate, and abrade the mucosal lining of the diverticulum. The abraded mucosa provides an entry site for bacteria, which proliferate rapidly within the obstructed diverticulum. The result is an acute inflammation that frequently causes perforation of the very thin diverticular wall. Microperforations may result in localized, "walled-off" areas of suppuration encompassing the perforated diverticular sac or may involve extensive abscess formation. Occasionally, free perforation into the abdominal cavity occurs, resulting in diffuse peritonitis. The symptoms of diverticulitis include fever; abdominal tenderness (generalized or localized to the involved segment of colon); dull, aching pain (generalized or localized to the left lower quadrant or suprapubic area); anorexia; and nausea. If free perforation occurs, symptoms of peritonitis will develop, including severe abdominal pain; acute, generalized abdominal tenderness; abdominal muscle rigidity and guarding; rebound tenderness; and hypoactive or absent bowel sounds. Occasionally the inflammation may extend to the ureter or to adjacent loops of small bowel, producing signs of ureteral or intestinal obstruction.

COMPLICATIONS

Peritonitis
Bleeding
Fistula formation
Ureteral obstruction
Intestinal obstruction

Complications of diverticulitis include sepsis, bleeding, fistula formation, ureteral obstruction, and intestinal obstruction. *Sepsis* results from extensive abscess formation or free perforation into the abdominal cavity, as has been discussed. *Bleeding* is a common complication of diverticular disease and ranges from mild to severe. Mild occult bleeding is thought to be caused by irritation of the granulation tissue frequently found at the mouth of the diverticular sacs. Massive bleeding results from erosion of the blood vessel adjacent to the diverticulum; it usually begins abruptly and frequently stops spontaneously. *Fistula formation* occurs as a result of serosal inflammation and may involve the bladder, the vagina, the ureter, loops of bowel, or the abdominal wall. *Ureteral obstruction* or *intestinal obstruction* may occur as a result of massive inflammation and edema; intestinal obstruction may also develop gradually as a result of several episodes of diverticulitis, with resultant fibrosis.

DIAGNOSTIC STUDIES AND FINDINGS

Diagnostic test	Findings
White blood cell count (WBC)	May show leukocytosis with a shift to the left in diverticulitis
Hemoglobin and hematocrit	May be low in patient with chronic or acute bleeding
X-ray (flat plate) of abdomen	May show free air under diaphragm with perforation into abdominal cavity; may show displacement of colonic lumen (with abscess)
Barium enema	Diverticular sacs; narrowing of colonic lumen; may show: irregular "sawtooth" appearance of bowel lumen (with circular muscle hypertrophy); thinning of haustral folds and shortening of colon; partial or complete obstruction; fistulous tract*
Colonoscopy	May or may not be able to visualize openings to diverticula; may be done to rule out carcinoma†
Intravenous pyelogram (IVP)	May be done to rule out ureteral obstruction

*Note: A barium enema usually is contraindicated during an acute episode of diverticulitis because of the potential for perforation. If a contrast study is to be done during an acute inflammation, water-soluble contrast (e.g., Gastrografin) usually is recommended.

†Note: Endoscopic procedures usually are contraindicated during acute episodes of diverticulitis because of the potential for perforation.

MEDICAL MANAGEMENT

GENERAL MANAGEMENT

Prediverticular disease: High-fiber diet (fresh fruits and vegetables, grains); bran therapy (1 tablespoon per day initially; titrated to produce one soft, formed stool per day or to relieve symptoms).

Diverticulosis: High-fiber diet (fresh fruits and vegetables, grains); some sources recommend omitting foods with large seeds or kernels; bran therapy (1 tablespoon per day initially; titrated to produce one soft, formed stool per day or to relieve symptoms).

Diverticulitis: Low-fiber diet until inflammation subsides; NPO status and IV fluid therapy when signs of peritonitis are present or during acute bleeding episodes; N/G intubation and suction when distention and vomiting are present; blood transfusions for replacement during massive bleeding episodes.

SURGERY

Colon resection with reanastomosis: (for repeated episodes of diverticulitis resulting in partial obstruction or for uncontrolled bleeding). Colon resection with proximal diverting colostomy and mucous fistula or Hartmann's pouch, followed later by takedown of colostomy and reestablishment of bowel continuity (for free perforation with peritonitis or localized perforation and abscess formation that does not respond to medical therapy). This may be referred to as a two-stage procedure. Diverting colostomy, followed later by resection of involved segment and end-to-end anastomosis, followed later by takedown of the colostomy. This is known as a three-stage procedure and is indicated for patients with perforation and abscess formation who fail to respond to medical therapy and who are too ill to tolerate a more definitive procedure at the time of initial surgery.

Diverting colostomy: may be required for management of obstruction; a more definitive procedure is postponed until the bowel can be decompressed and a preparatory regimen performed. The obstructed segment can then be resected and an end-to-end anastomosis constructed, with takedown of the colostomy.

Fistula repair: requires resection of the involved colon segment and closure of the fistulous tract; a temporary diverting colostomy may or may not be required.

MEDICAL MANAGEMENT—cont'd

DRUG THERAPY

Bulk laxatives (e.g., psyllium preparations) titrated to produce one soft, formed stool per day or to relieve symptoms (may be used for patients who do not tolerate or are unwilling to take bran).

Diverticulitis

Meperidine (Demerol) for analgesia: Dosage calculated according to patient's weight and tolerance (morphine is contraindicated because it causes increased segmentation and therefore increased intraluminal pressures).

Antibiotics until inflammation has resolved: Ampicillin (Amcill) 2 g daily or **cephalothin (Keflin)** 1-4 g daily in divided doses for mild diverticulitis (usually given parenterally). **Gentamicin (Garamycin)** or **tobramycin (Nebcin):** 3-5 mg/kg daily parenterally in divided doses, *and* **clindamycin (Cleocin):** 1.2-2.7 g daily parenterally in divided doses (up to 4.8 g daily may be given for life-threatening infection). These drugs are used for severe intraabdominal infection. **Cefoxitin (Mefoxin):** 3-12 g daily parenterally in divided doses (dosage depends on severity of infection). **Note:** Selection and dosage of antibiotics depend on the severity of infection and the occurrence of perforation. All antibiotics usually are continued for 7-10 days.

Vasopressin may be used to control bleeding (injected per angiographic catheter).

1 ASSESS

ASSESSMENT	OBSERVATIONS
Past and present patterns of bowel elimination	May report chronic constipation or constipation alternating with diarrhea; may report cramping abdominal pain before bowel movements; may report constipation at present
Usual pattern of fiber and fluid intake	May report chronic intake of low-fiber diet and refined sugars; may report limited fluid intake
Signs and symptoms of localized or generalized peritoneal inflammation	May report generalized abdominal pain or pain localized to left lower quadrant or to suprapubic area; pain may be described as intense or as dull and aching; may report anorexia or nausea; may have abdominal distention; abdominal tenderness may be noted on palpation and varying degrees of guarding may be present; may have rebound tenderness; palpable mass may be noted in left lower quadrant; may have diminished or absent bowel sounds
Evidence of lower intestinal bleeding	May report bloody stools; hematochezia may be present
Vital signs	Temperature may be elevated with diverticulitis; tachycardia and hypotension may be seen with massive bleeding or peritonitis
Evidence of fistula formation	May report stool or flatus per urethra or vagina; fecal drainage may be noted on abdominal wall

→ 〉 〉

2 DIAGNOSE

NURSING DIAGNOSIS	SUBJECTIVE FINDINGS	OBJECTIVE FINDINGS
Constipation related to low-fiber diet	Reports infrequent passage of hard, dry stools; may report pain related to bowel movements; may report chronic consumption of low-fiber diet	Stools are small caliber, hard, and dry; abdominal distention may be present
Altered renal, cerebral, cardiopulmonary, gastrointestinal, and peripheral tissue perfusion related to lower intestinal bleeding or perforation with peritonitis and sepsis	Reports feelings of dizziness; may report rectal bleeding or bloody stools; may report severe abdominal pain	Tachycardia; hypotension; fever; may have: abdominal distention; rectal bleeding or severe abdominal pain; "guarding" on palpation
Pain related to intraabdominal inflammation or chronic motility	Reports generalized abdominal pain or pain localized to suprapubic or left lower quadrant	Facial expression indicates pain; keeps knees flexed; guarding behavior during abdominal examination; restlessness

3 PLAN

Patient goals

1. The patient will establish regular elimination of soft, formed stools.
2. The patient will maintain normal perfusion of renal, cerebral, cardiopulmonary, gastrointestinal, and peripheral tissues.

3. The patient will be free of pain.

4 IMPLEMENT

NURSING DIAGNOSIS	NURSING INTERVENTIONS	RATIONALE
Constipation related to low-fiber diet	Monitor bowel movements for frequency, volume, and consistency.*	Continuous assessment of elimination patterns permits appropriate adjustments in the treatment plan.
	Provide (or instruct patient in) high-fiber diet *or* bran to produce soft, formed stools; administer bulk-forming laxatives as ordered.*	High-fiber diets and bran retain moisture in stool and also maintain bulk; bulky, soft stools distend the colon, promote peristaltic activity, and reduce the intraluminal pressure required for elimination; bulk laxatives have the same effect.
	Assure adequate fluid intake (six to eight 8-oz glasses daily).*	Adequate hydration prevents excessive drying of the stool and assures proper elimination of bulk agents.

*Note: These actions are not appropriate during acute episodes of diverticulitis: they should be initiated for patients with prediverticular disease or diverticulosis and for patients who have recovered from acute episodes of diverticulitis.

NURSING DIAGNOSIS	NURSING INTERVENTIONS	RATIONALE
	Encourage physical activity.*	Increased physical activity stimulates peri-
Altered renal, cerebral, cardiopulmonary, gastrointestinal, and peripheral tissue perfusion related to lower intestinal bleeding or perforation with peritonitis and sepsis	Measure bloody stools; monitor patient for increasing abdominal tenderness, rigidity, and distention.	Measuring stool volume helps quantify blood loss; increasing abdominal tenderness, rigidity, and distention may indicate perforation and peritonitis; acute blood loss causes hypovolemic shock unless adequate replacement is provided; perforation and peritonitis may cause septic shock.
	Monitor vital signs and urinary output for evidence of circulatory compromise (hypotension, tachycardia, tachypnea, and reduced urinary output).	Circulatory compromise is reflected by changes in B/P and urinary output; compensatory responses to circulatory compromise produce tachycardia and tachypnea.
	For patient with perforation and peritonitis: keep patient NPO and place N/G tube as ordered (or assist with placement); irrigate tube as needed to maintain patency.	Decompression of proximal bowel reduces distention and vomiting and prevents additional fecal spillage and peritoneal contamination.
	Administer antibiotics as ordered.	Antibiotics control bacterial proliferation and help eliminate intraabdominal infection, thus preventing or helping to correct sepsis and shock.
	Administer IV fluids and blood replacement as ordered; observe for transfusion reactions if blood is given.	Intravenous fluids are administered to maintain plasma volume; blood replacement may be required to replace RBCs and platelets during episodes of massive bleeding.
	If patient fails to respond to conservative therapy, prepare the patient for surgery or angiography.	Emergency surgery may be required to control bleeding or to manage perforation and peritonitis (e.g., resection and fecal diversion); angiography may be performed to determine bleeding sites and to administer vasopressin, which constricts mesenteric blood vessels.
Pain related to intraabdominal inflammation or chronic motility	For patient with acute diverticulitis: administer narcotic analgesics such as meperidine (Demerol) as ordered and needed for pain.	Intraabdominal infection causes peritoneal irritation, which results in severe abdominal pain; meperidine is the preferred analgesic, because morphine stimulates increased intraluminal segmentation and increased intraluminal pressure.
	For patient with diverticular disease without inflammation: administer bulking agents such as bran or psyllium products.	Bulk agents maintain soft, formed stools that are eliminated more easily and with less pressure; routine use of bulking agents may help correct the altered colonic motility and thus reduce the pain.

*Note: These actions are not appropriate during acute episodes of diverticulitis: they should be initiated for patients with prediverticular disease or diverticulosis and for patients who have recovered from acute episodes of diverticulitis.

5   EVALUATE

PATIENT OUTCOME	DATA INDICATING THAT OUTCOME IS REACHED
Patient has established regular elimination of soft, formed stools.	Patient reports regular elimination of soft, formed stools (daily or every other day).
Patient maintains normal perfusion of renal, cerebral, cardiopulmonary, gastrointestinal, and peripheral tissues.	Vital signs and urine output are normal; stools test negative for blood; abdomen is soft, nondistended, and nontender.
Patient is free of pain	Patient states that he no longer has cramping abdominal pain and abdominal tenderness.

PATIENT TEACHING

1. Explain the relationship between constipation, intraluminal pressure, and diverticular disease.
2. Explain the relationship between dietary bulk and fluid intake and constipation.
3. Instruct the patient in options for adding bulk to the diet: eating more fruits, vegetables, and grains, using bran, or using bulk laxatives. Explain the importance of adequate fluid intake in maintaining soft, formed stools and in promoting elimination of bulking agents.
   Explain that bran is extremely effective in restoring normal bowel function, and assess the patient's willingness to add bran. Explain that bran should be added gradually, beginning with 1 tablespoon a day and increasing the dose gradually until the desired results are obtained (soft, formed stool eliminated at regular intervals and relief of symptoms). Explain that it is normal to have increased amounts of flatus and some abdominal distention during the adaptation phase and that this is temporary.
4. Teach the patient with diverticulosis to avoid foods with kernels or large seeds.
5. Teach the patient the signs and symptoms of complications that should be reported to the physician: fever, abdominal pain and tenderness, abdominal distention, rectal bleeding.

Cholecystitis

Cholecystitis is an inflammation of the gallbladder (Figure 4-8); it is most commonly associated with cholelithiasis (Figure 4-9), or the presence of gallstones in the gallbladder (also known as gallstone disease). Cholecystitis may be acute or chronic.

EPIDEMIOLOGY

Cholecystitis is associated with gallstone disease in 95% of patients; the other 5% develop cholecystitis as a result of trauma, sepsis, vascular disease, or acquired immunodeficiency syndrome (AIDS). Gallstone disease is common in the United States and other developed countries, with an estimated incidence of 10% to 20%; the actual incidence is not known, because many patients are asymptomatic. There are two types of gallstones: cholesterol stones and pigmented stones. Cho-

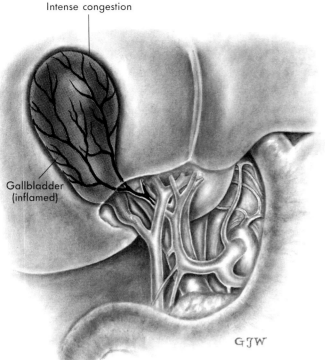

Intense congestion

Gallbladder
(inflamed)

GJW

FIGURE 4-8
Acute cholecystitis.

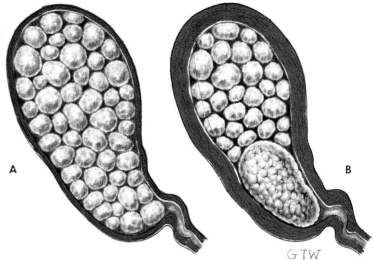

A

B

GJW

FIGURE 4-9
Cholelithiasis. **A,** Multiple faceted stones. **B,** Large and numerous small stones in chronic cholecystitis.

lesterol stones are by far the most common, accounting for 75% to 85% of cases of gallstones in the United States.

Several factors may play a role in the development of cholesterol gallstones, such as increased hepatic synthesis of cholesterol or decreased hepatic synthesis of bile salts, or both; the presence of pronucleating factors or the absence of antinucleating factors in the bile; and biliary stasis. Bile is composed primarily of water and three solid substances: cholesterol, bile salts, and phospholipids (lecithin). Cholesterol normally is insoluble in water, but it is rendered soluble in bile by its molecular association with bile salts and lecithin. Gallstones develop when there is an imbalance among the three solid components such that the volume of bile salts and lecithin is insufficient to solubilize the cholesterol; at this point the bile is said to be supersaturated with cholesterol, and precipitation may occur. Most commonly the imbalance involves an increased volume of cholesterol or a decreased amount of bile salts. Synthesis of cholesterol and bile salts is controlled by specific enzymes, and there is evidence that patients with cholesterol gallstone disease may have a dual defect that causes increased synthesis of cholesterol and decreased synthesis of bile salts. However, studies have shown that supersaturation of the bile with cholesterol does not in itself cause precipitation and gallstones; healthy people without gallstones also have supersaturated bile, at least intermittently. The determining element in gallstone de-

velopment is thought to be an excess of pronucleating factors (factors promoting precipitation) or a deficiency of antinucleating factors (factors inhibiting precipitation). Studies have shown that when bile from patients with cholesterol gallstones is mixed with bile from stone-free patients, gallstones develop; this supports the theory that a nucleating factor is present in the bile of patients with cholesterol gallstones. Moreover, studies comparing "normal" bile to the bile of patients with cholesterol gallstones have shown a delayed onset of precipitation, which supports the theory that an antinucleating factor is present in the bile of normal individuals. Biliary stasis can also contribute to gallstone formation. Gallbladder hypomotility is associated with the development of biliary sludge in the most dependent area of the gallbladder; biliary sludge consists of mucus and cholesterol crystals and is a precursor to gallstone formation.

Pigmented gallstones account for 15% to 25% of the cases of gallstones in the United States. These gallstones are composed primarily of bilirubin and other pigments, and they tend to develop when bilirubin and ionized calcium exceed their solubility levels and begin to precipitate. Thus pigmented gallstones may be found with conditions that cause an increase in unconjugated bilirubin, such as hemolysis and cirrhosis. These gallstones are also found in patients with biliary stasis; gallbladder mucus seems to contribute to the matrix of pigmented stones, and biliary sludge usually contains both bilirubin and mucus.

Table 4-3

RISK FACTORS AND PRESUMED MECHANISMS IN CHOLESTEROL GALLSTONE DISEASE

Risk factor	Presumed mechanism
Advancing age	?
Female sex	Possible effects of estrogens
Race (American Indians and whites)	Possible increased hepatic secretion of cholesterol and decreased production of bile salts
Ileal disease or resection	Reduced bile salt pool due to reduced absorption of bile salts in the terminal ileum
Obesity	Secretion of supersaturated bile
Pancreatitis	?
Pregnancy (intrahepatic cholestasis)	?
Oral contraceptives	Secretion of supersaturated bile
Total parenteral nutrition	Increased formation of sludge

Table 4-3 outlines risk factors for cholesterol gallstone disease and the presumed mechanisms.

PATHOPHYSIOLOGY

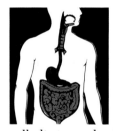 Gallstone disease is asymptomatic in many people, and treatment usually is not indicated for these individuals. Exceptions to this general rule include patients with nonfunctioning gallbladders, patients with stones larger than 2.5 cm in diameter, patients with diabetes or sickle cell disease who have documented gallstone disease, and patients with calcification of the gallbladder. Elective cholecystectomy may be recommended for these patients because of (1) the high risk of cholecystitis (in patients with nonfunctioning gallbladders or large stones), (2) the increased risk of mortality if emergency surgery is required (in patients with diabetes or sickle cell disease), and (3) the increased risk of gallbladder cancer (patients with calcified gallbladders).

Cholecystitis develops when one or more stones become impacted in the cystic duct; obstruction of the gallbladder causes biliary colic and an inflammatory response in the gallbladder. Most of the time the stone is dislodged, and the obstruction is relieved. Stones that are dislodged may pass through the biliary ducts into the intestine (with subsequent elimination in the stool) or may remain in the gallbladder. If the stone is dislodged, the inflammation gradually subsides and the only long-term effect is some residual fibrosis of the gallbladder wall. Some patients develop chronic cholecystitis, with repeated episodes of pain in the right up-per quadrant and nonspecific symptoms such as dyspepsia, heartburn, and nausea. These symptoms commonly are triggered by contraction of the gallbladder, which occurs in response to ingestion of fatty foods. Repeated episodes of cholecystitis may result in a fibrotic, nonfunctioning gallbladder; cholecystectomy usually is indicated for these patients.

If the stone is not dislodged, the inflammation intensifies. The gallbladder becomes distended and edematous, and the resulting vascular compromise may progress to severe ischemia, necrosis, and perforation; fortunately, this is uncommon.

Clinical signs and symptoms of acute cholecystitis include pain, right upper quadrant tenderness, anorexia, nausea, and vomiting. The pain may be generalized initially or may be located in the epigastric area, but it gradually localizes in the right upper quadrant; the pain may radiate along the right costal margin to the back or the tip of the scapula. The patient may also complain of dyspepsia and heartburn. Jaundice usually occurs if the common bile duct is obstructed by calculi. The severity and duration of the symptoms depend on the severity of the inflammation. If the stone is dislodged and the obstruction is relieved, the symptoms gradually resolve; however, if the obstruction is not relieved, the pain and tenderness become increasingly severe. Rebound tenderness may be present with advanced inflammation. Impending necrosis is evidenced by severe pain and tenderness, fever, chills, and leukocytosis; perforation should be suspected if the pain suddenly becomes generalized with rebound tenderness. Emergency surgery usually is indicated if the symptoms worsen or if there is evidence of impending or actual perforation.

Cholecystitis is primarily an inflammatory process; however, secondary bacterial invasion is possible, and bacteria can be cultured in about half of patients with acute cholecystitis. The invading organisms usually are normal intestinal flora.

Gallstone disease may also cause obstruction of the common bile duct by calculi; this is known as choledocholithiasis and is evidenced by biliary colic (right upper quadrant pain that radiates to the back or the tip of the scapula) and jaundice. Persistent obstruction of the common duct produces abnormal results on liver function tests. Surgical intervention usually is indicated.

COMPLICATIONS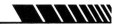

Empyema of the gallbladder (bacterial invasion of the bile)

Gangrene of the gallbladder

Perforation, localized or into the peritoneal cavity (localized perforation may be sealed off by migration of omentum into the area)

Cholecystenteric fistula (caused by perforation into an adjacent organ, such as the duodenum or hepatic flexure of the colon)

Gallstone ileus (caused by large stones that erode into the duodenum and cause intermittent obstruction)

DIAGNOSTIC STUDIES AND FINDINGS

Diagnostic test	Findings
White blood cell count (WBC)	Elevated with cholecystitis
Serum bilirubin	May be elevated with obstruction of common bile duct
Ultrasound study of gallbladder	Gallstones, thickening of gallbladder wall, enlarged gallbladder
Radioisotope scan (scintigraphy of gallbladder)	Visualization of liver and bile ducts; nonvisualization of gallbladder
X-ray (plain film) of abdomen	May show gallstones; used to rule out other abdominal processes; may show free air if perforation has occurred
Oral cholecystogram	May show stones or nonvisualization of gallbladder
Intravenous cholangiogram	May show stones in biliary system

MEDICAL MANAGEMENT

GENERAL MANAGEMENT

Mild cholecystitis with resolving symptoms: Dietary modifications (i.e., elimination of fatty foods and fatty liquids).

Acute cholecystitis: NPO; administration of IV fluids; insertion of N/G tube if abdominal distention, nausea, and vomiting are persistent.

SURGERY

Cholecystectomy with operative cholangiogram and common bile duct exploration as indicated: For patients with symptomatic gallbladder disease and selected patients with asymptomatic cholelithiasis.

Laparoscopic cholecystectomy: For patients with mild disease and no previous biliary or ulcer surgery.

Incisional or percutaneous cholecystostomy with tube decompression of gallbladder: For patients with acute cholecystitis who are very poor operative risks; cholecystectomy usually is performed at a later date, after the patient's condition has stabilized.

Continued.

MEDICAL MANAGEMENT—cont'd

DRUG THERAPY

Second-generation cephalosporin (e.g., cefamandole [Mandol]): 1-2 g q 4 h IV for patient with evidence of secondary bacterial invasion (i.e., leukocytosis, high fever).

Narcotic analgesic (e.g., meperidine [Demerol]) for severe pain: Dosage titrated according to patient's weight and response.

Antiemetics (e.g., promethazine [Phenergan]) to control nausea: 12.5-25 mg q 4-6 h as needed.

Chenodeoxycholic acid (CDCA): 13-16 mg/kg daily for up to 24 months for dissolution of cholesterol stones in a functioning gallbladder. **Note:** This drug works by reducing the cholesterol content of bile and increasing the bile salt pool, so that the bile becomes unsaturated. Current research indicates that this treatment is effective *only* for cholesterol stones smaller than 15 mm in diameter in a functioning gallbladder. Because supersaturation of the bile recurs within 1 to 3 weeks, continuous therapy may be required to prevent recurrence of gallstones.

Ursodeoxycholic acid (UDCA): 750 mg daily for up to 24 months for dissolution of cholesterol stones in a functioning gallbladder. **Note:** This drug works on the same principles as CDCA but is thought to be less hepatotoxic in comparable doses. It is indicated *only* for cholesterol stones in a functioning gallbladder and is most effective in thin patients, women, and patients with small or floating gallstones.

1 ASSESS

ASSESSMENT	OBSERVATIONS
Pain	May report pain in epigastric area or right upper quadrant that radiates through to back or tip of scapula; may describe pain as dull, aching, and constant; may report similar episodes of pain in past; may report onset of pain after ingestion of fatty foods or fluids; may report severe, generalized abdominal pain (if perforation has occurred)
Nausea and vomiting	May report anorexia, nausea, and vomiting corresponding with onset of pain
Vital signs	Fever may be present with cholecystitis; high fever (temperature over 38.89° C [102° F]) and chills may be seen with impending or actual perforation; tachycardia and hypotension may be seen with perforation, sepsis, and peritonitis
Color of skin and sclerae	Jaundice may be seen with obstruction of common bile duct
Abdominal tenderness	May have localized tenderness with rebound in right subcostal area; palpation of liver and gallbladder during inspiration may cause pain that interrupts inspiration (Murphy's sign); may have palpable mass in right upper quadrant (if localized perforation has occurred, with resultant migration of omentum); may have rigidity and guarding (if perforation and peritonitis have occurred)

2 DIAGNOSE

NURSING DIAGNOSIS	SUBJECTIVE FINDINGS	OBJECTIVE FINDINGS
Pain related to inflammatory process	Reports abdominal pain localizing to right upper quadrant; may state that pain radiates to back or scapular area; describes pain as dull, aching, constant	Restlessness; facial expressions reflecting pain; guarding on abdominal palpation; positive Murphy's sign; tenderness to palpation in right upper quadrant
High risk for fluid volume deficit related to vomiting	Reports persistent nausea and vomiting and feelings of dizziness and faintness; complains of dry mouth, thirst, weakness, and fatigue	Output exceeds intake; oliguria; increased urine concentration; dry mucous membranes; reduced skin turgor; postural hypotension; lethargy
Altered renal, cerebral, cardiopulmonary, gastrointestinal, and peripheral tissue perfusion related to perforation, peritonitis, and septic shock	Complains of sudden onset of severe, generalized abdominal pain	Abdominal rigidity and guarding on palpation; rebound tenderness; fever; hypotension; increasing abdominal distention; tachycardia

3 PLAN

Patient goals

1. The patient will have no abdominal pain or tenderness.
2. The patient will maintain a normal fluid and electrolyte balance.
3. The patient will maintain normal perfusion of renal, cerebral, cardiopulmonary, gastrointestinal, and peripheral tissues.

4 IMPLEMENT

NURSING DIAGNOSIS	NURSING INTERVENTIONS	RATIONALE
Pain related to inflammatory process	Assess pain (location, radiation, severity, nature) and patient's response to pain relief measures.	Characteristics of pain are clues to cause; increasing severity may indicate worsening inflammation; patient's response to pain relief measures governs modification of care plan.
	Administer analgesics (e.g., meperidine) as ordered and needed. Provide fat-free foods and fluids as permitted and tolerated.	Narcotic analgesics may be required to control severe pain. Ingestion of fats stimulates contraction of the gallbladder, which causes pain when inflammation is present.

→ > >

NURSING DIAGNOSIS	NURSING INTERVENTIONS	RATIONALE
High risk for fluid volume deficit related to vomiting and anorexia	Monitor patient's intake and output, including any emesis.	Output exceeding intake signals fluid volume deficit.
	Monitor patient for signs of hypovolemia (dry mucous membranes, oliguria, orthostatic hypotension, reduced skin turgor).	Prompt recognition permits early correction of fluid volume deficits.
	Administer antiemetics as ordered and needed.	Antiemetics reduce nausea and vomiting, thus reducing fluid losses and improving oral fluid intake.
	Provide fluid replacement as ordered and tolerated (PO or IV).	Maintaining fluid volume is essential to maintaining tissue perfusion.
Altered renal, cerebral, cardiopulmonary, gastrointestinal, and peripheral tissue perfusion related to perforation, peritonitis, and septic shock	Monitor patient for evidence of impending or actual perforation (increasing abdominal pain and tenderness, fever, leukocytosis, rebound tenderness).	Severe abdominal pain and tenderness, fever, and leukocytosis may indicate impending perforation; generalized abdominal pain and rebound tenderness may indicate perforation and peritonitis, which may precipitate septic shock.
	Monitor vital signs and urinary output for evidence of circulatory compromise (hypotension, tachycardia, tachypnea, and reduced urinary output).	Circulatory compromise is reflected by changes in B/P and urinary output; compensatory responses to circulatory compromise produce tachycardia and tachypnea.
	If patient has persistent vomiting and distention, keep NPO and place N/G tube as ordered (or assist with placement); irrigate tube as needed to maintain patency.	Removing gastric and duodenal secretions helps prevent gallbladder contraction and relieves vomiting and distention.
	Administer antibiotics as ordered.	Antibiotics are indicated if patient shows signs of bacterial invasion (fever, leukocytosis) to control infection and reduce inflammation.
	If symptoms of impending or actual perforation occur, prepare patient for surgery.	Emergency surgery is indicated to prevent perforation or control intraabdominal infection.

5 EVALUATE

PATIENT OUTCOME	DATA INDICATING THAT OUTCOME IS REACHED
Patient has no abdominal pain or tenderness.	Patient states that abdominal pain has resolved; palpation elicits no complaints of pain; there is no abdominal tenseness or guarding; patient no longer requires analgesics.
Patient maintains a normal fluid-electrolyte balance.	Intake and output are appropriately balanced; B/P and pulse are within normal limits; there are no signs or symptoms of fluid-electrolyte imbalance (e.g., weakness, dry mucous membranes, thirst, dizziness, concentrated urine); patient tolerates oral foods and fluids without pain, nausea, or vomiting.

PATIENT OUTCOME	DATA INDICATING THAT OUTCOME IS REACHED
Patient maintains normal perfusion of renal, cerebral, cardiopulmonary, gastrointestinal, and peripheral tissues.	Abdomen is soft and nondistended; there is no rebound tenderness or abdominal pain; patient's temperature, pulse, and B/P are normal.

PATIENT TEACHING

1. For an asymptomatic patient with documented cholelithiasis, explain that most patients remain asymptomatic and that cholecystectomy usually is not indicated unless symptoms occur. Teach the patient the signs and symptoms of cholecystitis that should be reported to the physician: abdominal pain and tenderness that increases in severity, fever, nausea, and vomiting.

2. For a patient with resolving cholecystitis, explain that the inflammation is caused by gallstones obstructing the gallbladder. Tell the patient that the gallstones usually become dislodged and that the symptoms then resolve. Explain that fatty foods and fluids should be avoided, since they may stimulate gallbladder contraction, thus increasing the inflammatory response and causing worsening or recurrence of symptoms. Provide a list of foods and fluids that have significant fat content.

3. For a patient who requires cholecystectomy (i.e., a patient with acute or chronic cholecystitis), explain the purpose of the procedure (to remove the diseased gallbladder and gallstones), and explain that the liver will continue to produce bile to support fat digestion. Explain preoperative and postoperative care procedures.

4. For a patient undergoing attempted pharmacologic dissolution of stones (e.g., patient with minimal symptoms who has cholesterol gallstones), explain the purpose of the medication and that long-term treatment is required to dissolve the gallstones.

Pancreatitis

Pancreatitis is an inflammation of the pancreas (Figure 4-10); it can be either acute or chronic.

EPIDEMIOLOGY

The term "acute pancreatitis" covers an entire spectrum of pathologic conditions of the pancreas, ranging from mild, usually self-limiting inflammation to severe inflammation that destroys pancreatic tissue and may be fatal. A number of pathologic conditions may cause or contribute to the development of pancreatitis, but the two most common causes are excessive alcohol intake and biliary tract disease.

Excessive alcohol intake has long been recognized as a major etiologic factor in the development of pancreatitis. The exact mechanism remains unknown, but three "theories" are being studied.

One theory is that the damage may occur as a result of pancreatic hypersecretion coupled with partial obstruction at Vater's ampulla, where pancreatic secretions empty into the duodenum. It has been established that alcohol stimulates increased production of gastric acid, which results in increased acidity of duodenal contents; this increased acidity causes the release of secretin, which stimulates the pancreas to produce large volumes of bicarbonate-rich fluid. Alcohol also causes increased resistance at Oddi's sphincter, which regulates the flow of secretions into the duodenum. It is hypothesized, therefore, that the increased secretion coupled with increased resistance at Vater's ampulla re-

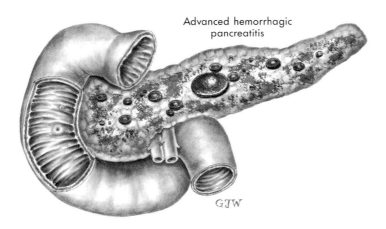

Advanced hemorrhagic pancreatitis

GJW

FIGURE 4-10
Acute pancreatitis.

sults in obstruction to flow, and that this may cause increased permeability within the pancreatic ducts, with resultant extravasation of pancreatic enzymes and damage to the pancreatic tissues. Another theory is that alcohol may cause precipitation of proteins and development of protein "plugs" in the pancreatic ducts; the resultant obstruction to flow is thought to cause increased permeability of the ductal wall, which permits extravasation of pancreatic enzymes and damage to the pancreatic tissues. The third theory is that the inflammation may be a result of hypertriglyceridemia, which is known to occur in many individuals who ingest large amounts of alcohol. It is theorized that the breakdown of the triglycerides may produce toxic levels of free fatty acids, which may damage the pancreatic acinar cells or the endothelial cells.

The mechanism by which biliary tract disease causes pancreatitis is also unknown. It is theorized that gallstones migrating through the common bile duct somehow cause reflux of bile into the pancreatic ducts, thus initiating the inflammation; studies have documented the presence of gallstones in the stools of about 90% of patients with gallstone-associated pancreatitis. Cholangiographic studies have shown a common channel between the pancreatic duct and the common bile duct in as many as 90% of patients with a history of pancreatitis related to gallstone disease; this channel is demonstrated in only 20% to 30% of patients with gallstone disease but no history of pancreatitis.

Additional etiologic factors for pancreatitis are listed in the box. Although the specific mechanisms of pancreatic damage are unknown, the common pathologic lesion seems to involve extravasation of activated enzymes into the pancreatic tissues, which results in varying degrees of autodigestion and tissue damage.

PATHOPHYSIOLOGY

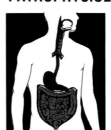

In most cases the inflammation is limited to varying degrees of interstitial edema; autodigestion of the pancreas does not occur in these mild cases. With pancreatitis caused by excessive alcohol intake, the onset of symptoms usually is about 12 to 24 hours after a heavy drinking episode. With gallstone-related pancreatitis, the symptoms commonly begin after a large meal. The primary clinical symptom in mild pancreatitis is abdominal pain, which usually is located in the midepigastric region and may radiate to the back; nausea and vomiting are common associated symptoms. These patients usually require only supportive care (i.e., pain control and fluid-electrolyte replacement).

Approximately 10% of patients with acute pancreatitis develop a fulminant form of the disease, characterized by autodigestion, hemorrhage, and necrosis of the pancreatic tissue. These patients require intensive supportive care and possibly surgical intervention for management of complications. Even with optimal management, the complication rate for these patients is high, and the mortality rate is about 30% to 50%.

The sequence of events leading to autodigestion has not been clearly identified. There is some evidence that autodigestion is initiated by obstruction of the acinar cells, which prevents the normal passage of the enzyme-containing granules into the pancreatic ducts. The enzyme-containing granules trapped within the cells may fuse with lysosomes in the cell, activating the enzymes. The activated enzymes can then initiate the autodigestive process. Limited pancreatic damage results in an acute illness that responds well to supportive therapy; extensive pancreatic damage commonly results in hemorrhagic and necrotic changes in the pancreatic tissue and in multiple related complications.

Pathologic changes that may be seen in acute pancreatitis include obstruction and distention of the pancreatic ducts, duodenal and bile duct obstruction caused by edema of the head of the pancreas, and extravasation of blood, pancreatic enzymes, and exudate into the retroperitoneal space, with resultant peritoneal irritation. Hypovolemia may occur as a result of protracted vomiting, third spacing of fluids within the bowel lumen (in response to peritoneal irritation), or loss of fluid through extravasation into the retroperitoneal space. Shock may result from a combination of factors such as hypovolemia and the release of substances that cause vasodilation and increased vascular permeability.

The predominant clinical findings in severe acute pancreatitis are the same as for mild pancreatitis: abdominal pain, nausea, and vomiting. However, the pain usually is more intense, and the vomiting may be severe and protracted. Additional signs and symptoms seen with severe pancreatitis include fever, tachycardia, epigastric tenderness, and abdominal distention. Bowel sounds may be hypoactive as a result of the ileus caused by the retroperitoneal inflammation. Hypotension and altered mental status may be seen if the disease has resulted in hypovolemia or shock. If complications are present, additional signs and symptoms may be seen.

The most common local complications include pancreatic phlegmon, pancreatic pseudocyst, and pancreatic abscess. Pancreatic phlegmon refers to a mass produced by the inflamed, necrotic pancreas, inflammatory infiltrates, and adjacent tissues; symptoms associated with pancreatic phlegmon include prolonged fever, abdominal pain and tenderness, prolonged leukocytosis, and an abdominal mass. Pancreatic pseudocyst refers to an accumulation of tissue debris, blood, fat droplets, and pancreatic secretions within areas of necrosis; the pseudocyst may develop within or adjacent to the pancreas. Pancreatic pseudocysts may be palpable as a mass in the upper abdomen or may be seen on ultrasound; serum amylase may be persistently elevated in these patients. Pancreatic abscess is the most serious local complication and represents bacterial invasion of the necrotic pancreatic debris. It may be difficult to distinguish pancreatic abscess from pancreatic phlegmon, because the signs and symptoms are the same and the only difference on computed tomography (CT) scan is the presence of extraluminal gas, which may or may not be visible. Pancreatic abscess requires prompt surgical intervention and is associated with a high mortality rate.

Major systemic complications include pulmonary disorders, cardiovascular complications, gastrointestinal hemorrhage, and metabolic complications. Psychiatric disorders have also been frequently reported in these patients.

Pulmonary complications occur in as many as 50% of patients with acute pancreatitis; atelectasis, pleural effusion, pneumonia, and adult respiratory distress syndrome (ARDS) are all commonly reported. Theories regarding the cause of pulmonary complications include the transudation of pancreatic enzymes through pores in the diaphragm, the effects of systemic substances produced in response to the disease, and abnormalities in surfactant induced by the disease. Cardiovascular complications include shock, disseminated intravascular coagulation (DIC), and pericardial effusion. Shock usually is caused by several factors, as was explained previously. Disseminated intravascular coagulation and pericardial effusion may be caused by proteolytic enzymes that have been released into the bloodstream. Gastrointestinal bleeding commonly results from coexisting peptic ulcer disease or from erosion of major blood vessels by the necrotic pancreatic process. Metabolic complications commonly reported include hyperglycemia and hypocalcemia. Hyperglycemia probably is caused by increased release of glucagon and reduced production of insulin; hypocalcemia may be due to binding of calcium by fatty acids in the inflammatory exudate or to reduced response to parathormone.

Mortality in acute pancreatitis varies from about 15% to almost 100%, depending on the severity of the disease. A prognostic guide has been used to predict the severity of the disease, using admission data and indicators obtained during the first 48 hours after admission. These prognostic indicators are outlined in the box on the next page. Mortality correlates with the number of positive indicators; patients with less than three positive indicators have essentially no mortality, whereas patients with seven or more positive indicators have almost 100% mortality.

Chronic pancreatitis is an inflammatory disease of the pancreas that results in progressive destruction of the gland and loss of the acinar cells, which leads to exocrine insufficiency. Chronic pancreatitis must be differentiated from recurrent pancreatitis; recurrent episodes of acute pancreatitis do not necessarily result in glandular destruction, which is the defining characteristic for chronic pancreatitis.

The causative factors for chronic pancreatitis are the same as for acute pancreatitis, but chronic alcoholism is the most common cause. Pathologic changes in the pancreatic tissue include protein plugs in the pancreatic ducts, reduced numbers of pancreatic islets and acinar cells, dilated ducts, and extensive fibrosis. Major clinical manifestations include abdominal pain, which may be severe, and signs of exocrine and endocrine insuffi-

---

PROGNOSTIC INDICATORS FOR A PATIENT WITH ACUTE PANCREATITIS (RANSON'S CLINICAL INDICATORS)

Signs on admission

Over 55 years of age
WBCs >16,000/mm^3
Serum glucose >200 mg/dl
Serum lactate dehydrogenase (LDH) >350 IU/L
Serum aspartate aminotransferase (AST or SGOT) >250 IU/L

Signs during first 48 h

Fall in Hct >10%
Rise in blood urea nitrogen (BUN) >5%
Serum calcium <8 mg/dl
Base deficit >4 mEq/L
Estimated fluid sequestration >6 L
Arterial oxygen pressure (Po$_2$) <60 mm Hg

Relation to morbidity/mortality

2 or fewer signs: 1% mortality
3-4 signs: 15% mortality
5-6 signs: 40% mortality
More than 6 signs: 100% mortality

---

ciency: steatorrhea, undigested muscle fibers in the stool, and hyperglycemia. Because the exocrine pancreas has tremendous reserve capacity, signs of exocrine and endocrine insufficiency do not usually appear until 90% or more of the pancreas has been destroyed.

The fibrosis associated with chronic pancreatitis may result in strictures of the common bile duct, which can cause bile duct obstruction. Pancreatic pseudocysts may occur with chronic pancreatitis and may be accompanied by pancreatic pleural effusions or pancreatic ascites. Pancreatic ascites and pleural effusions result from disruption of the pancreatic duct; an anterior disruption results in ascites, whereas a posterior disruption causes fluid accumulation in the retroperitoneal space, with the potential for mediastinal penetration and pleural effusions.

COMPLICATIONS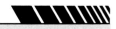

Acute pancreatitis

Local: Pancreatic phlegmon, pancreatic pseudocyst, pancreatic abscess, involvement of adjacent organs by necrotic process, obstructive jaundice, pancreatic ascites caused by disruption of pancreatic duct or leaking pseudocyst

Systemic: *Pulmonary:* pleural effusion, atelectasis, pneumonia, mediastinal abscess, hypoxemia, ARDS
Cardiovascular: pericardial effusion, electrocardiographic changes simulating myocardial infarction, thrombophlebitis, DIC, shock, sudden death resulting from shock
Gastrointestinal: hemorrhage resulting from associated peptic ulcer, variceal bleeding, portal vein thrombosis, or necrotic erosion into major blood vessels
Metabolic: hyperglycemia, hypocalcemia, hyperlipema
Renal: oliguria, azotemia, renal artery thrombosis, renal vein thrombosis
Central nervous system: psychosis, fat emboli
Fat necrosis: subcutaneous tissues, bone, other organs

Chronic pancreatitis

Common bile duct stricture and obstruction; pancreatic ascites; pancreatic pleural effusion; pancreatic pseudocyst; nutritional deficiencies: (steatorrhea); diabetes mellitus; pancreatic fistulas; splenic vein thrombosis

---

DIAGNOSTIC STUDIES AND FINDINGS

Diagnostic test	Findings
Serum amylase	Usually elevated to more than twice the upper limit of normal; elevated amylase levels are not diagnostic of pancreatitis because other conditions also cause elevated amylase levels and because amylase elevation does not consistently correlate with the severity of the pancreatic inflammation
Serum lipase	Frequently elevated; a more accurate indicator of pancreatic inflammation than serum amylase

DIAGNOSTIC STUDIES AND FINDINGS—cont'd

Diagnostic test	Findings
Serum lipids	May be elevated
Serum triglycerides	May be elevated
Isoamylase assay	Pancreatic isoamylase may be elevated
Liver studies	May be elevated, especially with gallstone-associated pancreatitis
Bilirubin	
Alkaline phosphatase	
Gamma-glutamyl transferase (SGGT)	
Alanine aminotransferase (SGPT)	
Aspartate aminotransferase (SGOT)	
Hematocrit (Hct)	Elevated levels may be seen with third spacing and hemoconcentration; decreased levels may be seen if hemorrhagic complications occur
White blood cell count (WBC)	Elevated levels common ($>10,000/mm^3$)
Serum glucose	May be elevated if endocrine function of pancreas is compromised (>180 mg/dl)
Serum calcium	Reduced levels may be seen (<8 mg/dl)
Blood urea nitrogen (BUN)	May be elevated (>45 mg/dl)
Arterial blood gases (ABGs)	Hypoxemia may be seen with pulmonary complications ($Po_2 < 60$ mm Hg)
Urinary amylase	Usually elevated ($>3,600$ U/24 h)
Amylase/creatinine clearance ratio	Usually elevated ($>6\%$)
X-ray (flat plate) of abdomen	May show cholelithiasis; nonspecific ileus; pancreatic calcifications; obliteration of the psoas margins as a result of retroperitoneal irritation; presence of air in the duodenal loop (secondary to localized ileus); dilated proximal jejunal loop localized in upper abdomen ("sentinel loop sign"); distention of colon to level of transverse colon with absence of air in the splenic flexure and distal colon ("colon cutoff sign")
Chest x-ray	Left pleural effusion, elevated left hemidiaphragm, and left basal atelectasis suggest acute pancreatitis; may also be used for differential diagnosis (e.g., left lower lobe pneumonia); may show pulmonary complications such as atelectasis, pneumonia, ARDS, and pleural effusions
Abdominal ultrasound study	May show pancreatic swelling, pancreatic edema, peripancreatic fluid collections, gallstones (presence of air- and fluid-filled loops of bowel reduce diagnostic accuracy of ultrasound)
Computed tomography (CT) scan	Pancreatic changes: enlargement, either focal or diffuse; edema; necrosis with liquefaction. Peripancreatic changes: fluid collections and blurring or thickening of surrounding tissue planes. May also be used to diagnose complications such as pancreatic phlegmon, pancreatic pseudocyst, and pancreatic abscess. *Note:* Accuracy of CT scan is improved with oral and intravenous contrast.
Magnetic resonance imaging (MRI) study	May provide more sophisticated imaging than CT and thus more accurate diagnosis of acute pancreatitis in the future
Upper gastrointestinal (GI) series	May show widening of the duodenal C loop, anterior displacement of stomach by enlarged pancreas or pancreatic pseudocyst; may be used to rule out perforated duodenal ulcer. **Note:** Not commonly used at present because findings are nonspecific.
Endoscopic retrograde cholecystopancreatography (ERCP)	May be used in recurrent or chronic pancreatitis to identify ductal changes or presence of calculi *Usually contraindicated in acute pancreatitis*
Fecal fat determination	Level may be elevated in chronic pancreatitis if exocrine insufficiency is present
Fecal analysis	May show excessive levels of fats, proteins, and undigested muscle fibers in chronic pancreatitis with exocrine insufficiency
Schilling test	May show impaired vitamin B_{12} absorption in patient with chronic pancreatitis and exocrine insufficiency
Secretin-cholecystokinin test	May show reduced levels of pancreatic enzymes produced in response to stimulus; indicated only for chronic pancreatitis with clinical exocrine insufficiency

MEDICAL MANAGEMENT

GENERAL MANAGEMENT—ACUTE PANCREATITIS

Mild form: NPO status; administration of IV fluids; resumption of oral foods and fluids when pain, tenderness, and ileus have resolved. **Note:** Premature resumption of oral intake has been associated with reactivation of the inflammation and formation of pancreatic abscesses.

Severe form: NPO status; N/G intubation and suctioning; administration of IV fluids and electrolytes to maintain fluid-electrolyte balance; TPN for patient unable to resume oral intake within about 1 wk (lipids contraindicated in patient with hyperlipidemia); measurement of intake and output to provide for accurate fluid replacement (insertion of indwelling catheter as necessary); invasive hemodynamic monitoring (e.g., Swan-Ganz or CVP catheter) for patient with hemodynamic instability; administration of blood or blood products as needed to replace blood losses in hemorrhagic states; administration of oxygen for patient with pulmonary complications resulting in hypoxemia; ventilator support for patient with respiratory distress syndrome; peritoneal lavage occasionally used to remove toxic peritoneal exudate in patient with early deterioration of clinical status (value of peritoneal lavage is controversial).

GENERAL MANAGEMENT—CHRONIC PANCREATITIS

Management of acute episodes as outlined above; dietary modifications as needed for patient with exocrine insufficiency (e.g., low-fat diet, supplementation with peptide-based formula); referral to alcohol treatment program for patient with alcohol-related pancreatitis; supportive counseling for patient and family in dealing with chronic illness.

SURGERY

Exploratory laparotomy: To rule out a surgically correctable disease with a potentially fatal outcome when the diagnosis is uncertain.

Laparotomy: With wide-sump drainage or laparotomy with debridement and open packing for management of pancreatic abscess.

Cholecystectomy and operative cholangiogram: For gallstone pancreatitis; surgical procedure usually is delayed until acute illness has subsided.

Ductal drainage procedures: (e.g., side-by-side pancreaticojejunostomy) for patient with chronic pancreatitis and dilated ducts.

Partial pancreatectomy: (e.g., proximal pancreaticoduodenectomy) or total pancreatectomy for patient with chronic pancreatitis and severe pancreatic fibrosis or several pseudocysts causing obstruction of the biliary tree.

DRUG THERAPY

Narcotic analgesics (e.g., meperidine [Demerol]):   As needed to control pain; dosage is titrated according to patient's weight and response to medication.

Antiemetics (e.g., promethazine [Phenergan], 12.5-25 mg IM q 4-6 h):   To control nausea and vomiting.

Insulin: As needed to maintain normoglycemia.

Antibiotics (e.g., ceftriaxone [Rocephin] or cephalothin [Keflin]):   As prophylaxis for severe pancreatitis or in combination with drainage procedures for management of pancreatic abscess; Rocephin 1-2 g daily, or Keflin, 2 g q 6 h IV.

H_2-receptor antagonists (e.g., cimetidine [Tagamet], 300 mg q 6 h):   As prophylaxis against gastrointestinal bleeding in patient with severe pancreatitis.

Antacids (e.g., Mylanta):   As prophylaxis against gastrointestinal bleeding for patient with severe pancreatitis.

MEDICAL MANAGEMENT—cont'd

Vasopressor agents: Such as dopamine (Intropin), 2-5 µg/kg/min, titrated to maintain B/P within established range.

Somatostatin (Sandostatin): May be given to inhibit secretion of pancreatic enzymes and gastric acid.

Pancrelipase (Viokase): 1 to 3 tablets with meals for patient with chronic pancreatitis and exocrine insufficiency.

---

1 ASSESS

ASSESSMENT	OBSERVATIONS
History	May report previous similar episodes; may have history of alcohol abuse or gallstone disease
Pain (location, nature, severity)	May report pain in epigastric region that radiates to back, pain in upper abdominal quadrants, or generalized abdominal pain; may describe pain as constant and boring or penetrating; severity may range from mild distress to severe pain; may report onset of pain after large meal (gallstone pancreatitis) or drinking binge (alcohol-related pancreatitis); may assume sitting and leaning position for partial relief; facial expressions may indicate pain; may be restless
Gastrointestinal function	May report nausea and vomiting; bowel sounds may be hypoactive; abdomen may be distended
Vital signs	May have fever; tachycardia; tachypnea; hypotension
Fluid-electrolyte balance	May have decreased skin turgor; oliguria; concentrated urine; dry mucous membranes; dizziness; weakness; confusion; pulse irregularities; tingling in hands and feet (fluid volume deficit, hyponatremia, hypokalemia, hypocalcemia)
Pulmonary function	May have tachycardia; tachypnea; diminished breath sounds; rales; shortness of breath; respiratory distress; confusion; cyanosis
Abdomen (inspection and palpation)	May be distended; with hemorrhagic pancreatitis may have bluish discoloration in periumbilical area (Cullen's sign) or flank area (Grey Turner's sign); may have muscle guarding and mild to severe tenderness on palpation; may have palpable mass (pancreatic phlegmon or pancreatic pseudocyst)

2 DIAGNOSE

NURSING DIAGNOSIS	SUBJECTIVE FINDINGS	OBJECTIVE FINDINGS
Pain related to pancreatic inflammation	Reports constant, penetrating abdominal pain (periumbilical, upper abdominal, or generalized) that may radiate to back	Facial expressions reflect pain; sits and leans forward; abdominal tenderness and guarding noted on palpation

→ > >

NURSING DIAGNOSIS	SUBJECTIVE FINDINGS	OBJECTIVE FINDINGS
Fluid volume deficit related to nausea and vomiting or to sequestration of fluids and electrolytes within lumen of bowel or peritoneal cavity	Reports nausea and vomiting; dry mouth, thirst, weakness, dizziness; may report tingling of hands and feet	Output exceeds intake; concentrated urine; reduced urinary output; dry mucous membranes; hypotension, tachycardia; reduced skin turgor
Altered renal, cerebral, cardiopulmonary, gastrointestinal, and peripheral tissue perfusion related to pancreatic abscess and peritonitis or to shock or bleeding	May complain of increasingly severe pain and of feeling anxious and short of breath	Hypotension, tachycardia, tachypnea; fever; oliguria; diaphoresis; respiratory distress; mental confusion; may have increasing abdominal tenderness and distention; may have bloody stools or evidence of intraabdominal bleeding (Cullen's sign or Grey Turner's sign)
Gas exchange, impaired related to atelectasis, pneumonia, or ARDS	Complains of difficulty breathing and shortness of breath; reports feelings of anxiety	Tachypnea, tachycardia; diminished breath sounds; rales; assumes sitting position; flaring of nostrils; cyanosis; mental confusion
Altered nutrition: less than body requirements related to nausea, vomiting, and malabsorption	Reports recent or continuous unplanned weight loss; may report frequent malodorous stools; complains of fatigue	Steatorrhea; muscle wasting; joint edema; dry, pluckable hair; dry, flaky skin; dry mucous membranes; lethargy
Coping, ineffective individual related to alcohol abuse	Reports excessive or continued consumption of alcohol or may deny alcohol abuse despite documented abuse	Difficulty setting appropriate goals; history of alcohol abuse; may deny relationship between alcohol intake and disease

3 PLAN

Patient goals

1. The patient will be free of abdominal pain and tenderness.
2. The patient will maintain a normal fluid and electrolyte balance.
3. The patient will maintain normal perfusion of renal, cerebral, cardiopulmonary, gastrointestinal, and peripheral tissues.
4. The patient will maintain normal gas exchange.
5. The patient will regain and maintain usual weight and ingest adequate nutrients daily.
6. The patient will establish effective strategies for coping with life stressors and illness.

4 IMPLEMENT

NURSING DIAGNOSIS	NURSING INTERVENTIONS	RATIONALE
Pain related to pancreatic inflammation	Monitor patient for increasing severity of pain and for response to analgesics.	Increasing severity of pain may indicate complications such as abscess formation; analgesics are titrated according to patient's response.

NURSING DIAGNOSIS	NURSING INTERVENTIONS	RATIONALE
	Administer analgesics such as meperidine (Demerol) as ordered and needed.	Severe pain requires narcotic analgesics; meperidine is preferred over morphine, which causes biliary spasm.
	Keep patient NPO until pain subsides; insert N/G tube (or assist with placement) as ordered; irrigate tube as needed to maintain patency.	Oral ingestion of nutrients stimulates pancreatic secretions, which may contribute to pancreatic injury; N/G suction may be used to reduce gastric drainage into the duodenum, which reduces the stimulus to pancreatic secretion.
	Administer somatostatin as ordered.	Somatostatin reduces pancreatic secretion and may help limit pancreatic injury.
Fluid volume deficit related to nausea and vomiting or to sequestration of fluids and electrolytes within lumen of bowel or peritoneal cavity	Monitor patient's intake and output, including any emesis.	Output exceeding intake indicates excessive fluid losses and the potential for fluid volume deficit.
	Monitor patient for signs of hypovolemia or electrolyte imbalance (e.g., dry mucous membranes, oliguria, orthostatic hypotension, reduced skin turgor, dizziness, confusion, and tingling in hands and feet).	Prompt recognition of fluid and electrolyte derangements permits early intervention and correction of deficits.
	Provide IV fluid replacement as ordered.	Maintaining fluid volume and electrolyte balance is essential to maintaining tissue perfusion and function.
	Administer antiemetics as ordered and needed.	Antiemetics reduce vomiting and thus reduce fluid losses.
Altered renal, cerebral, cardiopulmonary, gastrointestinal, and peripheral tissue perfusion related to hemorrhagic pancreatitis, gastrointestinal bleeding, pancreatic abscess and peritonitis, or shock	Monitor patient for indications of gastrointestinal bleeding or hemorrhagic pancreatitis, pancreatic abscess and peritonitis, or shock: bloody stools or emesis; bluish discoloration of flanks or periumbilical area; increasing abdominal pain and tenderness with fever; hypotension and tachycardia.	Acute blood loss may cause hypovolemic shock unless adequate replacement is provided; pancreatic abscess and peritonitis may precipitate septic shock; shock is a major cause of death in patients with pancreatitis.
	Monitor vital signs, urinary output, and Swan-Ganz or CVP catheter measurements (if applicable) for evidence of circulatory compromise: hypotension, reduced CVP and pulmonary artery pressure (PAP), tachycardia, tachypnea, and reduced urinary output.	Circulatory compromise is reflected by changes in B/P, CVP, PAP, and urinary output; compensatory responses to circulatory compromise produce tachycardia and tachypnea.
	Administer H_2-receptor antagonists (e.g., cimetidine) and antacids (e.g., Mylanta) as ordered (if patient has N/G tube, clamp tube for 20-30 min after administration).	H_2-receptor antagonists and antacids reduce gastric acidity and may help prevent gastrointestinal bleeding.
	Administer antibiotics as ordered (e.g., cephalothin).	Antibiotics are used to prevent or treat bacterial complications such as pancreatic abscess.

→ > >

NURSING DIAGNOSIS	NURSING INTERVENTIONS	RATIONALE
	Administer IV fluids and blood replacement as ordered; observe for transfusion reactions if blood is given.	IV fluids are administered to maintain plasma volume; blood replacement may be required to replace RBCs and platelets for patient with hemorrhagic complications.
	Administer vasopressor agents (e.g., dopamine) as ordered; titrate to maintain B/P within established range.	Vasopressors such as dopamine increase cardiac output and cause vasoconstriction to maintain B/P and tissue perfusion.
Gas exchange, impaired related to atelectasis, pneumonia, or ARDS	Monitor patient for signs of pulmonary complications: tachypnea, dyspnea, diminished breath sounds, rales, respiratory distress, cyanosis, confusion, and tachycardia.	Pulmonary complications are common in patients with pancreatitis and require prompt intervention to prevent serious morbidity or mortality.
	Administer oxygen as ordered and needed.	Oxygen administration helps correct hypoxemia, which improves tissue oxygenation and reduces dyspnea.
	For patient with worsening pulmonary status: prepare for and assist with endotracheal intubation and placement on ventilator.	Mechanical ventilatory support and positive end-expiratory pressure (PEEP) may be required for patient with ARDS.
Altered nutrition: less than body requirements related to nausea, vomiting, and/or malabsorption.	Monitor patient's weight, nutrient intake, and indicators of compromised nutritional status (e.g., hypoalbuminemia, joint edema).	Prompt recognition of nutritional deficits permits early intervention; correcting nutritional deficits helps prevent complications and improves patient's ability to heal and combat infection.
	Obtain order for TPN for patient with severe pancreatitis who cannot resume oral feedings within 1 wk or who has signs of malnutrition on admission.	TPN maintains protein stores and prevents complications associated with malnutrition.
	When patient can resume oral feedings, collaborate with patient and dietitian to provide high-calorie, high-protein diet based on patient's preferences.	Maintaining body weight and positive nitrogen balance reduces morbidity and improves health.
	For patient with chronic pancreatitis: observe for signs of exocrine insufficiency (e.g., weight loss, steatorrhea).	Chronic pancreatitis causes loss of exocrine gland function with resultant loss of enzyme production.
	For patient with chronic pancreatitis and signs of exocrine insufficiency: administer exogenous pancreatic enzymes (e.g., pancrelipase) as ordered	Exogenous enzymes are required for digestion of nutrients when disease destroys the exocrine pancreas (usually 90% destruction results in clinical signs of exocrine insufficiency).
	Monitor blood glucose levels, and administer insulin as ordered and needed.	Insulin production may be reduced in patients with severe acute pancreatitis or chronic pancreatitis; exogenous insulin is required for these patients to promote glucose metabolism and prevent metabolic derangements.

NURSING DIAGNOSIS	NURSING INTERVENTIONS	RATIONALE
Coping, ineffective individual related to alcohol abuse	Provide information about the relationship between excessive alcohol intake and pancreatitis.	So patient can make informed decisions about continued alcohol intake.
	Provide supportive counseling (e.g., reflective listening with therapeutic confrontation as indicated).	Supportive counseling helps patient explore feelings, identify major issues, and consider options for dealing with issues.
	Refer patient to local self-help support groups such as Alcoholics Anonymous.	Participation in self-help support groups reduces patient's sense of isolation, expands his or her support system, encourages development of new coping strategies, and has been demonstrated to be effective in modifying addictive behaviors.
	Offer professional counseling as an option.	Professional counseling helps patient confront and deal with issues.

5 EVALUATE

PATIENT OUTCOME	DATA INDICATING THAT OUTCOME IS REACHED
Patient has no abdominal pain or tenderness.	Patient states that pain has resolved; facial expressions do not indicate pain; abdominal palpation elicits no guarding or complaints of tenderness; patient requires no analgesics.
Patient maintains normal fluid-electrolyte balance.	Intake and output are balanced; urine is dilute; skin turgor is normal; B/P and pulse are within normal limits; mucous membranes are moist; patient has no symptoms of electrolyte imbalance such as dizziness, mental confusion, or tingling in hands and feet; patient tolerates oral foods and fluids without nausea or vomiting.
Patient maintains normal perfusion of renal, cerebral, gastrointestinal, cardiopulmonary, and peripheral tissues.	B/P, pulse, respiratory rate, and temperature are within normal limits; urine output is within normal limits; patient is alert and oriented; abdomen is soft, nondistended, and nontender; there is no evidence of gastrointestinal bleeding.
Patient maintains normal gas exchange.	Pulse and respiratory rates are within normal limits; breath sounds are clear; color is normal; patient is alert and oriented; there is no evidence of respiratory distress.
Patient has regained and maintains usual weight, ingests adequate nutrients on a daily basis.	Patient states that nausea and vomiting have resolved; he tolerates oral foods and fluids; patient has regained weight and maintains it to within 90% of usual weight; he has no steatorrhea and is normoglycemic.
Patient has established effective strategies for coping with life stressors and illness.	Patient acknowledges relationship between excessive alcohol ingestion and disease; he has identified need to omit alcohol; he has identified an effective support system and appropriate strategies for dealing with stress.

→ > >

PATIENT TEACHING

1. Explain the causes for this patient's pancreatitis, if known, and explain measures he can take to reduce the risk of recurrent attacks (e.g., forgoing alcohol if pancreatitis is alcohol related; treatment of gallstone disease if pancreatitis is gallstone related).
2. Teach the patient with chronic pancreatitis ways to reduce recurrent episodes of acute pancreatitis, i.e., avoid overeating, avoid alcohol, adhere to high-protein, moderate-fat diet.
3. Teach the patient with chronic pancreatitis and exocrine insufficiency the rationale and administration schedule for exogenous pancreatic enzymes. Teach the patient to monitor signs and symptoms of exocrine insufficiency (steatorrhea, weight loss, undigested muscle fibers in stool) and to report these signs and symptoms to the physician.
4. For the patient with endocrine insufficiency: teach the patient to monitor blood glucose, to administer insulin as ordered, to adhere to prescribed diet, and to recognize and respond to signs and symptoms of hypoglycemia or hyperglycemia.

Hepatitis

Hepatitis is a viral infection that primarily affects the liver; however, a number of extrahepatic manifestations may also occur, indicating that the disease is actually systemic. Hepatitis may be further classified according to causative agent (hepatitis A, hepatitis B, hepatitis C), duration (acute or chronic), and severity (acute or "classic," submassive hepatic necrosis, or fulminant disease with massive hepatic necrosis).

EPIDEMIOLOGY

Hepatitis causes significant morbidity and economic loss. The Centers for Disease Control estimates that there are 200,000 new cases of hepatitis B each year in the United States; 10,000 of these patients require hospitalization, and 10,000 to 20,000 become chronic carriers of the hepatitis B virus. (It is estimated that about 200 million people are carriers worldwide.) The financial impact of hepatitis B in the United States alone is thought to be about $750 million a year. These statistics must be interpreted in light of the fact that hepatitis B accounts for only 40% of all cases of hepatitis; thus the total impact is greater than these numbers reflect.

Hepatitis A, formerly referred to as "infectious" hepatitis, is transmitted through the fecal-oral route. It is more common in children and young adults and may occur in "epidemic" form as a result of food, water, or shellfish contamination. The virus is present in the stool of infected individuals during the last 2 weeks of the incubation period and until 2 weeks after the onset of clinical illness. There is no vaccine that protects against hepatitis A; however, administration of immune serum globulin after exposure can modify the severity of the disease. Infection with hepatitis A does not result in chronic liver disease and does confer lifelong immunity against the hepatitis A virus.

Hepatitis B, which formerly was known as "serum" hepatitis, is transmitted through both parenteral and nonparenteral routes. The mechanisms of transmission are not completely understood, but the surface antigen associated with the hepatitis B virus has been found in blood, breast milk, urine, saliva, nasopharyngeal washings, pleural fluid, feces, and semen. Parenteral exposure remains a major source of transmission, especially with the rising incidence of drug abuse; the hepatitis B virus can be transmitted in as little as 0.0005 ml of blood. A noninfectious vaccine has been developed that provides excellent protection against hepatitis B; prophylactic vaccination is recommended for all high-risk populations. (See the box for a list of groups at risk who should receive the vaccine.) Infection with hepatitis B may result in immunity or chronic liver disease or asymptomatic carrier status. There is evidence that asymptomatic carriers are at risk for reactivation of the

Table 4-4

COMPARISON OF HEPATITIS A, B, AND C

	Hepatitis A	Hepatitis B	Hepatitis C
Mode of transmission	Fecal-oral route	Contact with infected blood or body fluids	Parenteral and non-parenteral routes
Incubation period	14-42 days	50-180 days	14-150 days
Immunologic considerations	Does not result in chronic liver disease	May result in chronic liver disease (6%-10%)	May result in chronic liver disease (50%)
	No vaccine	Vaccine	No vaccine

disease during periods of immunosuppression. Asymptomatic carriers vary in their degree of infectivity.

The delta agent is a unique virus that requires the hepatitis B virus for its expression and that may modify the course of illness in patients who are coinfected (i.e., infected with both the hepatitis B virus and the delta agent). Coinfection usually produces an illness that is essentially the same as "classic" hepatitis B. Occasionally, however, coinfection can result in fulminant hepatitis; 20% to 50% of patients with fulminant hepatitis test positive for the delta agent. In addition, there is a strong correlation between chronic liver disease and coinfection; 60% to 80% of patients with chronic liver disease test positive for the delta agent. Most important, infection with the delta agent is thought to cause new disease in asymptomatic carriers or to accelerate clinical deterioration in patients with chronic hepatitis B.

The third type of hepatitis, formerly known as "non-A, non-B" hepatitis, is hepatitis C. Hepatitis C can be transmitted by either the parenteral or the nonparenteral route; it is the most common cause of posttransfusion hepatitis, accounting for 85% to 90% of cases. The nonparenteral routes of transmission are poorly understood at this time. A significant number of patients (50%) infected with hepatitis C develop chronic active liver disease; however, chronic liver disease in these patients is associated with a better prognosis than chronic liver disease from other causes. Some studies have shown an increased incidence of hepatocellular carcinoma in patients with chronic hepatitis C. Table 4-4 compares the three different types of hepatitis.

Chronic hepatitis occurs in two forms: chronic active hepatitis, also known as chronic active liver disease, and chronic persistent hepatitis. The diagnosis of chronic hepatitis is based on abnormalities in liver function tests and signs and symptoms of liver disease that persist for longer than 6 months.

GROUPS WHO SHOULD BE VACCINATED AGAINST HEPATITIS B

Health care workers
Renal dialysis patients
Institutionalized patients and their attending staff
Patients with hereditary or acquired disorders necessitating repeated transfusions
Patients with leukemia or other malignant disorders
Male homosexuals
Sexual partners of individuals who test positive for the hepatitis B surface antigen (HB_sAg)
Household contacts of HB_sAg carriers
Neonates of HB_sAg-positive mothers
Military and foreign service personnel assigned to areas where hepatitis B is endemic
Illicit drug users

Chronic active hepatitis is a serious illness that contributes significantly to morbidity and mortality associated with liver disease. Chronic active hepatitis may result from infection with hepatitis B or C. Certain drugs have also been shown to cause chronic active hepatitis. The most serious type of chronic active hepatitis is the idiopathic type, which is thought to be an autoimmune disorder. If untreated, chronic active hepatitis of autoimmune origin frequently progresses to cirrhosis, with an average survival period of only 4 to 5 years. However, most patients with idiopathic chronic active hepatitis respond well to treatment with corticosteroids. Patients with chronic hepatitic C experience a more gradual progression to cirrhosis (10-20 years). Steroids have not been effective, but interferon may benefit some patients.

Chronic persistent hepatitis is a much more benign disease and rarely progresses to cirrhosis; treatment is not required.

PATHOPHYSIOLOGY

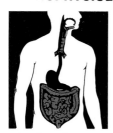

Viral hepatitis (Figure 4-11) ranges in severity from subclinical illness to fulminant disease; the most common pathologic patterns are "classic" viral hepatitis, submassive hepatic necrosis, and massive hepatic necrosis (fulminant hepatitis). The pathologic changes are the same, whether the causative agent is the hepatitis A, hepatitis B, or hepatitis C virus; however, some data indicate that the more severe pathologic patterns are more commonly seen with hepatitis B.

The signal lesion of hepatitis is necrosis of hepatocytes, with accumulation of inflammatory infiltrates and varying degrees of structural damage. With the "classic" pattern of viral hepatitis, necrosis is localized, there is diffuse inflammation, and some loss of the typical cord structure occurs. The inflammation can cause partial obstruction of the bile canaliculi, resulting in varying degrees of bile stasis and jaundice. Regeneration of hepatocytes begins within 48 hours of injury and is ongoing. With classic hepatitis there is no loss of lobular structure and no collapse of hepatic tissues. Submassive hepatic necrosis involves larger areas of necrosis known as "confluent necrosis"; a large number of hepatocytes are involved in the necrotic process, which results in severe inflammation, collapse of the hepatic tissues, and loss of the lobular structure. Fibrosis is commonly seen during the healing stages. "Massive hepatic necrosis" is the term used to describe extensive necrosis involving entire lobules; it usually is associated with fulminant liver failure.

Clinical symptoms range from mild to severe, depending on the extent of the underlying pathologic process. The "typical" presentation involves nonspecific prodromal symptoms followed by the appearance of jaundice. Common prodromal symptoms include anorexia, vague abdominal pain, nausea, vomiting, malaise, lethargy, fever, cough, myalgia, arthritis, urticaria, transient skin rashes, and abnormalities in taste and smell. The triad of headache, fever, and myalgia is particularly common during the prodromal phase of hepatitis A infections. The urine may become dark a few days before the onset of jaundice, as a result of bilirubinuria. The constitutional symptoms usually begin to subside after the jaundice appears. Jaundice commonly "peaks" around the second week of illness and typically is gone within 4 to 6 weeks. Classic physical findings include hepatomegaly and splenomegaly.

Variations on this typical clinical pattern include anicteric hepatitis, cholestatic hepatitis, and fulminant hepatitis. Anicteric hepatitis refers to hepatitis that does not produce jaundice. Many of these patients have

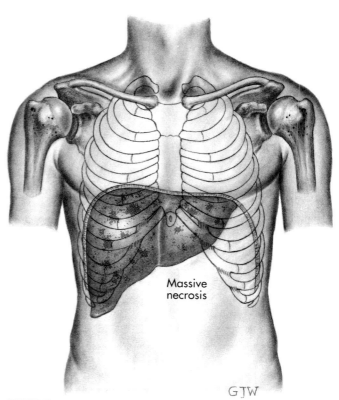

FIGURE 4-11
Acute viral hepatitis (fulminant hepatitis).

typical prodromal symptoms, but the diagnosis of hepatitis may be missed because jaundice is absent. Anicteric hepatitis does not necessarily follow a benign course; patients may have grossly abnormal liver function and even submassive hepatic necrosis. Patients who "suddenly" develop cirrhosis without any obvious cause may have had undiagnosed anicteric hepatitis.

Cholestatic hepatitis refers to viral hepatitis associated with signs and symptoms of biliary retention. These patients may have dark urine, deep jaundice, clay-colored stools, pruritus, and liver function test results consistent with obstructive disease. Pathologic features of cholestatic hepatitis include canalicular biliary stasis along with the classic features of hepatocyte damage. These patients may remain jaundiced for prolonged periods.

A small percentage of patients develop a more fulminant disease associated with submassive or massive hepatic necrosis. Clinical indicators include evidence of fluid accumulation (edema and ascites); signs of liver failure, such as hepatic encephalopathy (mental confusion, asterixis, fetor hepaticus), and rapid decrease in liver size. Laboratory studies reveal persistently high serum bilirubin levels and a prolonged prothrombin time that does not respond to vitamin K therapy. These patients have a higher mortality rate than patients with "classic" hepatitis.

Extrahepatic manifestations may also be seen, including such serious complications as cardiac disease, aplastic anemia, polyarteritis, pancreatitis, and renal disease. These complications are thought to result from deposition of immune complexes or viral damage affecting the involved organs.

Chronic active hepatitis is characterized by extensive intralobular or multilobular necrosis, accumulation of inflammatory infiltrates, loss of the normal hepatic structure, and significant fibrosis. Cirrhotic changes are evident in many patients by the time chronic active hepatitis is diagnosed. Chronic persistent hepatitis primarily involves inflammatory infiltrates; necrosis is limited, the hepatic structure is preserved, and little or no fibrosis develops. The clinical presentation and course are consistent with these pathologic changes; chronic active hepatitis is associated with progressive liver failure and possibly death, whereas chronic persistent hepatitis follows a benign course characterized chiefly by fatigue and hepatomegaly.

COMPLICATIONS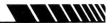

Fulminant liver failure
Cirrhosis
Extrahepatic complications: cardiac damage, pancreatitis, polyarteritis, renal damage, aplastic anemia

DIAGNOSTIC STUDIES AND FINDINGS

Diagnostic test	Findings
Serum antigen and antibody tests	
Hepatitis A antigen (HAAg)	Present in low levels in serum and stool of patients with hepatitis A; cleared rapidly, so negative results do not rule out hepatitis A
Hepatitis AAb	Positive IgM fraction indicates recent infection with hepatitis A; positive IgG fraction indicates previous infection (persists indefinitely)
Hepatitis B surface antigen (HB$_s$Ag)	Presence in serum indicates current infection with hepatitis B or past infection with carrier state
Hepatitis Be antigen (HB$_e$Ag)	Presence in serum indicates active and infective stage of hepatitis B; positively correlated with chronic active liver disease
Antibody to hepatitis B surface antigen (HB$_s$Ab)	Presence in serum indicates previous infection with hepatitis B and usually indicates immunity; also present after successful immunization against hepatitis B
Antibody to hepatitis B core antigen (HB$_c$Ab)	Presence in serum seen with previous or ongoing infection with hepatitis B; can be used to diagnose hepatitis B during lag phase between clearance of HB$_s$Ag and appearance of HB$_s$Ab, because HB$_c$Ab becomes positive fairly early in course of disease; high titers in chronic carrier state
Antibody to hepatitis Be antigen (HB$_e$Ab)*	Presence indicates low-grade infectivity and limited disease activity (hepatitis B); found predominantly in asymptomatic carriers
IgM anti-HB$_c$	High titers indicate acute infection with hepatitis B (titers persist for a few months after infection); low titers may be found in patients with chronic hepatitis B infection
Delta antigen	Presence indicates infection with delta agent
Antibody to delta agent (anti-δ)	Presence in serum indicates past or current infection with delta agent
Antibody to HCV (anti-HCV)	Presence in serum indicates infection with HCV
Liver function tests	
Serum bilirubin	Elevated levels commonly seen with icteric viral hepatitis (8-15 mg/dl); markedly elevated levels seen with cholestatic hepatitis (20-30 mg/dl); mild elevation may be seen with chronic persistent hepatitis
Serum alanine aminotransferase (ALT, SGPT)	Markedly elevated levels typically seen with acute hepatitis (>300 IU/L); may be elevated 1-2 wk before onset of jaundice
Serum aspartate aminotransferase (AST, SGOT)	Markedly elevated levels typically seen with acute hepatitis beginning 1-2 wk before onset of jaundice; marked elevation may be seen with chronic active hepatitis; moderately elevated levels may be seen with chronic persistent hepatitis

*Note: Hepatitis B core antigen (HB$_c$Ag) is found in the liver cells of patients with hepatitis B infection but cannot be detected in serum with current technology.

DIAGNOSTIC STUDIES AND FINDINGS—cont'd

Diagnostic test	Findings
Serum lactic dehydrogenase (LDH)	Elevated levels typically seen with acute hepatitis
Serum alkaline phosphatase	Normal or mildly elevated levels typically seen with acute hepatitis
Prothrombin time (PT)	Elevated levels may be seen with severe, fulminant disease and hepatic necrosis
Serum albumin	Decreased levels may be seen with severe, fulminant disease and hepatic necrosis
Serum ammonia	May be elevated with severe hepatic necrosis and encephalopathy
Urinalysis	Bilirubinuria typically present; proteinuria and hematuria may be seen with renal complications
Stool analysis for hepatitis A virus (HAV): radioimmunoassay, enzyme immunoassay, immune electron microscopy	Positive for 2-4 wk after exposure and until onset of clinical disease
Liver biopsy	Performed in patients who have symptoms or abnormal laboratory findings that are consistent with chronic liver disease and that persist for 6 mo: inflammatory infiltrates with minimal necrosis and fibrosis, typical of chronic persistent hepatitis, and marked necrosis with loss of normal lobular structure, typical of chronic active hepatitis

MEDICAL MANAGEMENT

GENERAL MANAGEMENT

"Classic" acute hepatitis: Activity restriction; low-fat, high-carbohydrate diet as tolerated during icteric phase; symptom control.

Fulminant disease with massive hepatic necrosis: Bed rest; IV fluids to maintain fluid-electrolyte balance; low-protein diet or nutritional support (enteral or parenteral) for patient unable to eat; enemas to reduce amounts of stool and colonic bacteria and thus reduce ammonia production; monitoring for bleeding or development of hepatic coma; fresh frozen plasma to correct coagulation defects.

Chronic active hepatitis: Activity restrictions based on patient's tolerance; low-fat, high-carbohydrate diet during episodes of jaundice; review of prescribed and over-the-counter medications with omission of drugs known to contribute to chronic active hepatitis (e.g., alpha-methyldopa, nitrofurantoin, isoniazid, sulfonamides, aspirin).

Chronic persistent hepatitis: No treatment needed; focus is on symptom control.

Note: Infection control measures must be observed for all patients with hepatitis; universal precautions are observed when handling blood or body fluids.

DRUG THERAPY

Vaccination against hepatitis B for high-risk groups (see box on page 157): Heptavax-B (initial dose, 1 ml IM; second dose, 1 ml IM 1 mo after initial dose; third dose, 1 ml IM 6 mo after initial dose. For patient with reduced immunity, schedule for three doses is the same but the dose is increased to 2 ml) or Recombivax (initial dose, 1 ml IM; second dose, 1 ml IM 1 mo after initial dose; third dose, 1 ml IM 6 mo after initial dose).
Note: Successful vaccination results in anti-HB_s titers of 10 mIU/ml or above; serologic testing before vaccination is recommended to identify those with negative titers who require vaccination. (Anti-HB_c identifies both carriers and those with immunity.)

For known or presumed exposure to hepatitis B (parenteral exposure, direct mucous membrane contact, sexual exposure, or oral ingestion involving HB_sAg-positive materials such as blood, plasma, or serum; infants born to mothers who are positive for HB_sAg): Hepatitis B immune globulin (Hep-B-Gammagee), 0.06 ml/kg IM as soon as possible after exposure and within 24 h if at all possible.

MEDICAL MANAGEMENT—cont'd

Recommendations for adults who have not been previously vaccinated against hepatitis B and who are exposed through (1) percutaneous (needle stick), ocular, or mucous membrane exposure to blood known or presumed to contain HB_sAg; (2) human bites by known or presumed HB_sAg carriers that penetrate the skin; or (3) intimate sexual contact with known or presumed HB_sAg carriers: Hepatitis B immune globulin as soon as possible after exposure (0.06 ml/kg IM) *and* initiation of vaccination with Heptavax or Recombivax as previously outlined, with initial dose given within 7 days of exposure.

Recommendations for adults who have been previously vaccinated against hepatitis B: Titer for anti-Hb_s checked promptly; if titer is above 10 mIU/ml (10 SRU), no treatment is required. If titer is below this level, administration of hepatitis B immune globulin as outlined above (0.06 ml/kg IM) and Heptavax or Recombivax 1 ml simultaneously at two different sites as soon as possible after exposure.

Postexposure prophylaxis for hepatitis A: Immune globulin 0.02-0.04 ml/kg IM within 2 wk of exposure (close personal contact with individual infected with hepatitis A).

Prophylaxis for individuals traveling to areas where hepatitis A is endemic: Immune globulin 0.02-0.04 ml/kg IM within 2 mo of travel; for prolonged travel, 0.06 ml/kg q 5 mo.

For fulminant hepatitis with encephalopathy: Neomycin sulfate, 4-12 g daily in divided doses PO, *or*, rectal administration of 200 ml 1% or 100 ml 2% solution retained for 30-60 min.

For chronic active hepatitis of autoimmune origin: Methylprednisolone (prednisone), 10-20 mg daily *or* methylprednisolone (prednisone), 10 mg daily in addition to azathioprine (Imuran), 50 mg daily for as long as 2 yr or even longer.

Antiemetics (e.g., promethazine [Phenergan]): As needed to control nausea and vomiting (prochlorperazine should be avoided).

Analgesics (e.g., acetaminophen): To control abdominal pain.

---

1 ASSESS

ASSESSMENT	OBSERVATIONS
History of exposure to hepatitis virus (acute hepatitis)	May report: similar illness in person with whom patient has had close contact; parenteral, ocular, mucous membrane, or sexual exposure to blood or body fluids of person with hepatitis B; recent blood transfusion (within past 6 mo); IV drug abuse; recent travel out of country
Prodromal symptoms (acute hepatitis)	May report: recent onset of anorexia; vague abdominal pain; fatigue; nausea; vomiting; fever; malaise; nasal congestion; cough; myalgia; transient skin rash; urticaria; alterations in smell and taste; weight loss
Jaundice	Sclerae and skin may appear jaundiced; urine may appear dark (tea colored); stools may appear clay colored; may complain of itching or may be seen chronically scratching

→ > >

ASSESSMENT	OBSERVATIONS
Abdominal examination	Palpation may elicit complaints of tenderness in right upper quadrant; hepatomegaly and splenomegaly may be evident; sudden reduction in liver size may be seen with severe necrosis
Evidence of hepatic failure	Ascites may be evident; evidence of bleeding may be seen (bruising, blood in urine or stool); may be confused, lethargic, or act inappropriately; asterixis may be present (flapping tremor of dorsiflexed hands)
Evidence of serious systemic complications (e.g., pulmonary edema, cardiac failure)	May hear rales in chest; pulse may be irregular, weak, or rapid; patient may complain of shortness of breath

2 DIAGNOSE

NURSING DIAGNOSIS	SUBJECTIVE FINDINGS	OBJECTIVE FINDINGS
High risk for infection related to exposure to hepatitis virus	Reports recent or potential exposure to hepatitis virus (e.g., needle stick; contact with blood or body fluids of infected person; travel to areas where virus is endemic)	Health care professional; renal dialysis patient; institutionalized patient or caregiver; patient requiring repeated transfusion; patient with leukemia; sexual partner of HB_sAg-positive individual; household contact of HB_sAg carrier; IV drug user; male homosexual; individual assigned to area where hepatitis is endemic
Fatigue related to liver inflammation	Complains of feeling tired and not having much energy; may report decreased activity tolerance and increased desire to rest and sleep	Appears tired; appears to limit activity
Altered nutrition: less than body requirements related to anorexia and nausea	Reports loss of appetite; may report alterations in taste and smell; may report nausea and vomiting	Reduced oral intake of food and fluids; weight is below usual
High risk for fluid volume deficit related to nausea and vomiting	Reports feelings of thirst, "dry mouth," dizziness, nausea, and vomiting	Reduced intake of oral fluids; intake less than output; oliguria; concentrated urine; vomiting; tachycardia; orthostatic hypotension; diminished skin turgor
Altered thought processes related to hepatic encephalopathy	Reports feelings of lethargy or euphoria	Disorientation; changes in personality (more aggressive or lethargic behavior); may progress to stupor and coma; asterixis may be seen
High risk for injury related to bleeding related to liver dysfunction	Reports prolonged bleeding with minor trauma	Epistaxis; blood in urine or stool; bruising

3 PLAN

Patient goals

1. Exposed individuals will remain free of hepatitis, and the patient will learn measures to prevent cross-infection.
2. The patient will be free of fatigue and able to resume usual activities.
3. The patient will regain or maintain usual weight and ingest adequate nutrients daily.
4. The patient will maintain a normal fluid and electrolyte balance.
5. The patient will be free of confusion and other signs of hepatic encephalopathy.
6. The patient will have no abnormal bleeding.

4 IMPLEMENT

NURSING DIAGNOSIS	NURSING INTERVENTIONS	RATIONALE
High risk for infection related to exposure to hepatitis virus	Encourage individuals at risk for hepatitis B to obtain vaccination with Heptavax or Recombivax.	Safe, effective vaccines are available that protect against hepatitis B; hepatitis B is associated with significant morbidity and can result in chronic liver disease.
	Help individuals with known or presumed exposure to hepatitis A or B to obtain appropriate prophylaxis: immune globulin for hepatitis A, hepatitis B immune globulin and Heptavax or Recombivax for hepatitis B.	Prompt administration of immune globulins provides passive immunity, which serves to prevent or modify the infection.
	Implement and instruct patient and significant others in appropriate infection control measures. Hepatitis A: gloves when handling stool, thorough handwashing after toileting or other personal care, proper disposal of stool and any items contaminated by stool, restrictions on food handling by infected individuals. Hepatitis B and C: gloves when handling blood or body secretions, single use and correct disposal of needles and syringes, separate eating and drinking utensils for infected individuals, appropriate disposal and disinfection procedures for items contaminated with blood or body fluids, condoms during sexual intercourse for individuals infected with hepatitis B (unless sexual partner has been immunized).	Patient, caregivers, and significant others must understand the mode of transmission and appropriate preventive measures to stop the spread of the virus.
Fatigue related to liver inflammation	For patient with evidence of submassive or massive hepatic necrosis (e.g., deep jaundice, marked abnormalities in liver function tests): maintain patient on bed rest. For patient with classic persistent hepatitis: restrict activity and provide additional rest according to patient's activity tolerance.	Bed rest reduces body's energy requirements and promotes liver's reparative process.

→ > >

NURSING DIAGNOSIS	NURSING INTERVENTIONS	RATIONALE
Altered nutrition: less than body requirements related to anorexia and nausea	Monitor patient's nutrient intake, nutrient losses through vomiting, and weight.	Positive nitrogen balance is essential for healing; early recognition of nutritional deficits permits prompt intervention.
	Administer antiemetics as ordered and needed.	Antiemetics reduce nausea and vomiting, thus promoting nutrient intake and reducing nutrient losses.
	During icteric phase: provide high-carbohydrate, low-fat diet as tolerated.	Jaundice indicates biliary stasis and thus reduced ability to digest fats; carbohydrates provide calories and energy needed for repair.
	For patient who cannot ingest adequate nutrients: collaborate with physician and nutritional support team to provide appropriate enteral or parenteral nutrition.	Adequate nutritional status is essential for liver repair.
	For patient with acute liver failure: low-protein diet or enteral formula.	A severely damaged liver cannot clear ammonia produced by bacterial action on proteins; elevated ammonia levels can result in encephalopathy.
High risk for fluid volume deficit related to reduced intake or excessive losses (vomiting)	Monitor patient for intake and output and signs and symptoms of fluid volume deficit: oliguria, dry mucous membranes, reduced skin turgor, orthostatic hypotension, and tachycardia.	Prompt recognition of fluid volume deficits permits early intervention.
	Administer antiemetics as ordered and needed.	Antiemetics reduce nausea and vomiting, thus reducing fluid loss and promoting intake.
	Provide fluid replacement as ordered and tolerated (oral or parenteral).	Fluid replacement is essential to maintaining blood volume and tissue perfusion.
Altered thought processes related to hepatic encephalopathy	Monitor patient for changes in level of consciousness, changes in behavior, or asterixis.	Changes in level of consciousness or behavior or development of asterixis (flapping tremor) are early signs of encephalopathy.
	Administer neomycin as ordered.	Neomycin reduces colonic bacteria; bacterial action on proteins produces ammonia, which causes encephalopathy.
	Maintain patient with severe liver necrosis on low-protein diet or formula.	Bacterial action on proteins produces ammonia, which causes encephalopathy; low-protein diets limit ammonia production.
	For patient with chronic active liver disease of autoimmune origin: administer prednisone or prednisone and azathioprine as ordered.	Long-term treatment with prednisone or prednisone and azathioprine controls chronic active liver disease and helps prevent progression.

NURSING DIAGNOSIS	NURSING INTERVENTIONS	RATIONALE
High risk for injury related to bleeding	Monitor patient for evidence of bleeding: hematuria, melena, epistaxis, and easy bruising.	Hematuria, melena, epistaxis, and bruising are indicators of bleeding, which may occur in severe liver failure because the liver fails to produce clotting factors.
	Administer fresh frozen plasma as ordered.	Fresh frozen plasma provides clotting factors.

5 EVALUATE

PATIENT OUTCOME	DATA INDICATING THAT OUTCOME IS REACHED
Exposed individuals are free of hepatitis, and patient can describe measures to prevent cross-infection.	Patient and caregivers can identify mode of transmission for hepatitis virus and use appropriate infection control measures; individuals at risk for hepatitis B have been vaccinated; individuals exposed to virus have obtained appropriate prophylaxis; patient's contacts do not have hepatitis.
Patient is free of fatigue and has resumed usual activities.	Patient has resumed usual life-style; she states that her fatigue has resolved and that she needs only her usual amount of rest.
Patient has regained or maintains usual weight and ingests adequate nutrients daily.	Weight is 90% or more of usual weight; patient consumes regular diet; patient states that anorexia, nausea, and vomiting have resolved and that her appetite is normal.
Patient maintains normal fluid-electrolyte balance.	Intake and output are balanced; patient has no signs or symptoms of fluid volume deficit (e.g., oliguria, orthostatic hypotension, dizziness, weakness, dry mucous membranes, thirst, diminished skin turgor); patient states that vomiting has resolved.
Patient is free of confusion and other signs of hepatic encephalopathy.	Patient remains alert and oriented; behavior is normal; there is no ascites or asterixis.
Patient has no abnormal bleeding.	Stools and urine are free of blood; gums and skin show no epistaxis or unusual bruising.

PATIENT TEACHING

1. Teach the patient, caregivers, and significant others how the hepatitis virus is transmitted, and instruct them in measures to prevent cross-infection. Hepatitis A: fecal-oral transmission; precautions include gloves when handling infected stool; thorough handwashing after toileting; no food preparation or handling by infected person; immune globulin for known exposure. Hepatitis B: mode of transmission is parenteral (mucous membrane, ocular, or skin break exposure to blood or body fluids of infected individual); precautions include gloves (and goggles if appropriate) when handling blood or body fluids,

→ > >

separate eating and drinking utensils for infected individual with proper disinfection, condoms during intercourse, vaccination for high-risk individuals and those in close contact with infected individual, and administration of hepatitis B immune globulin in addition to vaccination for known or presumed exposure. Hepatitis C: mode of transmission and precautions are the same as for hepatitis B; no vaccine is available.

2. Instruct the patient to get plenty of rest, to avoid strenuous activity, and to eat a high-calorie diet as soon as tolerated to promote healing within the liver. Instruct the patient to maintain a low-fat diet until the jaundice has resolved.

3. Teach the patient with chronic persistent hepatitis to space activities in order to limit fatigue; explain that this disease is not progressive and requires symptom management rather than treatment.

4. For the patient with chronic active liver disease: explain the progressive nature of the disease and the importance of continuous treatment; explain that certain drugs (e.g., aspirin) can cause liver damage, and emphasize the importance of checking with the physician before taking any medications (prescription or over the counter); instruct the patient to report any signs of worsening liver function to the physician promptly (e.g., abdominal swelling, bruising or bleeding, lethargy, or behavior changes). For the patient with chronic liver disease of autoimmune origin: explain the purpose, dosage, side effects, and importance of medications (prednisone or azathioprine or both), and emphasize that these drugs must be taken for prolonged periods and that they *must not* be discontinued suddenly.

Peritonitis

Peritonitis is an inflammation of the peritoneum (Figure 4-12). It may be classified as localized or generalized and as primary or secondary.

EPIDEMIOLOGY

Peritonitis is a serious inflammatory disorder; despite advances in supportive care and antibiotic therapy, the reported mortality is 18% to 60%. Mortality is especially high with peritonitis that occurs after abdominal or pelvic surgery; factors associated with increased mortality rates include advancing age and intraabdominal fecal contamination, such as occurs with perforation or anastomotic breakdown involving the colon.

Primary peritonitis is a peritoneal infection caused by bloodborne organisms or organisms arising from the genital tract, as opposed to infection resulting from peritoneal contamination by gastrointestinal secretions. Primary peritonitis is relatively rare, especially in adults. One cause of primary peritonitis is cirrhosis with ascites; about 25% of these patients develop bacterial infection of the ascitic fluid, usually with *Escherichia coli*. The infection is thought to be caused by the increased permeability of the bowel wall that results from portal hypertension; the increased permeability permits bacterial migration into the abdominal cavity.

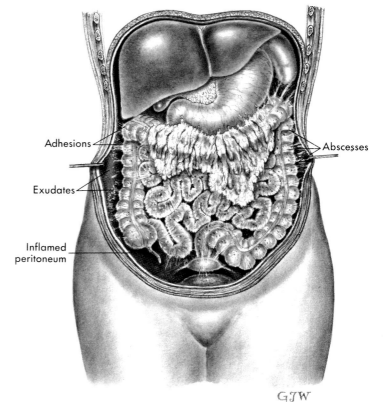

FIGURE 4-12
Acute peritonitis.

Additional causative factors include genitourinary infections that spread to involve the peritoneum, such as gonococcal salpingitis and *Chlamydia trachomatis* infections. A nonbacterial, granulomatous peritonitis can also occur, usually in response to such irritants as gauze fragments, dusting powders used on surgical gloves, and suture material.

Secondary peritonitis is a peritoneal inflammation resulting from contamination by gastrointestinal secretions. Common causes include the following:

- Acute infections and perforations involving intraabdominal organs (e.g., pancreatitis, appendicitis with rupture, perforated peptic ulcer, diverticulitis with perforation)
- Blunt or penetrating trauma to intraabdominal organs resulting in perforation and spillage of secretions (e.g., gunshot wounds or stab wounds involving small bowel or colon)
- Obstructive disorders of the bowel resulting in transudation of bacteria through the dilated ischemic bowel wall and potentially resulting in perforation and spillage of intestinal contents if the obstruction is not corrected (e.g., volvulus or strangulated hernia)
- Ischemic disorders affecting the bowel, with transudation of bacteria through the ischemic bowel wall followed by frank necrosis, perforation, and spillage of intestinal contents (e.g., mesenteric infarction)
- Postoperative peritonitis resulting from breakdown of anastomoses (e.g., colon resection with end-to-end anastomosis)

Postoperative peritonitis is fairly common and potentially fatal. It is more likely to occur when there is intraoperative spillage or when intestinal anastomoses are constructed under tension or with inadequate blood supply. Current recommendations are that compromised anastomoses be exteriorized (e.g., by constructing a temporary, double-barreled colostomy rather than a primary colonic anastomosis in a patient at risk).

Peritonitis is sometimes described as aseptic or septic; aseptic peritonitis refers to peritoneal inflammation caused by contamination with noninfected secretions, such as pancreatic fluid. However, bacterial invasion of any exudate eventually occurs, and the peritonitis becomes septic, or infected. The organisms commonly involved in peritonitis include the mixed flora of the intestinal tract and adjacent organs; gram-negative aerobes and anaerobes are the predominant organisms. Specific organisms commonly involved are *E. coli*, *Streptococcus faecalis*, *Pseudomonas aeruginosa*, staphylococci, *Klebsiella* sp., *Proteus* sp., *Bacteroides fragilis*, and *Clostridium* sp.

PATHOPHYSIOLOGY

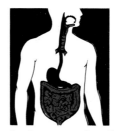 Bacterial proliferation within the abdominal cavity produces classic results; the peritoneal membrane becomes hyperemic and edematous, and large volumes of exudate are produced. The inflammatory exudate helps contain the infection, because it contains fibrin as well as leukocytes; the fibrin causes loops of bowel and segments of omentum to stick together, which helps to localize the inflammatory process, and the leukocytes begin phagocytosis of bacteria. However, the exudate may also contribute to the spread of infection, because it tends to disseminate throughout the abdominal cavity unless effective localization occurs early in the inflammatory process. Spread of the infection may also occur along the peritoneal membrane itself and by way of the lymphatics. The bacteria may also invade the bloodstream, causing septicemia; about 30% of patients with peritonitis have positive blood cultures, and studies have shown that bacteria are present in the bloodstream within 12 minutes after injection into the peritoneal cavity.

If the peritonitis is localized, the fluid losses into the abdominal cavity are limited and pathologic changes in the peritoneum and surrounding tissues remain localized. If, however, the peritonitis becomes generalized, large volumes of fluid may be lost into the abdominal cavity, and the inflammatory changes may involve the entire peritoneum and surrounding tissues.

Ileus is an invariable result of peritonitis. Although the exact cause is not known, it probably results from peristaltic inhibition by a combination of factors such as gaseous distention, fluid-electrolyte disturbances (e.g., hypokalemia), and sympathetic stimuli.

The outcome of the infectious process varies, depending on the cause and severity of the infection, the body's resistance, and the effectiveness of treatment. Optimally, the causative factors are corrected, the infection is controlled, and the inflammatory exudate is reabsorbed with no residual pathologic condition in the abdomen. If ischemic tissue is involved, adhesions may be produced, because new vessels sprout in response to ischemia, and the vascular ingrowth may convert the fibrinous exudate to fibrous adhesions. (If there is no vascular ingrowth, the fibrinous exudate usually is completely absorbed.) Incomplete control of the infection and incomplete absorption of the inflammatory exudate may result in formation of an inflammatory mass composed of the inflamed organ, adjacent loops of bowel, and segments of inflamed mesentery or omentum. The mass frequently is walled off from the rest of the abdominal cavity by dense adhesions. The mass eventually may resolve or may progress to formation of an abscess that requires drainage. Occasionally numerous inflammatory masses form, resulting in several abscesses and a chronic septic state that frequently is fatal.

The clinical manifestations also depend on the extent and severity of the underlying inflammation. Abdominal pain is the most consistent symptom; it may be gradual or abrupt in onset and may range from a dull ache to intense, unremitting pain. The pain may be generalized or localized to the area of the abdomen overlying the inflammation. Abdominal palpation elicits rigidity and complaints of tenderness in the areas of peritoneal inflammation. Nausea and vomiting commonly occur as a result of peritoneal irritation and ileus. Abdominal distention may be mild or severe; it re-

sults from the combined effects of ileus, gaseous distention of the bowel, and accumulation of inflammatory exudate within the abdominal cavity. Evidence of circulatory collapse may be seen in patients with septicemia or severe fluid losses (i.e., hypotension, tachycardia, oliguria, dry mucous membranes, and diminished skin turgor). The temperature is commonly elevated, although it may drop to subnormal if the patient's immune system is overwhelmed by fulminant peritonitis.

COMPLICATIONS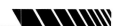

Septicemia
Formation of intraabdominal abscesses
Circulatory collapse (shock and death)

DIAGNOSTIC STUDIES AND FINDINGS

Diagnostic test	Findings
White blood cell count (WBC)	Usually elevated
Hematocrit (Hct)	May be elevated as a result of fluid loss and hemoconcentration
Serum electrolytes	Abnormalities may be seen as a result of fluid losses from vomiting (e.g., altered levels of potassium, sodium, and chloride)
Arterial blood gases (ABGs)	May show reduced levels of bicarbonate and carbon dioxide (metabolic acidosis with respiratory compensation)
Urinalysis	May be done to rule out pyelonephritis
Chest x-ray	May be done to rule out pulmonary sources of pain and distention (e.g., pneumonia or pleurisy)
X-ray (flat plate and upright) of abdomen	May show air fluid levels if obstruction is present; may show dilated loops of bowel (gaseous distention consistent with ileus); may show free air if bowel has perforated
Computed tomography (CT) scan of abdomen	May show abscess formation
Arteriography	May be done to rule out mesenteric infarction
Peritoneal aspiration with culture and sensitivity	May show cloudy peritoneal fluid; culture may reveal bacterial or fungal organisms

MEDICAL MANAGEMENT

GENERAL MANAGEMENT

Maintain patient on NPO status; N/G tube to suction; IV fluids to replace fluid and electrolyte losses; TPN; Swan-Ganz catheter or CVP line to monitor hemodynamic status; oxygen per nasal cannula as needed.

For patient with significant peritoneal contamination: Continuous peritoneal lavage with saline, saline-antibiotic solution, or dilute povidone-iodine solution.

SURGERY

Exploratory laparotomy to determine and remove the source of infection (e.g., resection of necrotic tissue, removal of inflamed organ, correction of obstruction, closure of perforation) or to drain abscesses and lavage peritoneal cavity.

MEDICAL MANAGEMENT—cont'd

DRUG THERAPY

Analgesics: (e.g., morphine) as ordered and needed for pain; antiemetics (e.g., promethazine) as ordered and needed for nausea and vomiting.

Broad-spectrum antibiotics to control infection: Aminoglycoside (e.g., gentamycin) or cephalosporin (e.g., cefuroxime) to control gram-negative organisms; metronidazole (Flagyl) to control anaerobes.

1 ASSESS

ASSESSMENT	OBSERVATIONS
Pain	May describe sudden or gradual onset of pain; may describe pain as generalized or may be able to localize pain; may describe pain as dull and aching or as severe and unrelenting; respirations may be shallow, and patient may complain of pain on deep inspiration; may keep knees bent; may exhibit guarding when abdomen is approached
Abdominal examination	May exhibit guarding and muscle rigidity; may complain of localized or generalized tenderness; rebound tenderness may be present; palpation in unaffected quadrants may cause pain in affected quadrant; bowel sounds may be hyperactive with tinkling, rushing sounds or may be diminished or absent; distention is present; tympanitic sound heard on percussion
Vital signs	Temperature may be elevated, normal, or subnormal; hypotension, tachycardia, and tachypnea may be present
GI function	May complain of anorexia, nausea, and vomiting; may report inability to pass gas or stool
Fluid-electrolyte balance	May exhibit signs of fluid volume deficit and electrolyte imbalance: orthostatic hypotension, tachycardia, oliguria, dry mucous membranes, diminished skin turgor, weakness, confusion

2 DIAGNOSE

NURSING DIAGNOSIS	SUBJECTIVE FINDINGS	OBJECTIVE FINDINGS
Pain related to peritoneal inflammation	Complains of generalized or localized abdominal pain; may describe pain as dull and aching or intense; complains of pain with deep breathing	Shallow respirations; abdominal guarding; keeps knees bent; facial expressions reflect pain; palpation elicits rigidity and complaints of tenderness; rebound tenderness may be present
Fluid volume deficit related to vomiting and third spacing	Complains of anorexia and nausea; reports vomiting; complains of dry mouth and thirst; may complain of dizziness and weakness	Vomiting; dry mucous membranes; diminished skin turgor; tachycardia; orthostatic hypotension; oliguria; concentrated urine; lethargy; confusion

→ › ›

NURSING DIAGNOSIS	SUBJECTIVE FINDINGS	OBJECTIVE FINDINGS
Altered renal, cerebral, cardiopulmonary, gastrointestinal, and peripheral tissue perfusion related to septicemia and shock	Reports feeling short of breath and anxious; may report increasing pain	Hypotension; tachycardia; tachypnea; diaphoresis; oliguria; fever; increasing abdominal distention and tenderness
Altered nutrition: less than body requirements related to anorexia, nausea, and vomiting	Reports nausea and vomiting	Actual weight is below 90% of usual weight; reduced oral intake of nutrients; vomiting

3 PLAN

1. The patient will be free of abdominal pain and tenderness.
2. The patient will maintain normal fluid and electrolyte balance.
3. The patient will maintain adequate perfusion of renal, cerebral, cardiopulmonary, gastrointestinal, and peripheral tissues.
4. The patient will attain and maintain usual weight and will ingest adequate nutrients daily.

4 IMPLEMENT

NURSING DIAGNOSIS	NURSING INTERVENTIONS	RATIONALE
Pain related to peritoneal inflammation	Monitor patient for increasing pain and for response to pain control measures.	Increasing pain indicates worsening of the inflammation; assessment of response to pain control measures permits modification of care plan as needed.
	Administer analgesics (e.g., morphine) as ordered and needed.	Narcotic analgesics are indicated to relieve severe pain.
	Help patient assume a position of comfort (e.g., knees flexed).	Positioning with knees flexed reduces traction on peritoneum and thus reduces pain.
Fluid volume deficit related to vomiting and third spacing	Monitor patient for intake and output and for signs of hypovolemia: dry mucous membranes, oliguria, orthostatic hypotension, diminished skin turgor, tachycardia.	Prompt recognition of fluid deficits permits early intervention.
	Administer antiemetics as ordered and needed.	Antiemetics reduce vomiting, thus reducing fluid losses.
	Keep patient NPO and place N/G tube as ordered (or assist with placement); irrigate tube as needed to maintain patency.	Decompression of stomach and proximal bowel reduces vomiting and permits accurate measurement of fluid losses.

NURSING DIAGNOSIS	NURSING INTERVENTIONS	RATIONALE
	Administer IV fluids as ordered.	IV fluids are administered to maintain plasma volume, which is essential for maintaining tissue perfusion.
Altered renal, cerebral, cardiopulmonary, gastrointestinal, and peripheral tissue perfusion related to septicemia and circulatory collapse (shock)	Monitor patient for increasing pain and tenderness and for signs and symptoms of septicemia and shock: fever, tachycardia, hypotension, diaphoresis, and shortness of breath.	Increasing pain and tenderness indicate worsening intraabdominal infection; fever, tachycardia, hypotension, diaphoresis, and shortness of breath indicate sepsis and shock; hypotension coupled with tachycardia and dropping temperature is a grave prognostic sign, whereas rising temperature coupled with slowly dropping pulse rate indicates localization of the infection.
	Help with placement of Swan-Ganz or CVP line as ordered; monitor hemodynamic parameters, and report abnormal findings promptly.	Accurate hemodynamic monitoring permits prompt intervention.
	Administer antibiotics as ordered.	Antibiotics eliminate bacteria and help control infection, thus reducing the potential for bacterial invasion of the bloodstream and septic shock.
	Carry out continuous peritoneal lavage as ordered.	Continuous peritoneal lavage helps rid the abdominal cavity of bacteria and bacterial debris, thus helping to control the infection.
	Administer oxygen by nasal cannula as ordered to patient with signs of hypoxia (e.g., shortness of breath, tachycardia).	Administration of oxygen increases the oxygen delivered to tissues.
	Notify physician of worsening clinical status, and prepare patient for surgery.	Emergency laparotomy may be required to correct underlying pathologic condition or to drain abscesses.
Altered nutrition: less than body requirements related to anorexia, nausea, and vomiting	Collaborate with physician and nutritional support team to provide TPN until patient can resume oral nutrient intake.	Nutritional support is needed to maintain positive nitrogen balance, which helps prevent complications and maintain immune system function.

5 EVALUATE

PATIENT OUTCOME	DATA INDICATING THAT OUTCOME IS REACHED
Patient has no abdominal pain or tenderness.	Patient states that abdominal pain and tenderness have resolved; he requires no analgesics; abdominal palpation elicits no guarding, rigidity, or tenderness.
Patient maintains a normal fluid-electrolyte balance.	Patient states that nausea has resolved; he tolerates oral food and fluids without vomiting; intake and output are balanced; there are no signs or symptoms of fluid volume deficit (e.g., oliguria, dry mucous membranes, diminished skin turgor, weakness, confusion); B/P and pulse are within normal limits.

→ > >

PATIENT OUTCOME	DATA INDICATING THAT OUTCOME IS REACHED
Patient has adequate perfusion of renal, cerebral, cardiopulmonary, gastrointestinal, and peripheral tissues.	Abdomen is soft, nondistended, and nontender; temperature, pulse, B/P, and respiratory rate are within normal limits; patient has no shortness of breath and is alert and oriented.
Patient has attained and maintains usual weight and ingests adequate nutrients daily.	Patient's weight is 90% or more of usual weight; he ingests oral food and fluids in adequate amounts without vomiting.

PATIENT TEACHING

1. Explain the rationale and specifics of the care plan; provide time for the patient and family to ask questions and discuss their concerns about the disease and the treatment plan.
2. If surgery is required, explain the planned procedure, as well as preoperative and postoperative care procedures.
3. If the patient is discharged with open wounds or drain sites, teach him and family members appropriate home care procedures.
4. If the patient is discharged with medications, explain their purpose, dosage, and any potential adverse reactions.

CHAPTER 5

Obstructive Disorders of the Gastrointestinal System

Intestinal Obstruction

Intestinal obstruction refers to failure of the intestinal contents to progress forward through the lumen of the bowel.

Intestinal obstructions may be categorized as functional or mechanical. Functional obstructions are caused by loss of peristalsis and are commonly referred to as *paralytic ileus*. Mechanical obstructions result from lesions that occlude the bowel lumen and are further classified as *simple* or *strangulated*. A simple mechanical obstruction involves only luminal obstruction, whereas a strangulated obstruction involves loss of luminal patency and obstruction of the blood supply to the involved bowel segment.

EPIDEMIOLOGY

Intestinal obstruction can occur at any age, although it is more common in middle-aged and elderly people. The etiologic factors vary, depending on the type of obstruction (i.e., functional or mechanical) and the age group; for example, fecal impaction is a fairly common cause of mechanical obstruction in older patients but is rare in other age groups.

The most common cause of *functional obstruction*, or ileus, is abdominal surgery. Although the exact mechanism of postoperative ileus is not well understood, it is thought to result from sympathetic nervous system inhibition of intestinal motility. Additional factors that may play a role in postoperative ileus include peritoneal irritation and hypokalemia. Studies have shown that postoperative ileus affects the different bowel segments to varying degrees. The small bowel is the first to recover motility; in fact, studies show that the small bowel regains motility as soon as fluids and gas reach the duodenum. Colonic motility returns within 24 to 48 hours after laparotomy, whereas gastric atony may persist for as long as 4 days. Since gastric motility is essential for transport of ingested nutrients into the duodenum, it is the stomach's recovery that determines the patient's ability to tolerate oral feedings.

It is well established that peritonitis always causes ileus; this is thought to result from several factors, including sympathetic stimulation, metabolic disturbances, and gaseous distention. There is no evidence that the inflammatory peritoneal exudate has a direct effect on intestinal motility. Retroperitoneal trauma may produce an ileus as a result of stimulation of the sympathetic nervous system, which acts to inhibit intestinal motility. Spinal cord injuries also cause an ileus, presumably because of trauma to the parasympathetic nerve fibers that stimulate motility. Metabolic disturbances such as uremia, myxedema, and hypokalemia are also associated with ileus; hypokalemia is by far the most common of these. Finally, large doses of anticholinergic drugs such as propantheline (Pro-Banthine) can inhibit peristalsis enough to cause a functional obstruction.

Mechanical obstructions most commonly occur in the small intestine (70% are small bowel obstructions, 30% are large bowel obstructions). The causative factors may be classified as intraluminal lesions, changes in the bowel wall, or extraluminal compression. Intraluminal lesions include fecal impactions, food bolus obstructions, and gallstones. Bowel wall lesions include strictures caused by inflammatory processes and bowel wall malignancies. Extraluminal factors include strangulated hernias, adhesions, and volvulus. The most common cause of mechanical obstruction is adhesions, which commonly develop after abdominal surgery. Strangulated hernias (inguinal and femoral) and bowel wall malignancies are also common etiologic factors for mechanical obstruction.

PATHOPHYSIOLOGY

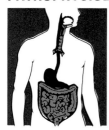

The primary pathophysiologic alteration associated with *functional obstruction*, or ileus, is loss of peristaltic activity; secondary alterations include gaseous distention of the intestine and fluid-electrolyte imbalances, which may occur as a result of vomiting, nasogastric suction, or third spacing of fluid into the intestinal lumen. Loss of peristaltic activity is evidenced by absence of bowel sounds and the patient's failure to pass flatus or stool via the rectum. Loss of peristaltic activity in turn causes accumulation of ingested and manufactured fluids and gases in the lumen of the bowel; this distention of the bowel is evidenced by abdominal distention. Severe, persistent ileus may cause extreme intestinal distention, which can impair the blood supply to the bowel wall and permit bacterial invasion; however, this degree of distention is much more likely to occur with mechanical obstruction than with functional obstruction. Accumulation of gastrointestinal secretions can also cause alterations in fluid and electrolyte balance; fluids that normally are reabsorbed are lost to the body as a result of vomiting, nasogastric suction, or sequestration within the lumen of the bowel. With severe distention the volume of fluid lost is even greater, because the capillaries begin to "leak" and allow transudation of fluid into the lumen of the bowel and the peritoneal cavity. Potential fluid-electrolyte abnormalities include fluid volume deficit, hypokalemia, and hyponatremia; loss of chloride can cause a compensatory increase in bicarbonate levels, resulting in alkalosis.

Clinical signs and symptoms typically include absence of bowel sounds, failure to pass flatus or stool per anus or stoma, and varying degrees of abdominal distention. Nausea and vomiting may occur, especially when the ileus is prolonged or the intraluminal distention is severe; in these cases, nasogastric decompression is necessary to reduce the distention and to provide accurate quantification of fluid losses. Signs and symptoms of fluid-electrolyte imbalance may be seen if intravenous replacement is inadequate or inaccurate.

Management of functional obstruction focuses on correcting the causative factors, maintaining the fluid-electrolyte balance, and controlling intestinal distention; the ileus usually resolves as the underlying process is brought under control, provided that no additional etiologic factors are superimposed (e.g., hypokalemia or a developing mechanical obstruction caused by fibrinous adhesions).

The initial event in mechanical obstruction is occlusion of the bowel lumen; secondary events include accumulation of intestinal secretions and ingested food and fluid in the lumen of the proximal bowel and increased peristaltic activity proximal to the obstruction. Tertiary events include fluid and electrolyte derangements, bacterial proliferation, and possible bowel wall ischemia, which in turn can lead to bacterial invasion of the bloodstream and even perforation of the bowel wall. Untreated mechanical obstruction can result in death from hypovolemia, sepsis, and peritonitis.

Fluid-electrolyte imbalance is a common complication of mechanical bowel obstruction. Normally 7 L of fluid is secreted into the lumen of the bowel daily and is then reabsorbed during the processes of digestion and absorption; in addition, the normal individual ingests about 2 L of fluid a day. Any interference with reabsorption can cause significant changes in the fluid and electrolyte balance. Mechanical obstruction causes loss of fluids and electrolytes, either through vomiting (or nasogastric suction) or through sequestration of massive volumes of fluid within the bowel lumen. The specific mechanism of fluid loss depends on the level of the obstruction. Proximal small bowel obstructions usually cause early copious vomiting and minimal intestinal distention, whereas distal small bowel obstructions produce early and massive intestinal distention but late vomiting. (Vomiting occurs when the bowel between the obstruction and the pylorus becomes so distended that the pylorus is obstructed.) Intestinal distention causes further interference with reabsorption and additional fluid loss; studies have shown that as the bowel progressively distends, its absorptive capacity decreases and its rate of secretion into the bowel lumen increases. In addition, the high intraluminal pressures cause obstruction of the capillary bed, and the capillaries begin to "leak" plasma into the bowel lumen and the peritoneal cavity. This loss of plasma proteins causes an osmotic "pull" that further promotes a fluid shift into the lumen of the gut and the peritoneal cavity. The fluid and electrolyte losses can be severe enough to induce hypovolemia, which if uncorrected causes circulatory collapse and death.

The stasis of intestinal secretions also causes bacterial overgrowth. Small bowel contents usually are sterile, partly because of gastric acidity, which eliminates many ingested organisms, and partly because of the normally rapid transit through the small bowel, which reduces bacterial proliferation. When stasis occurs, as with a mechanical obstruction, the limited bacteria in the small bowel fluid proliferate rapidly, and the small bowel fluid becomes progressively more "feculent" in nature. This explains the "fecal emesis" that occurs in long-standing mechanical obstructions; feculent emesis is not caused by regurgitation of colonic contents but by bacterial proliferation in the small bowel contents.

A potentially fatal complication of mechanical obstruction is bowel wall ischemia, which can result in bacterial invasion of the bloodstream and bowel wall perforation. Ischemia occurs when the intestinal distention becomes severe enough to produce intraluminal pressures that exceed capillary bed pressures; the result is venous congestion, rupture of arterioles, leakage of plasma into the intestinal lumen and peritoneal cavity, and increased permeability to intraluminal bacteria and toxins. Ischemic changes occur first in the mucosal and submucosal layers, but if uncorrected, the ischemia may progress to involve all layers of the bowel wall, and necrosis with perforation may result.

As was explained earlier, mechanical obstructions can be either *simple* or *strangulated;* strangulation occurs when the occlusive process involves the intestinal vasculature as well as the bowel lumen. Volvulus is an example of a strangulated, or "closed-loop," obstruction (Figure 5-1); strangulated hernias are another example. This type of obstruction can rapidly progress to perforation and peritonitis; the loss of blood supply causes severe ischemic changes, and the "closed loop" rapidly results in massive intestinal distention, which further impairs the intestinal circulation. One change associated with strangulation obstructions is early transudation of toxic intestinal contents across the ischemic bowel wall into the peritoneal cavity, which produces severe peritonitis and sepsis; the toxicity of the transudate is directly related to the proliferation of intestinal organisms and can be somewhat reduced by systemic antibiotic therapy.

The clinical manifestations of mechanical obstruction include colicky pain, hyperactive bowel sounds, vomiting, failure to pass stool and flatus per rectum or stoma, and abdominal distention. The colicky pain is a result of increased peristaltic activity proximal to the obstruction; the pain commonly occurs at intervals and frequently is described as "building to a peak, then sub-

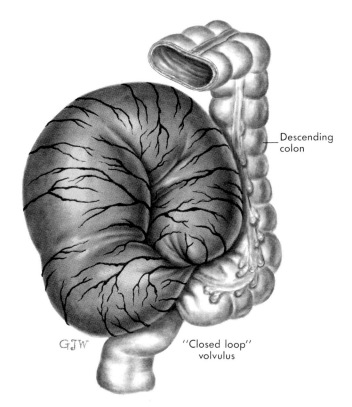

Descending colon

"Closed loop" volvulus

GJW

FIGURE 5-1
Volvulus of sigmoid (mechanical obstruction).

siding, then building again," which reflects the intermittent nature of peristalsis. With strangulation obstructions, the onset of pain usually is abrupt and the pain is severe. If the bowel perforates or becomes necrotic, the pain becomes intense, generalized, and unremitting. Auscultation reveals hyperactive or "tinkling" bowel sounds that are heard during peristaltic waves and that coincide with the cycles of pain. However, prolonged obstruction or obstruction complicated by peritonitis usually results in an ileus, with cessation of bowel sounds. Vomiting occurs as a result of accumulated intestinal contents; it occurs early in proximal obstructions and late in distal obstructions. Initially the emesis contains partially digested food; it then changes to watery, bile-stained intestinal fluid and finally becomes feculent as a result of bacterial proliferation. Failure to pass stool and flatus per rectum or stoma is a less consistent sign of mechanical obstruction; patients with proximal obstructions may continue to pass flatus and stool until the distal bowel is empty. The degree and location of abdominal distention provide a clue to the location of the obstruction; proximal jejunal obstruction causes epigastric distention, whereas distal ileal obstruction causes distention of the midabdomen that may be severe. Severe distention may in turn cause respiratory distress, since descent of the diaphragm is impeded.

Large bowel obstructions commonly are caused by progressive lesions such as malignancies or fecal impactions and tend to develop insidiously. As long as the ileocecal valve remains competent, intestinal distention is limited to the colon; because the small bowel is not involved, fluid-electrolyte abnormalities are uncommon, and vomiting occurs late if at all. However, the colon distention may be massive, and in extreme cases the cecum may actually perforate. Colon obstructions are characterized by failure to pass flatus or stool per rectum or stoma and by progressive, generalized abdominal distention. Colicky pain is not a typical feature of large bowel obstructions.

COMPLICATIONS

Fluid-electrolyte imbalance
Hypovolemia with circulatory collapse
Perforation
Intestinal ischemia and necrosis
Peritonitis secondary to perforation or to transudation of toxic contents across the ischemic bowel wall
Shock secondary to septicemia, hypovolemia, or peritonitis
Respiratory distress secondary to severe distention

DIAGNOSTIC STUDIES AND FINDINGS

Diagnostic test	Findings
Complete blood count (CBC)	Elevated white blood count (WBC) may be seen with strangulation, septicemia, or peritonitis; elevated Hb and Hct may be seen with hypovolemia due to hemoconcentration
Serum electrolytes and pH	Electrolyte abnormalities; common abnormalities include reduced levels of sodium, potassium, and bicarbonate; gastric losses may produce loss of chloride and a compensatory increase in bicarbonate; lowered pH (acidosis) may be seen with small bowel losses; elevated pH (alkalosis) may be seen with proximal obstruction causing gastric losses
Serum blood urea nitrogen	Elevated level may be seen with severe hypovolemia
Flat plate and upright films of abdomen	With functional obstruction (ileus): dilated loops of gas-filled bowel (small and large intestine) in supine position; air-fluid levels in upright position. With mechanical obstruction: dilated loops of gas-filled bowel above level of obstruction; air-fluid levels (in upright position) above level of obstruction
Contrast studies (barium meal with micropaque barium or barium enema)	Follow-through films (after barium meal) show point of obstruction; barium enema is used to identify point where colon is obstructed

MEDICAL MANAGEMENT

GENERAL MANAGEMENT

Functional obstruction (ileus): NPO status until peristalsis returns; nasogastric tube to suction for severe distention or vomiting; IV replacement of fluids and electrolytes.

Mechanical obstruction: NPO status; nasogastric or small bowel tube to suction for decompression of bowel proximal to obstruction; IV replacement of fluids and electrolytes; rectal enemas for attempted relief of partial colon obstruction.

SURGERY

Prompt surgical intervention is indicated for any strangulated (closed-loop) obstruction or any simple obstruction that fails to respond to conservative therapy; surgery should not be delayed unnecessarily in pa-

MEDICAL MANAGEMENT—cont'd

tients with mechanical obstruction because of the risk of necrosis and perforation. Surgery is *not* indicated for functional obstruction.

Exploratory laparotomy may be done to determine location and cause of obstruction.

Lysis of adhesions may be done for simple obstruction caused by adhesions.

Segmental bowel resection may be required to remove the obstructing lesion or to treat a strangulated obstruction with ischemic bowel changes (e.g., volvulus or strangulated hernia); ends of bowel may be brought to abdominal wall as a "double-barrelled" ostomy if end-to-end anastomosis is deemed risky; a second procedure is then required for takedown of stomas and reanastomosis of the bowel.

Diversion of fecal stream proximal to the obstruction may be required for decompression of the bowel or as the first stage in managing a constricting lesion in an unprepared bowel (e.g., transverse colostomy may be the first step in managing an obstructing sigmoid tumor); a second procedure is then required for resection of the constricting lesion, and a third procedure may be required if takedown of the ostomy is not completed during the second procedure.

DRUG THERAPY

Intravenous antibiotics for evidence of septicemia or peritonitis

Gentamicin: 3-5 mg/kg daily IV in three divided doses (dilute in 50-200 ml normal saline or D_5W); or ceftriaxone (Rocephin) 1-2 g daily IV.

Metronidazole (Flagyl): 15 mg/kg IV infused over 1 h; then 7.5 mg/kg IV q6h.

Narcotic analgesics (e.g., morphine sulfate): May be given to control pain once assessment has been completed.

---

1   ASSESS

ASSESSMENT	OBSERVATIONS
Medical-surgical history	May report previous abdominal surgery (mechanical obstruction)
Pain	May report sudden or gradual onset of severe, colicky pain (mechanical obstruction); may describe pain as "building to a peak" and then subsiding briefly before beginning again; may report abdominal "aching" or tenderness in addition to colicky pain
Gastrointestinal function	May report constipation alternating with diarrhea and change in caliber of stools (mechanical obstruction caused by colon tumor); may report anorexia, nausea, and vomiting (functional or mechanical obstruction); may report inability to pass stool or flatus (functional or mechanical obstruction)

ASSESSMENT	OBSERVATIONS
Abdomen	Inspection may reveal generalized distention (functional or mechanical obstruction) or localized swelling (hernia causing mechanical obstruction); auscultation may reveal absent bowel sounds (functional obstruction or late mechanical obstruction) or hyperactive, "tinkling" bowel sounds (mechanical obstruction); palpation may reveal tenderness, rebound tenderness, muscle guarding, or masses (mechanical obstruction)
Fluid-electrolyte balance	May report dry mouth, dizziness when standing, and weakness; output may exceed intake; inspection may reveal dry mucous membranes, sunken eyes, diminished skin turgor
Vital signs	Temperature may be elevated with sepsis or peritonitis; hypotension and tachycardia may be present with hypovolemia or septic shock; tachypnea may be present if distention interferes with respirations

2 DIAGNOSE

NURSING DIAGNOSIS	SUBJECTIVE FINDINGS	OBJECTIVE FINDINGS
Pain related to intestinal distention and ischemia	Complains of intermittent, colicky pain that may be intense	Facial expression indicates pain; restlessness; muscle guarding on abdominal palpation; tenderness on abdominal palpation
Fluid volume deficit (2) related to vomiting, nasogastric suction, or sequestration of fluids in bowel lumen	Reports dizziness and faintness; complains of dry mouth and thirst, weakness, and fatigue	Evidence of abnormal fluid losses (vomiting, nasogastric suction, abdominal distention); oliguria; increased urine concentration; dry mucous membranes; reduced skin turgor; postural hypotension; lethargy
Altered renal, cerebral, cardiopulmonary, gastrointestinal, and peripheral tissue perfusion related to septicemia, perforation, or necrosis of bowel	May complain of chills alternating with "feeling hot"; may complain of worsening abdominal pain	Fever; abdominal guarding and rebound tenderness; hypotension; tachycardia; increasing abdominal distention
Ineffective breathing pattern related to severe abdominal distention	Complains of difficulty breathing and shortness of breath	Tachypnea; diminished breath sounds; patient appears dyspneic and assumes sitting position; severe abdominal distention

3 PLAN

Patient goals

1. The patient will be free of abdominal pain and tenderness.
2. The patient will maintain a normal fluid and electrolyte balance.
3. The patient will maintain normal perfusion of renal, cerebral, cardiopulmonary, gastrointestinal, and peripheral tissues.
4. The patient's breathing pattern will be normal.

4 IMPLEMENT

NURSING DIAGNOSIS	NURSING INTERVENTIONS	RATIONALE
Pain related to intestinal distention and ischemia	Assess nature and severity of pain.	Characteristics of the pain provide clues about underlying pathologic condition; intermittent, colicky pain is consistent with mechanical obstruction; unrelenting pain may herald perforation or necrosis
	Administer analgesics (e.g., morphine) as ordered and needed.	Narcotic analgesics may be required to control severe pain.
Fluid volume deficit related to vomiting, nasogastric suction, or sequestration of intestinal secretions in bowel lumen	Monitor patient's intake and output (including emesis and N/G aspirate) and abdominal girth.	Output exceeding intake indicates fluid volume deficit; large amounts of fluid may be lost through vomiting, N/G suction, or third spacing of fluids in the bowel lumen (reflected by increasing distention).
	Monitor patient for signs of hypovolemia or electrolyte imbalance (e.g., dry mucous membranes, oliguria, orthostatic hypotension, extreme weakness).	Prompt recognition of fluid-electrolyte imbalance permits early correction of deficits.
	Provide IV fluid and electrolyte replacement as ordered.	Maintaining fluid volume and electrolyte balance is essential for tissue perfusion and neuromuscular function.
Altered renal, cerebral, cardiopulmonary, gastrointestinal, and peripheral tissue perfusion related to septicemia, perforation, or necrosis of bowel	Monitor patient for evidence of intestinal ischemia, impending or actual perforation, or septicemia (increasing abdominal pain and tenderness, fever, leukocytosis, rebound tenderness, hypotension, tachycardia).	Severe abdominal pain and tenderness, fever, and leukocytosis may indicate intestinal ischemia or impending perforation; generalized abdominal pain and rebound tenderness may indicate perforation and peritonitis, which may precipitate septic shock; fever, leukocytosis, hypotension, and tachycardia may indicate septicemia and septic shock.
	Keep patient NPO.	Oral food and fluids will cause further distention in the absence of peristalsis or the presence of mechanical obstruction.
	For patient with signs of mechanical obstruction, or functional obstruction with significant distention: place N/G tube as ordered (or assist with placement); irrigate tube as needed to maintain patency.	Decompression of the proximal bowel reduces intraluminal pressure and improves blood flow to bowel wall, thus reducing the potential for necrosis and perforation; decompression may permit spontaneous resolution of mechanical obstruction resulting from adhesions, because the decompressed bowel may be able to slip out of the obstructing adhesive band.
	Administer antibiotics as ordered.	Antibiotics are indicated for the patient with evidence of septicemia, ischemia, and impending or actual perforation to control bacterial proliferation and thus reduce production of bacterial toxins, which contribute to septic shock.

NURSING DIAGNOSIS	NURSING INTERVENTIONS	RATIONALE
	Monitor vital signs and urinary output for evidence of circulatory compromise (hypotension, tachycardia, tachypnea, and reduced urinary output).	Circulatory compromise is reflected by changes in B/P and urinary output; compensatory responses to circulatory compromise produce tachycardia and tachypnea.
	If symptoms of strangulation or impending or actual perforation occur, prepare patient for surgery.	Emergency surgery is indicated to prevent intestinal necrosis and perforation or to resect necrotic bowel and control intraabdominal infection.
Ineffective breathing pattern related to severe abdominal distention	Monitor patient for increasing abdominal distention and respiratory difficulties (tachypnea, dyspnea, cyanosis, confusion, shallow respirations, assumption of semierect position).	Increasing abdominal distention may cause respiratory distress by interfering with lung expansion; prompt recognition of respiratory distress permits early intervention.
	Institute measures to reduce abdominal distention (e.g., insertion, repositioning, or irrigation of N/G tube as ordered).	Eliminating abdominal distention promotes lung expansion and ventilatory function.
	Position patient with head of bed elevated.	Elevating the head of the bed reduces pressure on the diaphragm and enhances lung expansion.
	Administer oxygen as ordered and indicated.	Administering oxygen increases the blood oxygen level and reduces hypoxia.

5 EVALUATE

PATIENT OUTCOME	DATA INDICATING THAT OUTCOME IS REACHED
Patient has no abdominal pain or tenderness.	Patient states that abdominal pain has resolved; palpation elicits no complaints of pain; patient shows no abdominal guarding and no longer requires analgesics.
Patient maintains normal fluid and electrolyte balance.	N/G tube has been removed; patient tolerates oral food and fluids without nausea or vomiting; abdomen is not distended; intake and output are appropriately balanced; B/P and pulse are within normal limits; there are no signs or symptoms of fluid-electrolyte imbalance (e.g., weakness, dry mucous membranes, thirst, dizziness, concentrated urine, diminished skin turgor).
Patient maintains normal perfusion of renal, cerebral, cardiopulmonary, gastrointestinal, and peripheral tissues.	Patient's abdomen is soft and nondistended; there is no rebound tenderness or abdominal pain; temperature, pulse, and B/P are within normal limits.
Patient's breathing pattern is normal.	Patient has no shortness of breath; respiratory rate and depth are normal; there are no signs of hypoxia (e.g., cyanosis, confusion, tachycardia); abdomen is nondistended.

PATIENT TEACHING

1. Explain the reason for NPO status and for nasogastric or small bowel intubation (if applicable); instruct the patient in measures to reduce discomfort from nasogastric tube (e.g., oral rinses, lip lubrication, lozenges).
2. For the patient with functional obstruction: Explain that the bowel will regain normal motility and function when the underlying process (e.g., abdominal infection, postoperative trauma) has resolved.
3. For the patient with mechanical obstruction caused by adhesions in whom a trial of conservative therapy is planned: Explain that the purpose of the nasogastric or small bowel tube is to reduce swelling in the bowel so that it has a chance to slip through, and explain that surgery will be required if the obstruction does not resolve spontaneously.
4. For the patient with evidence of closed-loop (strangulated) obstruction or for the patient with mechanical obstruction that does not respond to conservative therapy: Explain the rationale for surgery, the planned surgical procedure, the potential for a temporary ostomy, and preoperative and postoperative care routines.

Gastric Cancer

Gastric cancer commonly refers to adenocarcinomas of the stomach. Adenocarcinoma is by far the most common gastric malignancy, accounting for about 95% of all cases. Other malignancies that may occur in the stomach include lymphomas and smooth muscle sarcomas.

EPIDEMIOLOGY

Gastric cancer is much less common in the United States today than it was in the past; it currently accounts for about 2% of all new cancer cases annually. However, it is much more common in other areas of the world, particularly Japan, where the incidence has remained consistently high. Men are twice as likely as women to develop gastric cancer, and the disease is most likely to develop between 50 and 70 years of age, with 60 being the "peak" age for both sexes.

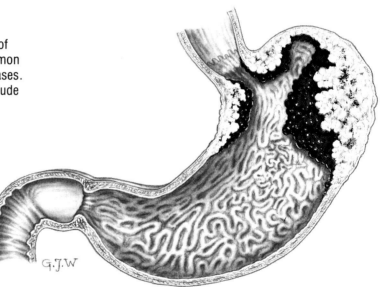

CARCINOMA OF STOMACH

Causative factors have not been clearly defined; however, the striking geographic differences in incidence strongly suggest environmental causes. The importance of environmental factors is further supported by the fact that emigrants from high-incidence to low-incidence countries show a significant decrease in the incidence of gastric cancer. One of the most important environmental factors is thought to be diet; a high-risk diet is thought to be high in complex carbohydrates, grains, and salt but low in animal fat, animal protein, salads, fresh, leafy green vegetables, and fresh fruit. The role of nitrates and nitrites is unclear; although there is evidence that nitrates and nitrites can be converted to carcinogenic nitrosamines in the presence of dietary salt, there is no clear correlation between nitrate consumption or exposure and gastric cancer. Fresh vegetables and fresh fruits are thought to play a protective role, at least partly because they contain high levels of vitamin C, which is known to be a nitrite scavenger. Other risk factors for gastric cancer are smoking and alcohol consumption.

Some medical conditions are associated with an increased incidence of gastric cancer, although they have not been shown to be "precursor conditions." Associated conditions include atrophic gastritis, pernicious anemia, partial gastrectomy, vagotomy and pyloroplasty, and gastric polyps. Gastric ulcers previously were considered possibly "premalignant," but current data do not support this relationship; the risk of gastric ulcers becoming malignant appears to be quite small.

PATHOPHYSIOLOGY

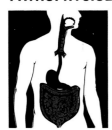 The pathologic effects of gastric cancer are related to obstruction of the gastric inlet or outlet, bleeding caused by tumor invasion of blood vessels, and metastasis affecting adjacent or distal structures. Unfortunately, gastric cancer may be asymptomatic until late in the disease; if symptoms are produced, they frequently are vague and likely to be confused with "indigestion" or peptic ulcer disease. This lack of symptoms frequently results in late diagnosis, which adversely affects the prognosis. As a result, massive screening programs have been undertaken in Japan, and these have been successful in identifying gastric tumors at an earlier point and in improving survival rates significantly. However, it is not economically feasible to initiate massive screening programs in countries with a low incidence of gastric cancer, such as the United States.

Obstructive symptoms may be produced by tumors in the cardiac or pyloric regions of the stomach. If the tumor is near the esophagogastric junction, the patient may experience increasing dysphagia, first for solids and later for liquids; dramatic weight loss may occur as a result of the inability to ingest adequate nutrients. Tumors near the pylorus initially may mimic the symptoms of peptic ulcers (e.g., epigastric pain, nausea, vomiting), but late symptoms are those of pyloric obstruction (early satiety, anorexia, nausea, vomiting). Bleeding may be caused by any gastric cancer. In some cases the bleeding may be occult and may go unnoticed until signs of anemia prompt a workup for occult bleeding. The bleeding can also be severe, as a result of erosion of major vessels; the patient experiences massive hematemesis or melena or both. If the tumor fails to cause obstruction or significant bleeding, the cancer may go undetected until metastasis to other organs produces symptoms.

Gastric cancers spread by the usual routes: direct invasion through the gastric wall into the peritoneum, lymphatic spread, and hematogenous spread. Initially the tumor spreads laterally in the submucosal layer; tumor cells can be found several centimeters away from the main lesion in tumors with an infiltrative growth pattern. Downward growth of the tumor results in penetration of the muscle layers and serosa; this penetration of the gastric wall is a negative prognostic sign. If the tumor penetrates to the serosal layer and the peritoneum, malignant cells may be released into the peritoneal cavity, which may result in peritoneal implants and pelvic tumors. About 60% of patients show invasion of regional lymph nodes at diagnosis; the prognosis depends on the number of nodes involved, but the 5-year survival rate for gastric cancer with lymph node involvement is in the 20% range. Hematogenous spread is to the liver, and patients with hepatic metastases have a very poor prognosis.

Staging systems commonly used for gastric cancer include the PHNS staging system used by the Japanese and the TNM system used in Europe and the United States (see inside back cover). In the Japanese system, the S factor, which reflects gastric wall penetration, is the most important prognostic factor.

Curative therapy for gastric cancer involves surgical resection; curative resections are indicated only for tumors confined to the stomach and local lymph nodes or for tumors involving adjacent structures that can be removed "en bloc." Chemotherapy and radiation may be used after resection to reduce recurrence. Palliative procedures may be indicated in advanced disease; for example, gastrojejunostomy may be performed to relieve gastric obstruction.

COMPLICATIONS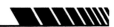

Hemorrhage
Obstruction (esophagogastric or pyloric)
Malnutrition
Metastasis

DIAGNOSTIC STUDIES AND FINDINGS

Diagnostic test	Findings
Hemoglobin and hematocrit	May be low in patient with occult bleeding
Liver function studies	May be elevated in patient with liver metastasis
Stool for occult blood	May be positive
Erythrocyte sedimentation rate	May be elevated
Carcinoembryonic antigen	May be elevated
Upper GI series (barium swallow with follow through)*	May show filling defect, polypoid mass, ulcerated mass, thickened gastric wall

DIAGNOSTIC STUDIES AND FINDINGS—cont'd

Diagnostic test	Findings
Esophagogastroscopy with biopsy and exfoliative cytologic study (brush or lavage cytologic study)	Malignancy may be visualized; gastric cells obtained for cytologic study may reveal malignancy; biopsy may reveal malignancy
Computed tomography (CT) scan	May provide preoperative staging information and may be used to estimate resectability; may show metastases
Magnetic resonance imaging	May be used to estimate resectability
Ultrasound (endoscopic) scan	May be used to assess depth of gastric wall penetration and to estimate resectability

Note: Both a barium study and endoscopy are recommended for diagnostic evaluation, since neither is 100% accurate in detecting gastric malignancies.

MEDICAL MANAGEMENT

GENERAL MANAGEMENT

IV fluid and electrolyte replacement may be indicated for patient who cannot ingest adequate fluids or who is bleeding; blood replacement may be indicated for patient with massive bleeding. Enteral feedings (e.g., jejunostomy tube feedings) or TPN may be indicated for a patient with obstructive malignancy to improve nutritional status before surgery; may also be used to maintain nutritional status after surgery in a patient who has undergone partial or total gastrectomy.

N/G tube to suction may be indicated to provide temporary gastric decompression in a patient with pyloric obstruction.

Radiation therapy may be administered after surgery.

SURGERY

Total gastrectomy with en bloc removal of spleen and omentum for lesion in proximal third of stomach; subtotal gastrectomy with omentectomy and removal of relevant nodes en bloc for lesion in distal two thirds of stomach.

Note: Additional structures (e.g., tail of pancreas) may be resected if necessary to achieve en bloc resection of tumor. Adequate margins of resection *must* be obtained and verified by frozen section; 5-cm clearance of tumor in all dimensions is considered adequate.

Gastrojejunostomy may be indicated for palliative management of unresectable obstructing tumor.

DRUG THERAPY

Combination chemotherapy may be given in conjunction with radiation therapy after surgery:

5-Fluorouracil (5-FU): 12 mg/kg IV for 4 days; 6 mg/kg IV on days 6, 8, 10, and 12; maintenance, 10-15 mg/kg weekly as single dose.

Doxorubicin (Adriamycin): 60-75 mg/m^2 q 3 wk, *or* 30 mg/m^2 on days 1-3 of 4-wk cycle.

Mitomycin C (Mutamycin): 2 mg/m^2 daily for 5 days, drug is then omitted for 2 days, and the cycle is repeated; *or* 20 mg/m^2 as a single dose and repeat in 6-8 wk.

1 ASSESS

ASSESSMENT	OBSERVATIONS
Medical history	May report pernicious anemia, chronic gastritis, or previous gastric surgery
Risk factors	May report routine alcohol consumption and cigarette smoking; may report diet high in complex carbohydrates, grains, and salt but low in animal fat, animal protein, leafy green vegetables, and fresh fruit
Tolerance of oral food and fluids	May report difficulty swallowing; may report vague epigastric distress; may report anorexia, nausea, vomiting; may report distaste for meat; may report persistent feelings of fullness
Nutritional status	May report recent weight loss; may exhibit signs of malnutrition (e.g., muscle wasting; fissures in corners of mouth; joint edema; dry, pluckable hair); may report severe dysphagia or frequent vomiting
Abdominal assessment	May reveal palpable mass, enlarged liver, palpable supraclavicular lymph nodes, ascites (physical findings usually are present only with advanced disease)
Emotional status and coping skills	May report mixed emotions (e.g., anxiety, fear, depression, anger, disbelief, optimism); may report inability to sleep or to complete ADLs; may report increased tension and conflict with family members; may report difficulty with decision making about health care and lack of understanding regarding treatment options

2 DIAGNOSE

NURSING DIAGNOSIS	SUBJECTIVE FINDINGS	OBJECTIVE FINDINGS
Impaired swallowing related to esophagogastric obstruction	Reports difficulty swallowing food and may report difficulty swallowing fluids; may report choking sensations	Limits oral intake to fluids or may refuse both solids and fluids; may experience choking
Altered nutrition: less than body requirements related to difficulty swallowing, anorexia, nausea, or vomiting	Reports recent weight loss; reports loss of appetite and distaste for meat; may report difficulty swallowing; may report feeling full with minimal intake; may report nausea and vomiting	Weight is below 85%-90% of usual weight; shows signs of malnutrition (e.g., pluckable hair, dry skin, fissures at corners of mouth, joint edema)
Anticipatory grieving related to diagnosis and prognosis	Reports feelings of sadness or depression; may report difficulty coping with or discussing feelings; may report altered sleep patterns; may verbalize feelings regarding threat to life	Appears withdrawn or depressed (e.g., cries frequently, limits verbal interaction and eye contact, sighs frequently, shows irritability)
Ineffective family coping related to diagnosis and prognosis	Patient and family members verbalize anxiety, difficulty handling issues related to illness and diagnosis, feeling overwhelmed, inability to share feelings	Patient and family demonstrate conflicting coping styles (e.g., denial on part of family when patient needs to discuss diagnosis and issues or vice versa); interactions marked by conflict; inappropriate response to issues and situation; failure to make decisions and follow treatment plan

NURSING DIAGNOSIS	SUBJECTIVE FINDINGS	OBJECTIVE FINDINGS
Fatigue related to nutritional compromise and anemia	Complains of feeling "tired all the time" and of being unable to perform usual activities; may complain of shortness of breath with exertion	Tachypnea and tachycardia develop after limited activity; patient limits activities and appears tired and listless

3 PLAN

Patient goals

1. The patient will be free of choking sensations.
2. The patient will attain and maintain his usual weight and will maintain an adequate nutrient intake.
3. The patient will be able to openly discuss his feelings about the diagnosis and prognosis and will demonstrate adaptive responses.
4. The patient and family will demonstrate effective coping and healthy interpersonal interactions.
5. The patient will be free of fatigue.

4 IMPLEMENT

NURSING DIAGNOSIS	NURSING INTERVENTIONS	RATIONALE
Impaired swallowing related to esophagogastric obstruction	Elevate the head of the bed for meals.	This facilitates swallowing.
	Monitor patient's ability to swallow, and modify his diet accordingly, (e.g., provide soft, well-hydrated foods with additional fluids [if tolerated], or limit oral intake to fluids if patient cannot tolerate solids).	Patients with tumors of the cardiac region are at risk for choking and aspiration if swallowed bolus of food cannot pass through the esophagogastric junction.
	For patient with partial obstruction who can tolerate solids: instruct patient to chew food well.	Thorough chewing reduces the size of swallowed food bolus and reduces the risk of choking or pain.
	For patient who cannot swallow fluids: keep patient NPO, and provide oral suction for use as needed.	Patients with complete esophagogastric obstruction are at risk for choking and aspiration.
Altered nutrition: less than body requirements related to difficulty swallowing, anorexia, nausea, or vomiting	Monitor patient's nutrient intake, nutrient losses (e.g., vomiting), and indicators of nutritional status (e.g., weigh weekly).	Inadequate nutrient intake, unusual nutrient losses, and indicators of compromised nutritional status must be identified and addressed to maintain positive nutritional status.
	Modify diet based on patient's preferences and tolerance (e.g., omit meat, provide soft foods and small, frequent feedings).	These modifications promote nutrient intake.
	Collaborate with physician to obtain nutritional consultation for patient with evidence of inadequate nutrient intake (e.g., weight loss, dietary intake <75% of prescribed diet).	Nutritional assessment provides accurate information about nutrient needs, which directs nutritional intervention.

→ > >

NURSING DIAGNOSIS	NURSING INTERVENTIONS	RATIONALE
	Collaborate with physician and nutrition support team to provide enteral or parenteral nutritional support for patient who cannot maintain adequate nutritional status with oral feedings.	To prevent malnutrition, alternatives to oral nutrition must be initiated if the patient cannot maintain nutritional status with oral nutrients.
Anticipatory grieving related to diagnosis and prognosis	Provide patient and family members time to discuss their feelings and concerns; encourage ventilation.	Exploring feelings and concerns is the first level of supportive counseling and facilitates the grieving process.
	Provide accurate information and clarification (when requested) about the disease and the treatment plan.	Information and clarification help the patient confront the diagnosis and understand the issues; seeking information is an action-oriented coping strategy.
	Reassure patient and family that conflicting, confusing, and negative emotions are normal and that expressing these feelings helps in dealing with grief (e.g., by talking, crying, yelling, thinking, or writing in a journal).	Recognizing that one's reactions are normal is reassuring and gives the patient "permission" to grieve.
	Refer patient to support groups or for counseling as indicated.	Support groups may be beneficial in reducing the patient's sense of isolation and increasing his support system; counseling is indicated for individuals with previous unresolved loss or difficulty dealing with feelings.
Ineffective family coping: compromised related to diagnosis and prognosis	Provide realistic information about the disease to family members, based on their readiness for information.	Information reduces the fear of the unknown and increases the ability to cope.
	Provide opportunities for family members to discuss their feelings, concerns, and frustrations in private (away from the patient).	Family members must adapt to changes in the patient's health status and to a potentially fatal outcome; they need an opportunity to ventilate their feelings and to confront their personal issues.
	Encourage family members to share their feelings and concerns with each other and with the patient.	Open communication reduces resentment and misunderstandings and improves the ability to cope with frustrations.
	If the patient cannot carry out his usual family roles, help him and family members renegotiate tasks so that the patient contributes as much as possible.	Renegotiating tasks maintains the patient's feeling of worth and reduces other members' overload and resentment.
	Suggest family counseling as an effective management approach.	Counseling supports family members in dealing effectively with the illness and their feelings.
	Encourage the patient and family to share recreational and pleasurable activities when possible.	Shared activities reduce stress and promote closeness, which improves the ability to cope.

NURSING DIAGNOSIS	NURSING INTERVENTIONS	RATIONALE
	Acknowledge negative feelings as normal and "OK."	Acknowledging the normality of negative feelings reduces guilt and enhances coping ability.
Fatigue related to nutritional compromise and anemia	Monitor patient's activity tolerance (i.e., assess for tachycardia, tachypnea, shortness of breath after activity).	Continuous assessment of activity tolerance permits appropriate modifications in activity and schedule.
	Space activities around scheduled rest periods.	Spacing activities reduces fatigue and improves activity tolerance.

5 EVALUATE

PATIENT OUTCOME	DATA INDICATING THAT OUTCOME IS REACHED
Patient is free of choking sensations.	Patient swallows food and fluids without difficulty and has no sensation of choking, *or* patient with obstructing lesion uses oral suction to handle secretions and has no choking sensations.
Patient has attained and maintains usual weight and adequate nutrition.	Weight is within 90% of usual weight; patient consumes at least 75% of prescribed diet or receives enteral or parenteral support; there are no signs of malnutrition (e.g., muscle wasting; fissures at corners of mouth; dry, pluckable hair; joint edema).
Patient can discuss feelings and concerns about diagnosis and prognosis and shows adaptive responses.	Patient verbalizes feelings and concerns openly; statements reflect understanding of diagnosis and treatment plan; patient can participate in decision making about treatment plan and is able to accept support from significant others, health team members, or both.
Patient and family demonstrate effective coping and healthy interpersonal interactions.	Patient and family members share their feelings with health team members and each other and can acknowledge negative feelings; they share pleasurable experiences and negotiate issues and concerns; they report reduced conflict and increased ability to deal with issues; they deal appropriately and realistically with treatment decisions.
Patient is free of fatigue.	Patient reports reduced fatigue and improved activity tolerance; he has no feelings of exhaustion, tachycardia, tachypnea, or shortness of breath after activity.

PATIENT TEACHING ■

1. Clarify and reinforce the physician's explanations about the diagnosis, prognosis, and treatment options or treatment plan.
2. Teach the patient measures to promote tolerance of oral foods and fluids (small, frequent feedings; soft, easily swallowed foods, thorough chewing).
3. Teach the patient the importance of maintaining optimum nutritional status, and help him plan a diet that is well tolerated and nutritious, *or* explain the reason for enteral or parenteral support, and instruct the patient and family in home maintenance (if applicable).
4. Explain the treatment plan (i.e., surgery, radiation, chemotherapy, symptom control, or a combination of these): rationale, specific treatment procedures or guidelines, and measures to promote treatment effectiveness and minimize adverse reactions.
5. Provide the patient and family with information about community resources such as local support groups and the American Cancer Society.

Colorectal Cancer

Colorectal cancer refers to malignancies involving the colon or rectum. Most of these tumors (about 95%) are adenocarcinomas; the remaining 5% are carcinoid tumors, leiomyosarcomas, and lymphomas. Squamous cell cancers may occur in the anal canal.

EPIDEMIOLOGY

Colorectal cancer is considered a disease of Western culture; the incidence is high in industrialized countries such as the United States and low in less developed countries such as those in Africa and Asia. This epidemiologic pattern suggests that environmental factors play a major role in the pathogenesis of colorectal cancer; the importance of environmental factors is further supported by the fact that emigrants migrating from low-incidence to high-incidence countries show an increased incidence of colorectal cancer as cultural assimilation occurs.

In the United States colorectal cancer is the second most common type of visceral malignancy; the probability of developing colorectal cancer by 70 years of age is about 4%. The incidence is somewhat higher among men than women, and cancer of the colon is about twice as common as cancer of the rectum.

Risk factors for colorectal cancer include polyposis syndromes, ulcerative colitis of more than 10 years' duration, Crohn's disease, and dietary factors. Polyposis syndromes predisposing to colorectal cancer include familial adenomatous polyposis (FAP), Turcot syndrome, and Gardner's syndrome. Familial adenomatous polyposis is the most common of these syndromes and is associated with a lifetime risk of developing colorectal cancer that approaches 100%. Recommendations for prevention include total colectomy for patients who are diagnosed with polyposis syndromes and routine screening (with air and contrast barium enema or colonoscopy) for children of patients with familial polyposis; screening should begin at 15 years of age and should be carried out at least annually until about 30 years of age. These screening recommendations are based on the fact that children of parents with polyposis have a 50% chance of developing the syndrome.

Ulcerative colitis and Crohn's disease are both associated with an increased risk of colorectal cancer, with ulcerative colitis being the more significant risk. The risk of colorectal cancer development in ulcerative colitis is cumulative; although it is low in the first 10 years after the onset of the disease, the incidence rises to about 20% in each subsequent decade. These patients require repeated screening beginning about 10 years af-

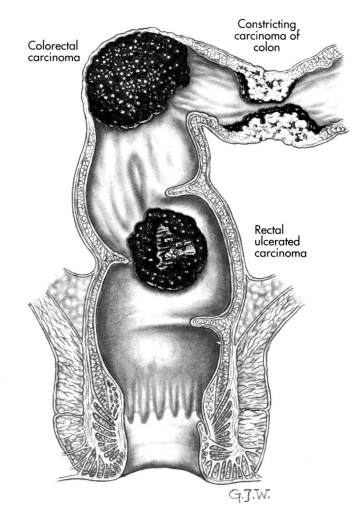

Colorectal carcinoma

Constricting carcinoma of colon

Rectal ulcerated carcinoma

G.J.W.

COLORECTAL CARCINOMA

ter onset of the disease; propnylactic proctocolectomy is recommended for any evidence of dysplasia. The incidence of colorectal cancer in patients with Crohn's disease is less clearly defined but is variably estimated to be between three and 20 times that of the general population.

Dietary factors are thought to be the key environmental factor contributing to the higher incidence of colorectal cancer in industrialized countries. Specifically, a diet high in saturated fat and meat and low in fiber is thought to contribute to the development of colorectal cancer; large amounts of saturated fat and meat may contribute to production of carcinogens, whereas fiber is thought to play a protective role, partly by diluting the fecal mass and any carcinogens and partly by altering the colonic flora and fecal pH, which may interfere with the production of carcinogens. Micronutrients such as beta-carotene and calcium may also play a protective role; the effects of diets that are low in fat, high in fiber, and that routinely include fruits and vegetables are currently under study.

Table 5-1

RECOMMENDED SCREENING FOR COLORECTAL CANCER

Screening procedure	Guidelines	Rationale
Digital rectal examination	Should be performed annually after age 40	Many colorectal cancers are located within reach of examining finger
Stool for guaiac	Should be performed annually after age 50	Earliest sign of colorectal cancer is painless, microscopic bleeding
	Serial specimens (3) recommended	Colorectal cancers bleed intermittently
	High-fiber "prep" diet recommended for 48-72 h before beginning specimen collection	Fiber may stimulate bleeding if cancer is present
	Omission of red meat and vitamin C recommended for 48-72 h before beginning test	Red meat and vitamin C can cause false-positive results
Proctosigmoidoscopy	Annually × 2 after age 50; then q 3-5 yr as long as two initial studies are normal and patient is asymptomatic	Proctosigmoidoscopy permits visual inspection of the rectosigmoid mucosa and prophylactic polypectomy if necessary

Whatever the causative factors, most colorectal cancers are thought to develop from adenomatous polyps. The relationship between adenomatous polyps and adenocarcinoma has been extensively studied, and considerable evidence supports the theory of an adenoma-carcinoma sequence. Although most polyps do not progress to cancer, the evidence is that most cancers do arise from polyps. This adenoma-carcinoma relationship is the basis for routine sigmoidoscopy and prophylactic polypectomy as screening measures for adults over 50 years of age and other high-risk individuals. The value of prophylactic polypectomy is underscored by the findings in one large study, in which routine colonoscopy and prophylactic removal of any identified polyps were shown to reduce the incidence of colorectal cancer to a fraction of that among the general population. Certain polyps seem to have greater malignant potential; these include adenomatous polyps that are sessile (rather than pedunculated), villous (rather than tubular), and large (bigger than 1.5 to 2 cm).

PATHOPHYSIOLOGY

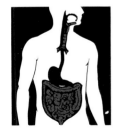
The pathologic effects of colorectal cancer involve intestinal obstruction; bleeding caused by tumor invasion of blood vessels, and the resulting anemia; and metastasis that affects adjacent or distal structures. Symptoms vary and are determined by the location of the lesion and the stage of the disease; the prognosis also varies and depends on the stage of the disease, specifically the involvement of lymph nodes and adjacent structures, the degree of cellular differentiation, and whether distant metastases are present. Unfortunately, early disease usually produces only minimal, vague symptoms, which delays diagnosis and adversely affects the prognosis.

The 5-year survival rate for localized lesions is 80% to 90%; once the disease has spread to adjacent structures and lymph nodes, the 5-year survival rate drops to 35% to 65%, and 5-year survival for patients with distant metastases is rare. These statistics emphasize the importance of routine screening of asymptomatic individuals and of public education regarding early symptoms of colorectal cancer. The American Cancer Society recommends routine screening for asymptomatic individuals beginning at 40 years of age, when the incidence of colorectal cancer begins to increase. Table 5-1 outlines recommended screening techniques, guidelines, and rationales. Public education is a continuing challenge; it focuses on the importance of early detection and the curability of most early lesions, and recommended screening measures and recognition of early signs of colorectal cancer. Education campaigns also stress the fact that colostomy is *not* usually necessary when lesions are detected early; most localized colorectal cancers can be cured with resection and reanastomosis.

Colorectal cancers can be categorized as right-sided lesions, left-sided lesions, and rectal lesions. Figure 5-2 compares the most common signs and symptoms according to location. Right-sided lesions are more commonly associated with significant blood loss, causing anemia and weakness; left-sided lesions are more likely to cause obstruction, because they tend to be constricting, "apple core" lesions. Rectal cancer may cause alternating constipation and diarrhea and a sense of incomplete emptying, or constant fecal urgency (tenesmus). **(For a color picture of adenocarcinoma see color plate 2 on p. x.)** Bleeding and pain can occur with any colorectal cancer, although the character and severity vary with location and the particular lesion. The American Cancer Society has identified the following as general warning signs for colorectal cancer: rectal bleeding, cramping abdominal pain, or a change in bowel habits.

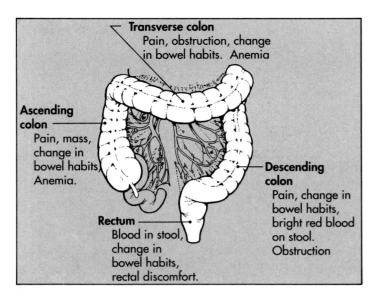

FIGURE 5-2
Signs and symptoms of colorectal cancer by location of primary lesion. Clinical manifestations are listed in order of frequency for each region (lymphatics of colon also shown). (From McCance and Huether.[36])

Any of these signs should prompt a thorough workup, including air with contrast barium enema and colonoscopy.

Colorectal cancer spreads by way of direct invasion, lymphatic invasion, and hematogenous invasion. Initially the tumor is confined to the mucosal and submucosal layers; as invasion progresses, it penetrates the deeper layers and finally the serosa and may then spread to adjacent structures and organs. Lymphatic spread may occur via the intramural lymphatics, which are located in the submucosal layer, or through the mesenteric lymphatics, which are adjacent to the mesenteric blood vessels. Lymphatic and hematogenous spread usually produces metastases in the liver or the lungs because of the patterns of venous and lymphatic drainage.

The two most commonly used staging systems for colorectal cancer are the Dukes' classification system and the system established by the American Joint Committee on Cancer; these two systems are compared in the text on the inside back cover.

Surgical resection is the mainstay of therapy for localized disease; it involves resection of the tumor itself with adequate margins and resection of the regional lymphatics and blood vessels. Surgical resection of isolated liver or lung metastases has been shown to improve survival, with a 20% "cure rate" when the metastatic lesions can be removed completely with free margins. Surgery may also be used for palliation; fecal diversions may be used to prevent or relieve obstruction, and resection of the primary tumor has been shown to improve both length of survival and quality of life in patients with disease that cannot be completely resected. The role of adjuvant therapy is receiving intensive study; new chemotherapeutic agents and new combinations of chemotherapy and radiation therapy recently have been found to reduce the recurrence rate and to improve survival in patients with residual or systemic disease. Radiation therapy is used before surgery to improve resectability and after surgery as adjuvant therapy for lesions involving adjacent structures or regional lymph nodes. Chemotherapy is used for patients with systemic disease and is being evaluated for potential benefit in patients with locally extensive disease; recent research indicates improved survival time for patients with locally invasive disease when adjuvant therapy includes chemotherapy as well as radiation.

COMPLICATIONS

Anemia
Intestinal obstruction
Death

DIAGNOSTIC STUDIES AND FINDINGS

Diagnostic test	Findings
Hemoglobin and hematocrit	May be low due to bleeding
Stool for occult blood (guaiac)	May be positive
Endoscopy (proctosigmoidoscopy or colonoscopy)	Malignant lesion or suspicious polyps; biopsy reveals malignancy
Barium enema with air and contrast	Filling defect or constricting "apple core" lesion
Computed tomography (CT) scan of liver, lungs, or brain	May reveal metastatic lesions
Liver studies	Abnormal results may be seen in patient with metastatic disease involving the liver
Intrarectal ultrasound scan	May reveal lymph node involvement

Diagnostic test	Findings
Carcinoembryonic antigen (CEA)	May be elevated in patient with colorectal cancer (some colorectal tumors secrete CEA); if preoperative level is elevated, serial CEA levels are obtained to monitor for recurrence (if preoperative level was high and level returned to normal after surgery, a subsequent rise usually indicates recurrence) *Note:* CEA is not an effective screening study, because not all colorectal tumors secrete the antigen

MEDICAL MANAGEMENT

GENERAL MANAGEMENT

For the patient with intestinal obstruction: NPO status, IV fluids, and N/G tube to suction.

For the patient with severe anemia: Administration of whole blood or packed RBCs may be required.

Radiation therapy may be administered preoperatively to improve resectability or postoperatively as adjuvant therapy to improve survival time.

SURGERY

Primary segmental resection with end-to-end anastomosis for resectable, nonobstructing lesion (e.g., right hemicolectomy for lesion in right colon; transverse colectomy for lesion in transverse colon; left hemicolectomy for lesion in descending colon; sigmoid resection for lesion in sigmoid colon; low anterior resection of rectum for lesion in proximal two thirds of rectum).

Abdominoperineal resection of rectum with end sigmoid colostomy for lesion in distal one third of rectum (when unable to obtain adequate margins of resection [i.e., 2 cm distal to tumor] without removing or destroying anal sphincter).

Temporary diverting colostomy followed by segmental resection, end-to-end anastomosis, and takedown of colostomy for obstructing lesion. (Temporary colostomy provides decompression of obstructed bowel and allows bowel preparation before resection.)

Temporary colostomy may be done in conjunction with low anterior resection to provide fecal diversion while low rectal anastomosis heals; colostomy is closed once anastomosis has healed.

Colostomy or ileostomy may be performed as palliation for unresectable obstructing lesion.

En bloc resection of adjacent organs and structures attached to malignant tumor (e.g., small bowel loops, uterus, coccyx) is indicated for curative surgical resection.

Oophorectomy is recommended for women with locally invasive colorectal cancer (to reduce recurrence).

DRUG THERAPY

5-FU (5-fluorouracil): 12 mg/kg daily IV for 4 days; 6 mg/kg daily on days 6, 8, 10, and 12; maintenance, 10-15 mg/kg weekly; may also be given as infusion into portal vein.

Leucovorin calcium (Citrovorum): May be given to permit higher doses of 5-FU.

Mutamycin (Mitomycin): 2 mg/m^2 daily for 5 days; omit for 2 days, and repeat cycle; *or* 20 mg/m^2 as single dose, and repeat in 6-8 weeks.

Note: Stop drug if platelets are <75,000/mm^3 or WBC is <3,000/mm^3.

Floxuridine (FUDR): IV, 0.1-0.6 mg/kg daily for 4 days; intraarterial, 0.1-0.6 mg/kg daily for 1-6 wk; hepatic artery, 0.4-0.6 mg/kg daily for 1-6 wk.

Levamisole is a new drug that was found in a large trial to reduce recurrence by 41% and the death rate by 33% when given in conjunction with 5-FU.

1 ASSESS

ASSESSMENT	OBSERVATIONS
Family and medical history	May report family members with polyposis syndromes; may report history of ulcerative colitis, Crohn's disease, or colorectal polyps
Risk factors	May report diet high in fat and meat and low in fiber, fruits, and vegetables
Bowel function	May report increasing problems with constipation, alternating constipation and diarrhea, or change in caliber of stool (may describe stool as "pencil size" or "ribbonlike"); may report rectal bleeding or blood-streaked or tarry stools; may report complete obstipation (inability to pass stool) and increasing abdominal distention (with obstructing lesion); may report feelings of incomplete evacuation or a constant sense of fecal urgency
Activity tolerance	May report increasing fatigue, shortness of breath with exertion, inability to complete usual activities
Pain	May report cramping abdominal pain, rectal pain, or abdominal and low back pain
Rectal examination	May reveal palpable lesion in rectal vault
Abdominal assessment	May reveal palpable mass or enlarged liver (with advanced disease and liver metastasis); may reveal distention (with obstruction)
Emotional status and coping skills	May report mixed emotions (e.g., anger, anxiety, fear, depression, disbelief, optimism); may report inability to sleep or complete ADLs; may report increased tension and conflict with family members; may report difficulty making decisions about health care. May lack understanding of options

2 DIAGNOSE

NURSING DIAGNOSIS	SUBJECTIVE FINDINGS	OBJECTIVE FINDINGS
Constipation related to obstructing lesion	Reports constipation or difficulty getting bowels to move; reports alternating bouts of constipation and diarrhea; may report total inability to pass stool; may report frequent use of laxatives or enemas to produce bowel movements	Small-caliber stools; abdominal distention
Diarrhea related to obstructing lesion or effects of pelvic radiation	Reports diarrhea alternating with constipation *or* frequent loose stools	Frequent loose stools that may have a foul odor (obstructing lesion)
Pain related to intestinal distention or malignant invasion of neural structures	Reports cramping abdominal pain, abdominal and lower back pain, or rectal pain	Facial expressions reflect pain; assumes knees-flexed position
Fatigue related to anemia or pelvic radiation	Complains of feeling tired all the time and of being unable to complete usual activities; may complain of shortness of breath with exertion	Tachypnea and tachycardia following limited activity; patient limits activities and appears tired and listless

NURSING DIAGNOSIS	SUBJECTIVE FINDINGS	OBJECTIVE FINDINGS
Anticipatory grieving related to diagnosis and prognosis	Reports feelings of sadness or depression; may report difficulty coping with or discussing feelings; may report altered sleep patterns; may verbalize feelings about threat to life	Appears withdrawn or depressed (e.g., cries frequently, limits verbal interaction and eye contact, sighs frequently, shows irritability)
Ineffective family coping related to diagnosis and prognosis	Patient and family members verbalize feelings of anxiety, difficulty handling issues related to illness and diagnosis, feeling of being overwhelmed, and inability to share feelings	Patient and family demonstrate conflicting coping styles (e.g., denial on part of family when patient needs to discuss diagnosis and issues or vice versa); interactions marked by conflict; inappropriate response to issues and situation; failure to make decisions and follow treatment plan

3 PLAN

Patient goals

1. The patient will have regular bowel movements and no constipation.
2. The patient will have bowel movements of normal consistency and frequency.
3. The patient will have no abdominal, rectal, or low back pain.
4. The patient will have no feelings of fatigue.
5. The patient will be able to openly discuss his feelings about the diagnosis and prognosis and will demonstrate adaptive responses.
6. The patient and family will demonstrate effective coping and healthy interpersonal interactions.

4 IMPLEMENT

NURSING DIAGNOSIS	NURSING INTERVENTIONS	RATIONALE
Constipation related to obstructing lesion	Monitor frequency, consistency, and volume of bowel movements.	Early detection of constipation permits prompt intervention.
	Encourage adequate fluid and fiber intake.	Fiber and fluid produce a soft, easily eliminated stool and promote peristalsis.
	Encourage physical activity as tolerated.	Activity promotes peristalsis.
	Administer laxatives and enemas as ordered and needed.	Laxatives and enemas promote peristalsis and produce a more fluid stool; fluid stools are more easily eliminated with a partially obstructing lesion.
	For patient with complete obstipation and increasing abdominal distention: prepare patient for surgery.	Emergency surgery is required to relieve obstruction and provide for fecal diversion.

→ > >

NURSING DIAGNOSIS	NURSING INTERVENTIONS	RATIONALE
Diarrhea related to obstructing lesion or effects of pelvic radiation	Measure and record volume and consistency of diarrheal stools.	This permits determination of the volume of fluid lost.
	Monitor fluid intake and urine output.	Output (stool and urine) exceeding intake and reduced urine output are indicators of fluid volume deficit.
	Provide fluid replacement (PO or IV) as ordered and tolerated.	Replacement of fluids is essential to maintain plasma volume and tissue perfusion.
	For patient with diarrhea related to pelvic radiation: encourage "constipating" foods such as pasta, rice, cheese, and dairy products.*	Certain foods and fluids have a thickening effect on stool consistency.
	For patient with diarrhea related to pelvic radiation: administer antidiarrheals as ordered (e.g., loperamide, diphenoxylate, or bulk agents); *Note:* Instruct patient not to take OTC antidiarrheal agents such as Pepto-Bismol unless approved by his physician.*	Antidiarrheal drugs may be beneficial for patients with radiation-induced diarrhea, because they reduce intestinal motility or help to thicken the stool (bulk agents); bismuth-containing drugs (e.g., Pepto-Bismol) are not recommended, since the bismuth, a metallic agent, may act to concentrate radiation in the bowel lumen.
	For patient with radiation-induced diarrhea: instruct patient to avoid enemas and colostomy irrigations.	Enemas and colostomy irrigations stimulate peristalsis and increase diarrhea.
	Provide perianal skin protection: sealants to intact skin; moisture barrier cream to intact, erythematous, or denuded skin.	Sealants and moisture barrier ointments provide protective coatings and help prevent perianal breakdown.
Pain related to intestinal distention or malignant invasion of neural structures	Monitor patient for type and severity of pain.	Type and severity of pain provides clues to cause (e.g., severe cramping pain may indicate worsening obstruction).
	Administer analgesics as ordered and needed.	Analgesics help to control severe pain.
	For patient with obstipation and worsening distention: keep patient NPO; insert N/G tube to suction as ordered (or assist with insertion).	Withholding oral intake reduces distention and pain; N/G intubation provides proximal decompression, which reduces distention and pain.
Fatigue related to anemia or pelvic radiation	Monitor patient's activity tolerance (i.e., assess for tachycardia, tachypnea, or shortness of breath following activity).	Continual assessment of activity tolerance permits appropriate modifications in activity and schedule.
	Space activities with scheduled rest periods.	Spacing activities reduces fatigue and improves activity tolerance.

*Constipating foods and antidiarrheal drugs are contraindicated for the patient with an obstructing lesion causing alternating constipation and diarrhea, because reducing intestinal motility or thickening the stool may precipitate obstipation and complete obstruction.

NURSING DIAGNOSIS	NURSING INTERVENTIONS	RATIONALE
	Administer whole blood or packed RBCs as ordered; monitor for transfusion reaction.	Whole blood or packed RBCs may be required to correct severe anemia.
Anticipatory grieving related to diagnosis and prognosis	Provide patient and family members time to discuss their feelings and concerns; encourage ventilation.	Exploring feelings and concerns is the first level of supportive counseling and facilitates the grieving process.
	Provide accurate information and clarification (when requested) about the disease and the treatment plan.	Information and clarification help the patient confront the diagnosis and understand the issues; seeking information is an action-oriented coping strategy.
	Reassure patient and family that conflicting, confusing, and negative emotions are normal and that expressing these feelings is helpful in dealing with grief (e.g., by talking, crying, yelling, thinking, or writing in a journal).	Recognizing that one's reactions are normal is reassuring and gives the patient "permission" to grieve.
	Refer patient to support groups or for counseling as indicated.	Support groups may be beneficial in reducing the patient's sense of isolation and increasing his support system; counseling is indicated for individuals with previous unresolved loss or difficulty dealing with feelings.
Ineffective family coping related to diagnosis and prognosis	Provide family members with realistic information about the disease according to their readiness for information.	Information reduces the fear of the unknown and increases the ability to cope.
	Provide opportunities for family members to discuss their feelings, concerns, and frustrations in private (away from the patient).	Family members must adapt to changes in the patient's health status and to a potentially fatal outcome; they need an opportunity to ventilate their feelings and to confront their personal issues.
	Encourage family members to share their feelings and concerns with each other and the patient.	Open communication reduces resentment and misunderstandings and improves the ability to cope with frustrations.
	If patient cannot carry out usual family roles, help him and family renegotiate tasks so that the patient contributes as much as possible.	Renegotiating tasks maintains patient's feelings of worth and reduces other members' overload and resentment.
	Suggest family counseling as an effective management approach.	Counseling supports family members in dealing effectively with the illness and their feelings.
	Encourage patient and family to share recreational and pleasurable activities when possible.	Shared activities reduce stress and promote closeness, which improves the ability to cope.
	Acknowledge negative feelings as normal and "OK."	Acknowledging the normality of negative feelings reduces guilt and enhances coping ability.

→ > >

5   EVALUATE

PATIENT OUTCOME	DATA INDICATING THAT OUTCOME IS REACHED
Patient has regular bowel movements and has no constipation.	Patient reports regular bowel movements of soft to formed consistency *or* states that he can eliminate stool by means of laxatives and enemas; patient's abdomen is soft and non-distended.
Patient's bowel movements are of normal consistency and frequency.	Patient reports that diarrhea is resolved; stools are soft or, if stools are liquid, frequency of stools is normal.
Patient has no abdominal, rectal, or low back pain.	Patient states that pain has resolved or is well controlled; his facial expressions do not reflect pain.
Patient has no feelings of fatigue.	Patient reports reduced fatigue and improved activity tolerance; patient has no feelings of exhaustion, tachycardia, tachypnea, or shortness of breath following activity.
Patient can discuss feelings and concerns about diagnosis and prognosis and shows adaptive responses.	Patient verbalizes feelings and concerns openly; his statements reflect understanding of the diagnosis and treatment plan; patient takes part in decision making about treatment plan and can accept support from significant others, health team members, or both.
Patient and family demonstrate effective coping and healthy interpersonal interactions.	Patient and family members share their feelings with health team members and each other; they acknowledge negative feelings and are able to share pleasurable experiences and to negotiate issues and concerns; they report reduced conflict and increased ability to deal with issues, and they deal appropriately and realistically with treatment decisions.

PATIENT TEACHING

1. Clarify and reinforce the physician's explanations about the diagnosis, prognosis, and treatment options or treatment plan.
2. Teach the patient measures to maintain normal bowel elimination (i.e., measures to prevent constipation or control diarrhea).
3. Explain the treatment plan (i.e., surgery, radiation, chemotherapy, symptom control, or a combination of these): rationale, specific treatment procedures or guidelines, and measures to promote the regimen's effectiveness and minimize adverse reactions.
4. If applicable, explain the purpose and basic management of colostomy, and refer the patient to the enterostomal therapy (ET) nurse for in-depth management.
5. Provide the patient and family with information about community resources such as support groups (e.g., United Ostomy Association for patient with colostomy) and the American Cancer Society.

Pancreatic Cancer

Pancreatic cancer refers to malignancies affecting the exocrine pancreas; most of these tumors (about 75%) are adenocarcinomas.

EPIDEMIOLOGY

The incidence of pancreatic cancer is rising steadily; in the United States it is more common than cancer of the stomach, with about 27,000 new cases reported each year. It is more common in men than in women (1.7:1 ratio) and in blacks than in whites. Most patients are over 60 years of age, with the peak incidence occurring between 70 and 80 years of age. It is more lethal than any other malignancy, with a death rate of about 95%.

The etiology of pancreatic cancer is unknown, although heavy cigarette smoking has been shown to increase the risk as much as fivefold. The disease seems to be more common in Western cultures, suggesting that high-fat diets are a risk factor. Some studies have suggested that the risk is higher for persons in certain occupations (e.g., chemists, metal workers, and gas plant workers), and for persons with chronic pancreatitis, diabetes, and cirrhosis; however, these are preliminary findings that have not been confirmed.

PATHOPHYSIOLOGY

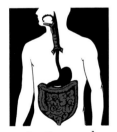

Pancreatic cancer tends to be a silent disease until it has already metastasized; early symptoms usually are mild and nonspecific. The lack of defined symptoms, coupled with the retroperitoneal location of the pancreas and its inaccessibility to palpation and direct radiologic examination, make early diagnosis extremely difficult. As a result, most patients (86%) have demonstrable metastatic disease at the time of diagnosis. The lateness of diagnosis is a key factor in the extremely high mortality rate.

The triad of symptoms most commonly seen with pancreatic cancer is abdominal or back pain, weight loss, and jaundice. The most common symptom is pain; the location, severity, and characteristics of the pain vary, depending on the location of the malignancy and the stage of the disease. Lesions in the head of the pancreas commonly cause midepigastric and right upper quadrant pain, with radiation to the back; the pain usually is described as steady, dull, and aching. Lesions in the body of the pancreas cause midabdominal pain, whereas lesions in the tail produce pain that localizes to the left upper quadrant. The pain may be described as colicky, dull,

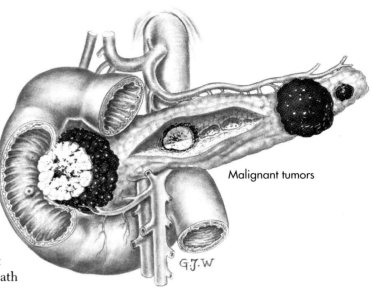

Malignant tumors

CARCINOMA OF PANCREAS

aching, boring, or sharp and intermittent. Severe, unrelenting pain suggests extension of the malignancy into the retroperitoneal tissues and nerve plexuses. The pain of pancreatic cancer may be temporarily relieved or reduced by leaning forward in the sitting position.

Weight loss, the second most common symptom, may be caused by anorexia and nausea or by the effects of obstruction of the common bile duct and pancreatic duct, which results in impaired digestion of fat and protein. Additional symptoms that may occur include weakness and fatigue, early satiety, vomiting, and diarrhea; early satiety, postprandial fullness, nausea and vomiting, and gastrointestinal bleeding (with resultant anemia and weakness) all relate to erosion of the duodenal mucosa by the malignancy.

The most common physical finding is jaundice, which is caused by invasion or obstruction of the common bile duct. Additional physical findings include hepatomegaly, visible or palpable enlargement of the gallbladder, abdominal tenderness, and occasionally an abdominal mass. Tumor invasion of the splenic artery may produce a bruit in the periumbilical area or left upper quadrant.

Pancreatic cancer is classified as stage I (confined to the pancreas), stage II (involving regional lymph nodes), or stage III (distant metastases present). As noted earlier, distant metastasis is present at initial diagnosis in most cases. The most common site of metastatic disease is the liver; other common sites include the peritoneum and the lungs. In addition to distant metastasis, the tumor may extend locally to involve adjacent structures such as the stomach, biliary tree, and small intestine.

Treatment of pancreatic cancer currently involves primarily surgical resection; curative procedures involve radical resection of all structures involved in the malignant process and reconstruction of the gastrointestinal tract, whereas palliative procedures are designed to relieve obstruction and provide some degree of symptom control. Radiation therapy and chemotherapy may be used as adjuvant therapy. Although the current long-term survival rate is extremely low, there are encouraging reports of improved survival among select groups of patients undergoing radical surgical procedures and new combinations of radiation and chemotherapy.

COMPLICATIONS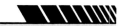

Biliary obstruction	Malnutrition
Gastrointestinal bleeding	Diabetes mellitus
Pancreatic exocrine insufficiency	Death

DIAGNOSTIC STUDIES AND FINDINGS

Diagnostic test	Findings
Hemoglobin and hematocrit	May be lowered due to gastrointestinal bleeding
Stool for occult blood	May be positive in patient with GI bleeding
Stool for fat and protein	May be positive
Liver function tests	May be abnormal (elevated bilirubin and enzymes; decreased albumin)
Carcinoembryonic antigen	May be elevated
Upper gastrointestinal series	May show extrinsic compression of the duodenum or infiltration of duodenal mucosa; may be used to rule out other disorders of upper GI tract
Ultrasound scan	May reveal lesion, especially if it is >2 cm and is located in head of pancreas; lesions in body and tail of pancreas are more difficult to detect with ultrasound *Note:* Endoscopic ultrasound can detect lesions <20 mm in diameter
Computed tomography (CT) scan	May show change in size or contour of gland; may show edema, atrophy, or dilation of pancreatic duct
Selective angiography	May reveal infiltrative hypovascular lesions or may show arterial displacement by tumor (uncommon); may show arterial occlusion and narrowing in advanced disease; may be used to determine resectability and to identify major vessels before surgery
Endoscopic retrograde cholangiopancreatography (ERCP) (diagnostic procedure of choice in most centers)	Used to distinguish between pancreatitis and pancreatic carcinoma; permits aspiration of pancreatic juice for cytologic studies
Percutaneous transhepatic cholangiography (PTC)	May reveal partial or complete obstruction of common bile duct just above pancreatic head (in cancer of the head of the pancreas); permits aspiration for cytologic studies
Percutaneous pancreatic biopsy under radiologic guidance	Provides definitive diagnosis without open surgical procedure

MEDICAL MANAGEMENT

GENERAL MANAGEMENT

IV fluid and electrolyte replacement for patient with nausea and vomiting precluding adequate oral intake.

Administration of whole blood or packed RBCs for patient with severe anemia caused by GI bleeding.

High-calorie, low-fat diet for patient with weight loss and fat intolerance.

Nutritional support (enteral or parenteral) for malnourished patient to restore positive nitrogen balance before surgery.

Radiation therapy (intraoperative, external beam, or interstitial implants) as adjuvant or palliative therapy.

Endoscopic placement of biliary stents to prevent biliary obstruction.

Continued.

MEDICAL MANAGEMENT—cont'd

SURGERY

Exploratory laparotomy to provide accurate diagnosis and determine resectability.

Pancreaticoduodenectomy for periampullary lesions (tumors located around Vater's ampulla) and cancers of the head of the pancreas (when there is no evidence of distant metastasis). (Involves resection of distal stomach, gallbladder, distal common bile duct, duodenum, and proximal pancreas; reconstruction involves choledochojejunostomy, pancreaticojejunostomy, and gastrojejunostomy.)

Total pancreatectomy is performed in some centers for cancers of the head of the pancreas.

Biliary bypass procedures are indicated for patients with unresectable disease and biliary obstruction: cholecystojejunostomy *or* cholecystectomy with choledochojejunostomy, *or* percutaneous placement of biliary stents.

Chemical splanchnicectomy (with ethyl alcohol or phenol): To control pain.

Distal pancreatectomy for lesions of the body or tail of the pancreas.

DRUG THERAPY

Narcotic analgesics (e.g., morphine sulfate): As needed to control pain.

Antiemetics (e.g., promethazine): As needed to control nausea and vomiting.

Fluorouracil (5-FU): 12 mg/kg daily IV for 4 days; 6 mg/kg daily on days 6, 8, 10, and 12; maintenance, 10-15 mg/kg weekly as single dose (adjuvant therapy).

Streptozocin (Zantosar): 500 mg/m^2 for 5 days q 6 wk until desired response; alternate with 1,000 mg/m^2 for 2 wk (adjuvant therapy).

Vitamin K: Before surgery, to restore normal clotting (for patient with malabsorption of fat-soluble vitamins).

Broad-spectrum antibiotics: Preoperatively for patient undergoing surgical resection.

Insulin and pancreatic enzymes (e.g., Cotazym): May be required for patient who has had total pancreatectomy or who develops exocrine and endocrine insufficiency.

---

1 ASSESS

ASSESSMENT	OBSERVATIONS
Pain	May report epigastric and right upper quadrant pain that is steady, dull, aching, and radiates to back (lesions in head of pancreas); may report pain in midabdominal area (lesions in body of pancreas) or left upper quadrant (tail of pancreas); may describe pain as colicky, dull, boring, aching, or sharp; may sit and lean forward to obtain partial relief; facial expressions may reflect pain
Nutritional status	May report recent weight loss; present weight may be less than 85%-90% of usual weight; may report early satiety, postprandial fullness, anorexia, nausea, and vomiting; may limit nutrient intake; may have fatty stools; may exhibit signs of glucose intolerance (thirst, increased urine output); may exhibit signs of malnutrition (e.g., muscle wasting; dry, sparse hair; joint edema)

→ > >

ASSESSMENT	OBSERVATIONS
Activity tolerance	May complain of reduced activity tolerance, fatigue, shortness of breath and exhaustion following limited activities; may exhibit reduced activity tolerance (e.g., tachycardia and tachypnea following limited activity)
Evidence of biliary obstruction	Skin and sclerae may appear jaundiced; stools may appear clay colored; urine may appear tea colored; may complain of pruritus
Abdominal assessment	Inspection may reveal visibly enlarged gallbladder; palpation may reveal enlarged liver, enlarged gallbladder, or palpable pancreatic mass (in slender individuals); abdominal tenderness may be evident on palpation
Emotional status and coping skills (patient and family)	May report mixed emotions (e.g., anxiety, fear, depression, anger, disbelief, optimism); may report inability to sleep or complete ADLs; may report increased tension and conflict with family members; may report difficulty making decisions about health care and may demonstrate lack of understanding of options; may exhibit denial related to diagnosis

2 DIAGNOSE

NURSING DIAGNOSIS	SUBJECTIVE FINDINGS	OBJECTIVE FINDINGS
Pain related to malignant invasion of neural structures	Complains of abdominal pain that may radiate to back; may describe pain as dull and aching, colicky, or sharp and intermittent	Facial expressions reflect pain; sits and leans forward to obtain relief
Altered nutrition: less than body requirements related to anorexia, nausea, vomiting, and malabsorption	Reports recent weight loss; complains of early satiety and postprandial fullness, anorexia, nausea, or vomiting; may report fatty, foul-smelling stools	Weight is less than 85%-90% of usual weight; ingests less than 75% of diet; may exhibit signs of malnutrition (e.g., muscle wasting; joint edema; dry, sparse hair)
Fatigue related to anemia	Complains of feeling tired all the time and of being unable to complete usual activities; may complain of shortness of breath with exertion	Tachypnea and tachycardia following limited activity; limits activity and appears tired and listless
Anticipatory grieving related to diagnosis and prognosis	Reports feeling sad or depressed; may report difficulty coping with or discussing feelings; may report altered sleep patterns; may verbalize feelings about threat to life	Appears withdrawn or depressed (e.g., cries frequently, limits verbal interaction and eye contact, sighs frequently, shows irritability)
Ineffective family coping related to diagnosis and prognosis	Patient and family members verbalize feelings of anxiety, difficulty handling issues related to illness and diagnosis, feeling overwhelmed, and inability to share feelings	Patient and family demonstrate conflicting coping styles (e.g., denial on part of family when patient needs to discuss diagnosis or vice versa); interactions marked by conflict; inappropriate response to issues and situation; failure to make decisions and follow treatment plan

3 PLAN

Patient goals

1. The patient will be free of abdominal pain, or pain will be well controlled.
2. The patient will attain and maintain his usual weight and will maintain an adequate nutrient intake, or he will have no nausea or vomiting.
3. The patient will be free of fatigue.
4. The patient will be able to openly discuss his feelings about the diagnosis and prognosis and will demonstrate adaptive responses.
5. The patient and family will demonstrate effective coping and healthy interpersonal interactions.

4 IMPLEMENT

NURSING DIAGNOSIS	NURSING INTERVENTIONS	RATIONALE
Pain related to malignant invasion of neural structures	Monitor pain for location, character, and severity.	Location, character, and severity of pain provide information about disease progression and effectiveness of pain control measures.
	Help patient find a comfortable position.	Sitting and leaning forward frequently provides partial pain relief for patients with pancreatic cancer.
	Administer analgesics as ordered and needed.	Narcotic analgesics frequently are required to control the pain associated with pancreatic cancer.
	Collaborate with physician to establish effective analgesia.	Additional pain control measures may be needed to control pain.
Altered nutrition: less than body requirements related to anorexia, nausea, vomiting, and malabsorption	Monitor patient's nutrient intake, nutrient losses (e.g., vomiting), and indicators of nutritional status (e.g., weigh weekly).	Inadequate nutrient intake, unusual nutrient losses, and indicators of compromised nutritional status must be identified and addressed to maintain positive nutritional status.
	Collaborate with physician and nutritional support staff to provide enteral or parenteral nutritional support for patient scheduled for resection who exhibits signs of malnutrition (e.g., weight loss, muscle wasting).	Positive nitrogen balance is essential to promote healing and prevent postoperative complications; therefore nutritional deficits must be corrected before surgery.
	Provide low-fat diet as tolerated for patient with evidence of biliary obstruction (e.g., jaundice) or fat intolerance (e.g., fatty stools in patient who has had major resection or who has advanced disease).	Biliary obstruction reduces the patient's fat tolerance due to loss of bile flow to the duodenum; exocrine pancreatic insufficiency (due to glandular destruction or to massive pancreatic resection) results in fat intolerance due to loss of pancreatic enzymes.
	Administer pancreatic enzymes (e.g., Cotazym) as ordered (i.e., for patient who has undergone massive pancreatic resection).	Exogenous administration of pancreatic enzymes is needed to promote nutrient digestion in the patient who has undergone massive pancreatic resection.

NURSING DIAGNOSIS	NURSING INTERVENTIONS	RATIONALE
	Monitor patient for signs of glucose intolerance (e.g., excessive thirst, polyuria, elevated blood glucose).	Patient who has undergone massive pancreatic resection may develop diabetes mellitus due to loss of pancreatic islet cells.
	Administer insulin as ordered and needed.	Exogenous insulin is required for patients who cannot produce adequate amounts of endogenous insulin to prevent or correct metabolic derangements.
	For patient with terminal disease: provide oral foods and fluids as desired and tolerated.	The goal of terminal care is to provide comfort.
	Administer antiemetics as ordered and needed.	Antiemetics reduce nausea and vomiting and help improve nutrient intake.
Fatigue related to anemia	Monitor patient's activity tolerance (i.e., assess for tachycardia, tachypnea, shortness of breath following activity).	Continual assessment of activity tolerance permits appropriate modifications in activity and schedule.
	Space activities with scheduled rest periods.	This reduces fatigue and improves activity tolerance.
	Administer whole blood or packed RBCs as ordered.	Whole blood or packed RBCs may be given to correct severe anemia resulting from GI bleeding; correcting anemia improves activity tolerance.
	Help patient make appropriate adjustments in activity levels and expectations as physical status changes.	Adjusting expectations and activity levels based on physiologic status reduces frustration and fatigue.
Anticipatory grieving related to diagnosis and prognosis	Give patient and family members time to discuss their feelings and concerns; encourage ventilation.	Exploring feelings and concerns is the first level of supportive counseling and facilitates the grieving process.
	Provide accurate information and clarification (when requested) about the diagnosis, prognosis, and treatment plan.	Information and clarification help the patient and family confront the diagnosis and prognosis and understand the issues; seeking information is an action-oriented coping strategy.
	Reassure patient and family that conflicting, confusing, and negative emotions are normal and that expressing these feelings is helpful in dealing with grief (e.g., by talking, crying, yelling, thinking, or writing in a journal).	Recognizing that one's reactions are normal is reassuring and gives the patient and family "permission" to grieve.
	Refer patient and family to support groups or for counseling as indicated.	Support groups may be beneficial in reducing the patient's and family's sense of isolation and providing additional support; counseling provides assistance in dealing with issues and feelings.

NURSING DIAGNOSIS	NURSING INTERVENTIONS	RATIONALE
Ineffective family coping related to diagnosis and prognosis	Provide realistic information about the disease to family members according to their readiness for information; provide opportunities for family members to discuss their feelings, concerns, and frustrations in private (away from the patient).	Information reduces the fear of the unknown and increases the ability to cope; family members must adapt to changes in the patient's health status and to a probably fatal outcome; they need an opportunity to ventilate their feelings and to confront their personal issues.
	Encourage family members to share their feelings and concerns with each other and the patient.	Open communication reduces resentment and misunderstandings and improves the ability to cope with frustrations.
	Suggest family counseling as an effective management approach.	Counseling supports family members in dealing effectively with the illness and their feelings.
	Encourage the patient and family to share recreational and pleasurable activities when possible.	Shared activities reduce stress and promote closeness, which improves the ability to cope.
	If patient cannot carry out usual family roles, help him and family renegotiate tasks so that the patient contributes as much as possible.	Renegotiating tasks maintains patient's feelings of worth and reduces other members' overload and resentment.
	Acknowledge negative feelings as normal and "OK."	Acknowledging the normality of negative feelings reduces guilt and enhances coping ability.

5   EVALUATE

PATIENT OUTCOME	DATA INDICATING THAT OUTCOME IS REACHED
Patient has no abdominal pain; or pain is controlled.	Patient states that pain is gone or well controlled; facial expressions do not reflect pain; patient appears relaxed and comfortable.
Patient has attained and maintains usual weight and ingests adequate nutrients, or has no nausea/vomiting.	Weight is within 90% of usual; patient ingests and tolerates at least 75% of prescribed or regular diet and has no signs of malnutrition (e.g., muscle wasting; dry, sparse hair; joint edema); *or* patient states that nausea and vomiting are absent or are well controlled by medication.
Patient is free of fatigue.	Patient reports reduced fatigue and improved activity tolerance; patient has no feelings of exhaustion and no tachycardia, tachypnea, or shortness of breath following activity; *or* patient plans and spaces activities appropriately according to tolerance.
Patient can discuss his feelings and concerns about the diagnosis and prognosis and shows adaptive responses.	Patient verbalizes feelings and concerns openly; his statements reflect understanding of the diagnosis, prognosis, and treatment plan; he participates in decision making about the treatment plan and accepts support from significant others, health team members, or both.

→ › ›

PATIENT OUTCOME	DATA INDICATING THAT OUTCOME IS REACHED
Patient and family demonstrate effective coping and healthy interpersonal interactions.	Patient and family members share their feelings with health team members and each other; they acknowledge negative feelings and are able to share pleasurable experiences and negotiate issues and concerns; they report reduced conflict and increased ability to deal with issues, and they deal appropriately and realistically with treatment decisions.

PATIENT TEACHING

1. Clarify and reinforce the physician's explanations about the diagnosis, prognosis, and treatment options or treatment plan.
2. Explain the treatment plan (i.e., surgery, radiation, chemotherapy, symptom control, or a combination of these): rationale, specific treatment procedures or guidelines, and measures to promote the regimen's effectiveness and minimize adverse reactions.
3. For the patient with pancreatic insufficiency: Instruct the patient in administration of insulin and pancreatic enzymes.
4. Provide the patient and family with information about community resources such as local support groups, the American Cancer Society, home health care, and hospice organizations.

Cancer of the Liver

Cancer of the liver includes both primary and secondary (metastatic) malignancies. About 80% of primary liver cancers are hepatocellular carcinomas, also known as hepatomas; these tumors develop in the hepatocytes. Cholangiocarcinomas (tumors arising in the bile ducts) account for about 15% of primary lesions; the other 5% are hepatobiliary carcinomas or sarcomas.

EPIDEMIOLOGY

Primary liver cancers are rare in the United States, although they are common in other parts of the world. Hepatocellular carcinoma is common in Asia and Africa, possibly because of the prevalence of *Aspergillus flavus*, a mold found on spoiled corn, peanuts, and grain, which produces the carcinogen aflatoxin. Cholangiocarcinoma is common in areas where liver fluke infestation is prevalent, although the mechanism by which this infestation causes cancer is unknown.

In the United States primary liver cancer is more common in blacks than in whites and in men than in women; it most commonly occurs between 40 and 60 years of age. Although the etiology has not been established, there is a close association between the development of hepatocellular carcinoma and the presence of chronic liver disease, particularly cirrhosis and

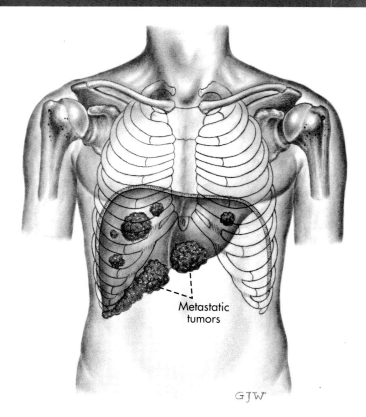

Metastatic tumors

GJW

HEPATIC CARCINOMA

chronic active hepatitis. Another risk factor is the presence of a liver cell adenoma; this is a benign lesion that is most common in women of menstrual age and that has been associated with use of oral contraceptives. Although the lesion is benign, it does sometimes become malignant and therefore should be resected or carefully monitored for malignant changes.

Most liver cancers in the United States are metastatic lesions. The most common site for primary lesions is the colon or rectum; additional sources include the pancreas, stomach, breasts, and lungs.

PATHOPHYSIOLOGY

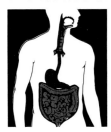 Hepatocellular carcinomas most commonly appear as a single large mass with or without satellite lesions; less commonly they occur as multiple nodules, and occasionally the disease is diffuse, with multiple small nodules scattered throughout the liver. The lesions may be confined to one lobe of the liver or may involve both lobes; the extent and location of the tumors are important factors in determining resectability. Cholangiocellular carcinomas usually are solitary lesions that develop along the bile duct and extend into the liver tissue.

Diagnosis of liver cancer typically is delayed until late in the course of the disease, when expansion of the tumor causes pain. Early symptoms usually are nonspecific and include nausea, vomiting, and dull pain or pressure in the right upper quadrant. Signs of hepatocellular carcinoma in a patient with cirrhosis include increasing jaundice and anorexia; if the tumor causes obstruction, the patient may develop ascites and other signs of worsening portal hypertension. Cholangiocellular carcinoma usually causes pain, anorexia, and weight loss; jaundice may occur as a result of bile duct obstruction. Occasionally liver tumors necrose and rupture, resulting in massive bleeding.

Liver cancer spreads initially to the hepatic veins and then to the lungs and bones.

The prognosis for individuals with liver cancer is poor. Surgical resection offers the only possibility of cure, and only 30% to 40% of patients with primary liver tumors have surgically resectable disease (defined as tumor confined to one lobe or a resectable area of the liver in a patient whose general condition is good and who has no evidence of metastases, severe cirrhosis, or marked impairment of liver function). For patients with resectable primary liver cancers, the 5-year survival rate is about 34%; for patients with resectable metastatic lesions, the 5-year survival rate is 20% to 30%. Patients with unresectable lesions receive palliation through chemotherapy, radiation, and hepatic artery ligation.

COMPLICATIONS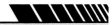

Metastatic disease	Hemorrhage
Biliary obstruction and jaundice	Malnutrition
Portal hypertension	Death

DIAGNOSTIC STUDIES AND FINDINGS

Diagnostic test	Findings
Serum alkaline phosphatase	Commonly elevated with hepatocellular carcinoma
Serum glutamic-oxaloacetic transaminase (AST)	Commonly elevated with hepatocellular carcinoma
Serum glutamic-pyruvic transaminase (ALT)	Commonly elevated with hepatocellular carcinoma
Serum bilirubin	May be elevated; marked elevations may indicate unresectable disease
Serum albumin	May be reduced in patient with cirrhosis or liver failure
Alpha-fetoprotein	May be elevated with hepatocellular carcinoma
Carcinoembryonic antigen	Elevated level may be seen with metastatic disease arising from GI tract
Chest x-ray	May reveal elevated diaphragm consistent with hepatomegaly; may reveal pulmonary lesions if metastasis has occurred
Ultrasound scan	Reveals solid lesions and distinguishes between cystic and solid tumors; cannot distinguish benign from malignant lesions
Computed tomography (CT) scan	May reveal metastatic lesions from colon or rectum (metastases are denser than primary liver tumors or normal liver tissue)
Magnetic resonance imaging (MRI) study	May be used to differentiate liver tumors from cavernous hemangiomas and to evaluate relationship of hepatic veins to tumor masses in preparation for surgical resection
Arteriography	May show changes in vessels consistent with presence of tumors (e.g., dilation, distortion, or displacement of vessels or pooling of dye in tumor area); may be used to determine arterial anatomy before resection
Liver biopsy	Reveals tumor type
Lung scan	Done to rule out metastases; surgical resection is contraindicated with metastasis
Bone scan	Done to rule out metastases; surgical resection is contraindicated with metastasis
Coagulation profile (for preoperative evaluation)	May be abnormal (prolonged clotting)

MEDICAL MANAGEMENT

GENERAL MANAGEMENT

For patient with resectable lesion scheduled for surgery:

Parenteral or enteral nutritional support as needed to correct nutritional deficits.

Administration of enemas to reduce ammonia-producing bacteria.

For patient with unresectable disease:

Oral, enteral, or parenteral nutritional support as needed to maintain nutritional status during treatment with chemotherapeutic agents.

Radiation therapy (limited to 2,000-3,000 rad) for palliation of painful liver cancers.

IV fluids and whole blood or packed RBCs as needed for patient with massive bleeding.

IV albumin as indicated for hypoalbuminemia and edema.

SURGERY

Curative resection for patient who meets criteria for resection:

Resectable lesion (i.e., confined to one lobe or a resectable area of the liver; not involving the vena cava or porta hepatis).

No cirrhosis, ascites, or jaundice.

Acceptable liver function.

No evidence of metastatic disease.

Good physical condition.

Hepatic artery ligation to induce tumor regression in patient with unresectable malignancies (this procedure contraindicated in patient with cirrhosis, ascites, or jaundice).

Paracentesis for management of severe ascites.

DRUG THERAPY

Vitamin K: May be given before surgery to support normal clotting.

Oral antibiotics (e.g., Neomycin): May be given before surgery to reduce ammonia-producing bacteria in colon.

IV antibiotics may be given during and after surgery to prevent or control infection.

Diuretics: May be given to control edema.

Narcotic analgesics (e.g., morphine sulfate): As needed to control pain.

Antiemetics (e.g., promethazine): As needed to control nausea and vomiting.

Fluorouracil (5-FU): IV, 12 mg/kg daily for 4 days; 6 mg/kg daily on days 6, 8, 10, and 12; maintenance, 10-15 mg/kg weekly as single dose (should not exceed 800 mg a day with daily dose or 1 g a week with weekly dose).

Note: Fluorouracil may also be given via portal venous infusion pump or hepatic artery infusion; infusion via hepatic artery has caused severe gastritis and biliary sclerosis.

Combination chemotherapy may be tried; agents used include methotrexate, cyclophosphamide (Cytoxan), vinblastine, and nitrogen mustard.

1 ASSESS

ASSESSMENT	OBSERVATIONS
Medical history	May report history of alcohol abuse, cirrhosis, or hepatitis; may report history of GI malignancy
Pain	May report pain in right upper quadrant; palpation may elicit complaints of tenderness in right upper quadrant
Nutritional status	May report anorexia, nausea, vomiting, and recent weight loss (weight may be less than 85%-90% of usual weight); may show signs of nutritional depletion (e.g., muscle wasting, joint edema)
Abdominal assessment	Inspection may reveal ascites; percussion and palpation may reveal hepatomegaly; palpation may elicit tenderness in right upper quadrant
Evidence of liver dysfunction	Skin and sclerae may appear jaundiced; may have ascites, signs of portal hypertension (e.g., prominent veins on abdominal wall), and evidence of impaired clotting (e.g., bruising, petechiae)
Emotional status and coping skills	May report mixed emotions (e.g., anxiety, fear, depression, anger, disbelief, optimism); may report inability to sleep or complete ADLs; may report increased tension and conflict with family members; may report difficulty making decisions about health care, and may lack understanding of options; may exhibit denial

2 DIAGNOSE

NURSING DIAGNOSIS	SUBJECTIVE FINDINGS	OBJECTIVE FINDINGS
Pain related to malignant involvement of neural structures	Complains of pain and tenderness in right upper quadrant	Facial expressions reflect pain; palpation elicits complaints of tenderness; muscle guarding may be noted on palpation
Altered nutrition: less than body requirements related to anorexia, nausea, and vomiting	Reports anorexia and recent weight loss; may report nausea and vomiting	Weight is less than 85%-90% of usual weight; ingests less than 75% of ordered diet; may show signs of malnutrition (e.g., muscle wasting, joint edema, fissures at corners of mouth)
Fluid volume excess related to liver dysfunction and hypoalbuminemia	Reports swelling in feet, legs, and abdomen; may report shortness of breath	Edema and ascites are evident; dyspnea may be evident
Activity intolerance related to anemia	Complains of feeling tired all the time and of being unable to complete usual activities; may complain of shortness of breath with exertion	Tachypnea and tachycardia following limited activity; patient limits activity and appears tired and listless
Anticipatory grieving related to diagnosis and prognosis	Patient or family reports feelings of sadness or depression; may report difficulty coping with or discussing feelings; may report altered sleep patterns; may verbalize feelings about threat to life	Appears withdrawn or depressed (e.g., cries frequently, limits verbal interaction and eye contact, sighs frequently, shows irritability); may exhibit denial

NURSING DIAGNOSIS	SUBJECTIVE FINDINGS	OBJECTIVE FINDINGS
Ineffective family coping related to diagnosis and prognosis	Patient and family members verbalize feelings of anxiety, difficulty handling issues related to illness and diagnosis, feeling overwhelmed, and inability to share feelings	Patient and family demonstrate conflicting coping styles (e.g., denial on part of family when patient needs to discuss diagnosis and issues or vice versa); interactions marked by conflict; inappropriate response to issues and situation; failure to make decisions and follow treatment plan

3 PLAN

Patient goals

1. The patient will have no pain, or the pain will be well controlled.
2. The patient will attain and maintain his usual weight and will maintain an adequate nutrient intake, or he will have no nausea or vomiting.
3. The patient will have no edema or ascites, or edema and ascites will be controlled.
4. The patient will show improved activity tolerance or will adapt his activities appropriately based on tolerance.
5. The patient and family will be able to openly discuss their feelings about the diagnosis and prognosis and will demonstrate adaptive responses.
6. The patient and family will demonstrate effective coping and healthy interpersonal interactions.

4 IMPLEMENT

NURSING DIAGNOSIS	NURSING INTERVENTIONS	RATIONALE
Pain related to malignant invasion of neural structures	Monitor pain for character and severity.	Characteristics of pain provide information about disease progression and effectiveness of pain control measures.
	Administer analgesics as ordered and needed; collaborate with physician to ensure effective pain control.	Narcotic analgesics frequently are required to control pain associated with cancer.
Altered nutrition: less than body requirements related to anorexia, nausea, and vomiting	Monitor patient's nutrient intake, nutrient losses (e.g., vomiting), and indicators of nutritional status (e.g., weigh daily or weekly).	Inadequate nutrient intake, unusual nutrient losses, and indicators of compromised nutritional status must be identified and addressed to maintain positive nutritional status.
	Collaborate with physician and nutritional support staff to provide enteral or parenteral nutritional support for patient scheduled for resection or chemotherapy and who shows signs of nutritional deficits (e.g., weight loss, muscle wasting).	Positive nitrogen balance is essential to promote healing, maintain immunocompetence, and prevent complications related to surgery or chemotherapy; therefore nutritional deficits must be corrected before treatment or surgery.
	Provide low-fat diet as tolerated for patient with evidence of biliary obstruction (e.g., jaundice).	Biliary obstruction reduces the patient's fat tolerance because of loss of bile flow to the duodenum.
	Administer antiemetics as ordered and needed.	Antiemetics improve nutrient intake by controlling nausea and vomiting.

NURSING DIAGNOSIS	NURSING INTERVENTIONS	RATIONALE
	For patient with terminal disease: provide oral foods and fluids as desired and tolerated.	The goal of terminal care is to provide comfort.
Fluid volume excess related to liver dysfunction and hypoalbuminemia	Monitor patient for increasing edema, ascites, or both.	Prompt recognition of fluid volume excess permits early intervention.
	Administer albumin as ordered.	Albumin increases oncotic pressure in blood vessels and acts as an osmotic diuretic.
	Administer diuretics as ordered.	Diuretics reduce intravascular volume by reducing reabsorption in the renal tubules and increasing urinary output.
	Elevate head of bed for patient with ascites and dyspnea.	Elevating the head of the bed increases diaphragmatic excursion and reduces shortness of breath.
	For patient with severe ascites: prepare patient for paracentesis and assist as needed.	Paracentesis removes excess ascitic fluid.
Activity intolerance related to anemia	Monitor patient's activity tolerance (i.e., assess for tachycardia, tachypnea, and shortness of breath following activity).	Continual assessment of activity tolerance permits appropriate modifications in activity and schedule.
	Space activities with scheduled rest periods.	Spacing activities reduces fatigue and improves activity tolerance.
	Help patient make appropriate adjustments in activity level and expectations as physical status changes.	Adjusting expectations and activity level based on physiologic status reduces frustration and fatigue.
	Administer whole blood or packed RBCs as ordered.	Whole blood or packed RBCs may be given to correct severe anemia resulting from massive bleeding; correcting anemia improves activity tolerance.
Anticipatory grieving related to diagnosis and prognosis	Give patient and family members time to discuss their feelings and concerns; encourage ventilation.	Exploring feelings and concerns is the first level of supportive counseling and facilitates the grieving process.
	Provide accurate information and clarification (when requested) about the diagnosis, prognosis, and treatment plan.	Information and clarification help the patient and family confront the diagnosis and prognosis and understand the issues; seeking information is an action-oriented coping strategy.
	Reassure patient and family that conflicting, confusing, and negative emotions are normal and that expressing these feelings is helpful in dealing with grief (e.g., by talking, crying, yelling, thinking, or writing in a journal).	Recognizing that one's reactions are normal is reassuring and gives the patient and family "permission" to grieve.

→ > >

NURSING DIAGNOSIS	NURSING INTERVENTIONS	RATIONALE
	Refer patient and family to support groups or for counseling as indicated.	Support groups may help reduce patient's and family's sense of isolation and provide additional support; counseling provides help in dealing with issues and feelings.
Ineffective family coping related to diagnosis and prognosis	Provide realistic information about the diagnosis and prognosis to family members based on their readiness for information; provide opportunities for family members to discuss their feelings, concerns, and frustrations in private (away from the patient).	Information reduces the fear of the unknown and increases the ability to cope; family members must adapt to changes in the patient's health status and to a potentially fatal outcome; they need an opportunity to ventilate their feelings and to confront their personal issues.
	Encourage family members to share their feelings and concerns with each other and the patient.	Open communication reduces resentment and misunderstandings and improves the ability to cope with frustrations.
	Suggest family counseling as an effective management approach.	Counseling supports family members in dealing effectively with the illness and their feelings.
	Encourage patient, family to share recreational, pleasurable activities if possible.	Shared activites reduce stress and promote closeness, which improve ability to cope.
	If patient cannot carry out usual family roles, help him and family renegotiate tasks so that patient contributes as much as possible.	Renegotiating tasks maintains the patient's feelings of worth and reduces other members' overload and resentment.
	Acknowledge negative feelings as normal and "OK."	Acknowledging the normality of negative feelings reduces guilt and enhances coping ability.

5   EVALUATE

PATIENT OUTCOME	DATA INDICATING THAT OUTCOME IS REACHED
Patient has no pain, or pain is well controlled.	Patient states that pain has been relieved or is well controlled; facial expressions do not reflect pain; patient appears relaxed and comfortable.
Patient has attained and maintains his usual weight and ingests adequate nutrients, or patient has no nausea or vomiting.	Weight is within 90% of usual weight; patient ingests and tolerates at least 75% of prescribed or regular diet and has no signs of malnutrition (e.g., muscle wasting, joint edema, fissures at corners of mouth); *or* patient states that nausea and vomiting have resolved or are well controlled by medication.
Patient has no edema or ascites, or edema and ascites are controlled.	Inspection reveals no edema or ascites; patient states that swelling in legs, feet, and abdomen has been eliminated, *or* edema and ascites are stable, and patient has no dyspnea.

PATIENT OUTCOME	DATA INDICATING THAT OUTCOME IS REACHED
Patient shows improved activity tolerance, or has adapted his activities appropriately based on tolerance.	Patient reports reduced fatigue and improved activity tolerance; patient does not experience feelings of exhaustion, tachycardia, tachypnea, or shortness of breath following activity; *or* patient plans and spaces activities appropriately based on tolerance.
Patient and family can discuss their feelings and concerns about the diagnosis and prognosis and show adaptive responses.	Patient and family members verbalize feelings and concerns openly; their statements reflect understanding of the diagnosis, prognosis, and treatment plan; they participate in decision making about the treatment plan; patient accepts support from significant others, health team members, or both.
Patient and family demonstrate effective coping and healthy interpersonal interactions.	Patient and family members share their feelings with health team members and each other; they acknowledge negative feelings and share pleasurable experiences; they negotiate issues and concerns and report reduced conflict and increased ability to deal with issues; they deal appropriately and realistically with treatment decisions.

PATIENT TEACHING

1. Clarify and reinforce the physician's explanations about the diagnosis, prognosis, and treatment options or treatment plan.
2. Explain the treatment plan (e.g., surgery, chemotherapy, radiation, symptom control, or a combination of these): rationale, specific treatment procedures or guidelines, and measures to promote the regimen's effectiveness and minimize adverse reactions.
3. Provide the patient and family with information about community resources such as local support groups, the American Cancer Society, home health care, and hospice care.

Cirrhosis of the Liver

Cirrhosis is a chronic degenerative disease of the liver that disrupts liver structure and function. Cirrhosis may be categorized according to cause (e.g., alcoholic cirrhosis, biliary cirrhosis, postnecrotic cirrhosis, or metabolic cirrhosis).

EPIDEMIOLOGY

Cirrhosis is a leading cause of death in the United States. Alcoholic cirrhosis is the most common type and typically is seen in middle-aged men. Biliary cirrhosis may occur as a complication of collagen diseases (primary biliary cirrhosis) or as a result of prolonged biliary

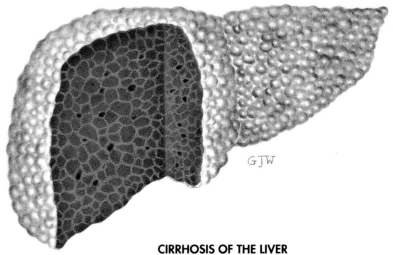

CIRRHOSIS OF THE LIVER

obstruction (secondary biliary cirrhosis). Postnecrotic cirrhosis occurs as a complication of chronic liver disease, such as hepatitis, and metabolic cirrhosis is associated with rare metabolic defects.

Alcoholic cirrhosis, also known as Laënnec's cirrhosis and fatty cirrhosis, is caused by the toxic effects of chronic alcohol abuse on the liver. The metabolism of alcohol produces acetylaldehyde, and excessive amounts of acetylaldehyde can significantly alter the function of hepatocytes. The severity of liver damage is directly related to the amount and duration of alcohol abuse. Surprisingly, most alcoholics do not develop cirrhosis; the disease occurs in only about 25%. The factors that cause cirrhosis to develop in some alcoholics but not in others have not yet been defined.

Alcoholic cirrhosis is a progressive disease comprising three phases. The first phase is characterized by fatty infiltration, which occurs because the damaged hepatocytes are less able to oxidize fatty acids. As a result, ingested fats and lipids mobilized from adipose tissue are incompletely oxidized and deposited in the liver. This process is reversed if alcohol consumption is eliminated; however, continued alcohol abuse may result in progression to the second phase, an inflammatory process known as alcoholic hepatitis. This phase is characterized by degeneration and necrosis of the liver cells (hepatocytes) and by infiltration of the damaged tissue with leukocytes and lymphocytes. The inflammation and degeneration trigger nodular regeneration and fibrosis (third phase), the hallmarks of cirrhosis.

Primary biliary cirrhosis occurs when the bile ducts become inflamed and damaged, possibly as a result of autoimmune mechanisms; these changes are followed by fibrosis and nodular regeneration. Secondary biliary cirrhosis develops as a result of prolonged biliary obstruction, which causes increased pressure in the hepatic duct, biliary stasis, and damage to the portal ducts and surrounding tissues. The end result is the nodular regeneration characteristic of cirrhosis.

Postnecrotic cirrhosis and metabolic cirrhosis are also caused by chronic liver damage resulting in fibrotic regenerative changes.

PATHOPHYSIOLOGY

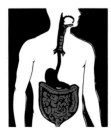

Whatever the specific cause, cirrhosis occurs as a result of regenerative changes subsequent to repetitive liver injury. Injury ranges from limited necrosis of liver cells to destruction of entire lobules, with collapse of the reticulin framework in the area or areas of necrosis. The repair process involves production of connective tissue (collagen) to bridge the gaps in the liver structure and regeneration or hypertrophy of the hepatocytes. The replacement of the underlying liver structure with con-

nective tissue produces anatomic distortions that alter the structure of the liver. These anatomic distortions have a particular impact on the vascular structure; whereas the normal liver structure involves perfusion of each lobule of sinusoids by both the hepatic artery and the portal vein, areas of regeneration are perfused only by the hepatic artery. This reduction in blood flow increases the vulnerability of the regenerating tissue (or "nodule") and also increases resistance in the portal venous system. When there is marked destruction of liver tissue with resultant fibrosis and anatomic distortions, the obstruction to portal venous 'flow can be severe enough to produce portal hypertension.

Limited amounts of liver damage do not alter liver function studies, because the liver possesses tremendous reserve capacity; liver function studies are not altered until most of the liver tissue has been destroyed and replaced by scar tissue. Clinical signs of liver failure begin to appear when the liver's ability to perform its numerous functions is impaired by the reduction in functioning hepatocytes, or when the resistance to portal venous flow results in symptomatic portal hypertension. Portal hypertension initially is a "silent" complication of cirrhosis; it becomes symptomatic when it becomes severe enough to cause other complications (i.e., esophageal varices, ascites, edema, and hepatorenal syndrome).

Portal hypertension occurs when the anatomic distortions in the liver tissue obliterate or constrict enough of the vascular channels to produce abnormal resistance to portal inflow. This abnormal resistance causes increased pressure in the veins that normally drain from the intestinal tract into the portal vein and then into the liver. (Normal pressure in the portal vein is about 8 mm Hg; in a patient with portal hypertension, it may be as high as 20 to 30 mm Hg.) The obstruction to venous flow from the intestine into the liver causes the development of collateral venous channels that "bypass" the liver and drain directly into the systemic circulation. The most common site for development of collateral vessels is in the distal esophagus (between the gastric vein, which drains into the portal system, and the azygos vein, which drains into the superior vena cava); collaterals can develop in other areas as well. For example, a patient with an intestinal stoma may develop collateral vessels between the abdominal wall and the portal system. (**For a color picture of caput medusae see color plate 7 on p. x.**) These collateral channels sometimes are large enough to effectively decompress the portal system; more commonly, the collaterals are poorly supported, thin-walled vessels prone to varicosities.

Variceal bleeding is the most lethal complication of portal hypertension. Esophageal and gastric varices are the most common site of variceal bleeding, because these vessels are located in the submucosal layer and therefore are prone to erosion. Approximately 50% of patients with cirrhosis develop varices, but only about 20% of those with varices ever bleed. Nonbleeding varices are asymptomatic and may go undiagnosed, but even if they are diagnosed, there is no well-defined management approach. Patients with known varices may be given medications to control gastric acidity, since reflux esophagitis is one factor thought to trigger bleeding. Other initiating factors may be minor trauma or sudden increases in portal pressure; most likely bleeding is initiated by some combination of the known trigger factors. Variceal bleeding usually is sudden in onset and can be massive; 30% to 80% of patients die as a result. Emergency management of variceal bleeding includes iced lavage, intravenous infusion of vasopressin, and balloon tamponade (e.g., with a Sengstaken-Blakemore tube); an emergency esophagogastroduodenoscopy may be done to confirm the source of the bleeding, since these patients are also prone to upper gastrointestinal bleeding from gastritis and peptic ulcer disease. Definitive management usually involves injection sclerotherapy or a portal-systemic shunt to decompress the portal system. Although injection sclerotherapy and portal-systemic shunts have been effective in reducing the incidence of variceal bleeding, the long-term survival rate remains very poor due to the underlying liver disease. The reported 5-year survival rates range from 0 to 35%. Studies have failed to demonstrate any survival benefit from prophylactic shunting; the benefits of prophylactic sclerotherapy currently are under study. One challenge with prophylactic therapy is the need to identify patients who are likely to bleed from their varices and who are therefore appropriate candidates for prophylaxis; one classification scheme has been devised that includes factors such as the size of varices and functional liver status/hepatic reserve. The results of these studies will help direct future management of patients with known varices.

The mechanisms underlying the formation of ascites are complex and not completely understood. Ascitic fluid is composed primarily of liver lymph, which is high in protein, and intestinal lymph, which is low in protein. The two primary factors in the development of ascites appear to be increased resistance to blood flow in the liver (portal hypertension) and increased retention of sodium and water by the kidneys. Portal hypertension contributes to the development of ascites in two ways:

1. Increased resistance to blood flow in the liver causes large amounts of plasma to leak out of the sinusoids into the perivascular lymphatics, thus tremendously increasing the production of lymph in the liver; this causes dilation of the lymphatics draining the liver, which precipitates leakage of high-protein lymph into the abdominal cavity. (Liver lymph is very high in protein, because the sinusoidal membranes are very permeable and allow free transport of protein out of the vascular space and into the lymphatics.) The high-protein lymph creates an osmotic gradient that further increases fluid leakage into the abdominal cavity.

2. The increased vascular resistance and resulting vasocongestion cause plasma to leak out of the vascular compartment into the liver tissues and then into the abdominal cavity. The resistance to portal flow also causes "back pressure" in the intestinal vasculature, which precipitates edema of the bowel wall and further leakage of fluid into the abdominal cavity.

The second major causative factor in the development of ascites, sodium and water retention, results from a reduction in renal blood flow, which probably is precipitated by the hepatorenal syndrome. The reduction in renal blood flow precipitates a compensatory increase in the production of aldosterone and antidiuretic hormone, which causes persistent retention of sodium and water. The resulting increase in intravascular volume adds to the vascular congestion and development of ascites.

Another factor that may contribute to the development of ascites in a patient with cirrhosis is the reduced production of albumin by the hepatocytes; hypoalbuminemia reduces the intravascular oncotic pressure and further increases extravasation of fluid into tissue spaces. The mechanisms contributing to ascites are outlined in Figure 5-3.

Symptomatic treatment of ascites includes administration of diuretics and albumin, paracentesis, and placement of a peritoneovenous shunt (between the abdominal cavity and the internal jugular vein) to provide continuous redistribution of the ascitic fluid to the systemic circulation. Definitive management of ascites involves correcting the underlying portal hypertension (e.g., portal-systemic shunt) or, for the patient with advanced liver disease, liver transplantation. A patient with ascites is at risk of developing bacterial peritonitis. Causative organisms usually include *Escherichia coli*, pneumococci, and beta-hemolytic streptococci; treatment involves intravenous administration of appropriate antibiotics.

Edema in a cirrhotic patient is caused by the increased intravascular volume that results from sodium and water retention and the reduced oncotic pressure caused by hypoalbuminemia.

Hepatorenal syndrome is another complication of cirrhosis that is thought to result from portal hypertension. Hepatorenal syndrome is categorized as type I or type II. Type II, the more common form, is caused by a redistribution of blood flow that shunts blood away

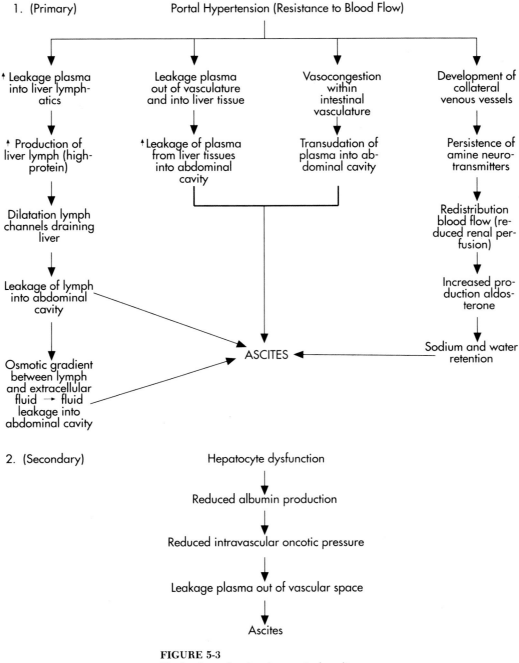

FIGURE 5-3
Mechanisms for development of ascites.

from essential organs such as the kidneys and into the peripheral and splanchnic circulation; this redistribution is thought to be caused by the persistence of amine neurotransmitters that normally are inactivated by the liver and that "bypass" the liver as a result of collateral blood flow. These neurotransmitters cause dilation of the vessels in the periphery (as opposed to the relative constriction normally maintained by norepinephrine). As a result, renal perfusion is reduced, which reduces glomerular filtration and activates the renin-angiotensin mechanism; the result is increased sodium and water reabsorption and intrarenal shunting of blood away from the cortex, with eventual development of oliguria and azotemia. Therapy is directed toward increasing renal perfusion; if renal perfusion is normalized, renal function usually returns to normal. Type I hepatorenal syndrome is caused by hypovolemia secondary to persistent ascites; treatment is directed toward resolution of the ascites and restoration of intravascular fluid volume.

In addition to the complications related to portal hypertension, cirrhotic liver disease is characterized by disorders related to loss of hepatocyte function. The most important of these disorders result from compromise of the liver's ability to produce and transport bile, synthesize proteins and clotting factors, and detoxify metabolic by-products and drugs.

Bile production and transport may be affected by diminished hepatocyte function or by obliteration of the normal biliary ductal system. Diminished hepatocyte function results in hepatocellular jaundice, which is characterized by reduced conjugation of the bilirubin molecule and increased serum levels of indirect (unconjugated) bilirubin. Obliteration of bile ducts produces obstructive jaundice; in this case the hepatocytes are able to conjugate the bilirubin molecule, but the bile is not excreted into the intestine and instead enters the serum as a result of rupture of the dilated bile ducts. In obstructive jaundice the serum level of direct (conjugated) bilirubin is elevated. Many patients with cirrhosis have a combination of hepatocellular and obstructive jaundice, which is characterized by increased levels of both direct (conjugated) and indirect (unconjugated) bilirubin. Compromised bile production and excretion causes jaundice and pruritus (which is the result of elevated plasma levels of bile acids); it also compromises digestion and absorption of fats and fat-soluble vitamins.

The liver normally plays an important role in synthesis of proteins and clotting factors. Compromised synthesis of plasma proteins causes hypoalbuminemia, which contributes to edema and ascites through reduced intravascular oncotic pressure. Compromised synthesis of clotting factors causes bleeding disorders. Reduced synthesis of prothrombin and other clotting factors may be due to loss of hepatocytes or to diminished absorption of vitamin K (which is essential for synthesis of prothrombin and factors VII, IX, and X) secondary to obstructive jaundice. The liver also synthesizes fibrinogen and factor V; these are not vitamin K dependent. In addition, thrombocytopenia may result from hypersplenism or recent alcohol ingestion. Coagulopathies caused by obstructive jaundice can be treated effectively by administration of vitamin K; coagulopathies caused by hepatocyte dysfunction require administration of whole blood or fresh frozen plasma. Factor V is contained only in fresh whole blood or fresh frozen plasma and cannot be provided through use of banked blood. Folic acid can help reverse thrombocytopenia resulting from recent alcohol ingestion.

One of the liver's most important functions is detoxification of many drugs and metabolic by-products. Loss of this function renders the patient much less able to tolerate drugs that are detoxified by the liver; the dosage and frequency of administration of such drugs must be modified for these patients. Loss of normal detoxification also reduces the patient's ability to tolerate certain dietary substances, such as protein. The most dangerous complication caused by loss of the liver's detoxification function, hepatic encephalopathy, is related to protein metabolism.

Hepatic encephalopathy is a disorder of protein metabolism and excretion. It is characterized by cerebrocortical compromise, and there is a wide spectrum of severity, ranging from diminished intellectual function to coma. Encephalopathy may occur "spontaneously" as a result of end-stage liver disease or following a portalsystemic shunt, or it may be "induced" by factors that increase the protein load, such as variceal bleeding. The exact etiologic mechanism for hepatic encephalopathy is not known. For years ammonia was considered the primary cerebral "toxin"; however, there is poor correlation between ammonia levels and degree of encephalopathy. Currently it is believed that several byproducts of the alterations in protein metabolism may contribute to encephalopathy; ammonia and aromatic amino acids are among those under study. Normally the liver converts products of protein metabolism, such as ammonia, into urea, which is eliminated by the kidneys; encephalopathy is most likely to develop in patients whose ability to synthesize urea after a protein load is reduced by 50% or more. Early clinical indicators of developing encephalopathy include alterations in personality and behavior and diminished intellectual function; later manifestations range from asterixis (flapping tremor) and agitation to drowsiness and variable levels of confusion, with eventual progression to coma if the encephalopathy is not corrected. Treatment involves correcting reversible factors (e.g., azotemia or gastrointestinal bleeding), restricting protein intake (the level of restriction depends on the severity of the encephalopathy), and using laxatives and enemas to purge the gut of ammonia sources (e.g., blood and stool) and ammonia-producing bacteria.

An additional complication of cirrhotic liver disease is malnutrition, which may be manifested by muscle wasting and a cachectic appearance; the malnutrition results from metabolic derangements and from reduced nutrient intake, which is common in alcoholism and in liver disease (as a result of anorexia and nausea). Attention to nutritional deficits is an important component of management for these patients.

As is evident from this brief overview, cirrhotic liver disease is a very complex disorder with numerous complications. For a patient with early disease (e.g., fatty liver), the treatment focus is on eliminating the toxins, such as alcohol; if hepatotoxins can be eliminated, the liver can regenerate. The only definitive management for a patient with severe liver disease is liver transplantation. Short of this, treatment focuses on managing the many clinical manifestations and complications related to portal hypertension, hepatocellular dysfunction, or both.

COMPLICATIONS

Portal hypertension	Hepatorenal syndrome
Esophageal varices	Congestive heart failure
Ascites	Hepatic encephalopathy
Bacterial peritonitis	Malnutrition
Edema	Clotting disorders

DIAGNOSTIC STUDIES AND FINDINGS

Diagnostic test	Findings
Serum bilirubin	May be elevated; high level of direct bilirubin may indicate obstructive jaundice; high level of indirect bilirubin may indicate hepatocellular jaundice
Urine bilirubin	May be elevated in obstructive jaundice
Urine urobilinogen	May be elevated in hepatocellular jaundice; absence indicates severe biliary obstruction
Aspartate aminotransferase (AST; formerly SGOT, serum glutamic-oxaloacetic transaminase)	Commonly elevated in liver inflammation or injury*; dramatic reduction may indicate fulminant hepatocellular failure
Alanine aminotransferase (ALT; formerly SGPT, serum glutamic-pyruvic transaminase)	Commonly elevated in liver inflammation or injury*; dramatic reduction may indicate fulminant hepatocellular failure
Alkaline phosphatase	Commonly elevated with biliary obstruction
Serum 5'-nucleotidase	Commonly elevated with biliary obstruction
Serum albumin	Commonly low
IgA	May be elevated with alcoholic cirrhosis
IgM	May be elevated with biliary cirrhosis
Prothrombin time	Commonly prolonged, due to either biliary obstruction or hepatocellular disease
Serum ammonia (NH$_3$)	Commonly elevated with encephalopathy
Serum amino acids	Abnormal levels common with encephalopathy
Blood urea nitrogen and creatinine	May be elevated in patient with hepatorenal syndrome
Complete blood count	Hb and Hct may be reduced in patient with GI bleeding; anemia and thrombocytopenia may be seen in patient with hypersplenism
Serum electrolytes	May be abnormal
Serum glucose	May be elevated or decreased
Flat plate and upright film of abdomen	May reveal hepatosplenomegaly; if ascites is present, may reveal abdominal haziness and widely separated intestinal loops
Abdominal ultrasound scan	May reveal intraabdominal fluid if ascites is present (will detect as little as 100 ml of free fluid)
Paracentesis	Done to confirm ascites (normal findings on fluid analysis are: specific gravity <1.016; protein concentration <2.5 g/dl; cell count <300/L [mononuclear]); with peritonitis, findings are reversed: high specific gravity, high protein, >500 polymorphonuclear leukocytes/L.
Barium swallow	May reveal esophageal or gastric varices
Esophagogastroduodenoscopy	Done to determine site of bleeding; may reveal esophageal or gastric varices or gastritis or peptic ulcerations
Angiography (percutaneous transhepatic portography)	Done to diagnose esophageal varices and to visualize portal venous circulation
Portal venous pressure and wedged hepatic venous pressure (venography)	Elevated in patient with portal hypertension
Liver scan	May show diffuse changes typical of cirrhosis
Percutaneous needle biopsy	Done to confirm diagnosis of cirrhosis and to determine severity of disease; may show fatty infiltration (early disease) or severe degeneration and scarring (advanced disease)
Endoscopic retrograde cholecystopancreatography (ERCP)	May reveal biliary tract obstruction (in patient with secondary biliary cirrhosis)
Electroencephalography	May be abnormal in patient with encephalopathy

*Degree of elevation may not correlate well with extent of hepatic damage, especially in alcohol-associated disease.

MEDICAL MANAGEMENT

GENERAL MANAGEMENT

Elimination of alcohol intake.

High-protein, high-calorie diet: (1.1 g protein/kg ideal body weight/24 h* plus 35 nonprotein calories/kg) given orally, enterally, or parenterally.

*Protein load is reduced for patient with hepatic encephalopathy.

For patient with ascites/edema: Sodium restriction (250-500 mg daily); fluid restriction (1,000 ml daily) if serum sodium is <130 mEq/L; bed rest to support liver function and diuresis; paracentesis for severe or persistent ascites; Swan-Ganz or central venous pressure (CVP) monitoring for patient with hemodynamic instability being diuresed or aggressively treated for ascites.

For patient with hepatic encephalopathy (mild): Tap water enemas until clear; low-protein, high-carbohydrate diet (15-20 g low-ammonia or all-vegetable protein) until encephalopathy has been reversed; then protein in diet is gradually advanced (by 5-10 g daily) until patient can tolerate 0.5-0.7 g of high-quality, low-ammonia protein/kg ideal body weight daily.

For patient with hepatic encephalopathy (severe): Tap water enemas until clear; N/G intubation and suction as needed to decompress stomach and prevent vomiting and aspiration; endotracheal intubation as needed to protect airway and maintain ventilation; NPO status; IV replacement of fluids and electrolytes.

For patient with GI bleeding (e.g., bleeding esophageal varices): NPO status; N/G intubation with iced saline or tap water lavage; IV administration of fluids and electrolytes; administration of whole blood as needed; insertion of triple-lumen, double-balloon tube for tamponade of bleeding varices.

SURGERY

Paracentesis to control ascites.

LeVeen or Denver peritoneovenous shunt for continuous reinfusion of persistent ascites.

Endoscopic sclerotherapy to control bleeding esophageal varices.

End-to-side portacaval shunt to correct portal hypertension.

Side-to-side portacaval shunt to correct portal hypertension and ascites (provides for portal decompression and outflow tract for retrograde flow of portal blood).

Distal splenorenal shunt for partial portal decompression and control of esophageal varices.

Liver transplantation for patient with severe hepatocellular failure.

DRUG THERAPY

Vitamins and trace minerals

Vitamin K (Synkayvite): 5-10 mg IV or IM every other day for three doses to correct clotting abnormalities.

For patient with ascites and edema: *Spironolactone (Aldactone):* 100 mg daily; *hydrochlorothiazide (Hydrodiuril):* 50-100 mg daily in addition to spironolactone for more resistant ascites; *furosemide (Lasix):* 40 mg daily (in combination with spironolactone) for ascites resistant to spironolactone/hydrochlorothiazide combination; *salt-poor albumin:* 40 g daily per IV infusion.

For patient with bacterial peritonitis: *Cefamandole:* 500 mg-2 g IV q 4 h.

For patient with hepatic encephalopathy: *Neomycin:* 1-1.5 g PO qid until encephalopathy has resolved; then 2-3 g daily while protein is increased until patient can tolerate protein without developing encephalopathy; *lactulose* titrated to maintain two to three stools a day in patient with chronic encephalopathy.

Continued.

MEDICAL MANAGEMENT—cont'd

For patient with hepatorenal syndrome: *Levodopa (Levopa):* Up to 1.5 g PO daily (preceded by antacid) to increase vascular resistance.

For patient with bleeding varices: *Vasopressin by continuous IV infusion:* 0.4-0.9 U/min until bleeding stops; then dosage is decreased by 0.1-0.2 U/min q 12 h (bolus dose of 20 U in 500 ml of D_5W may be given in emergency).

Propranolol (Inderal): For long-term prophylaxis in managing bleeding varices when initial bleeding is too mild to justify surgical intervention.

Cimetidine (Tagamet): To reduce gastric acidity (and reflux esophagitis) in patient with gastritis/ulcer disease or esophageal varices.

Insulin: as needed to control hyperglycemia.

1 ASSESS

ASSESSMENT	OBSERVATIONS
History	May report history of alcohol abuse, collagen disease, gallstones, pancreatitis, hepatitis, or inherited metabolic disorder (e.g., Wilson's disease)
Nutritional status	May report recent weight loss; may report anorexia, nausea, and vomiting; weight may be less than 85% of usual weight; may have signs of malnutrition (e.g., muscle wasting; fissures at corners of mouth; thin, dry skin)
Abdominal assessment	Inspection may reveal evidence of ascites (generalized abdominal distention, increased abdominal girth, prominent abdominal veins radiating from umbilicus); palpation may reveal abnormally large or small liver that feels hard, enlarged spleen (with portal hypertension), evidence of ascites (fluid wave), or tenderness (bacterial peritonitis); percussion may reveal shifting dullness (with ascites); auscultation may reveal diminished bowel sounds (with ascites or peritonitis)
Jaundice	Skin and sclerae may appear jaundiced; patient may report dark urine and clay-colored stools (obstructive jaundice) and pruritus
Gastrointestinal bleeding	May report bloody emesis and bloody or tarry stools (small or large volume); stools or emesis or both may test positive for occult blood
Vital signs	May reveal hypotension and tachycardia (with bleeding or hepatorenal syndrome); tachypnea (with severe ascites); and fever (with peritonitis)
Renal function	Patient may report swelling and weight gain; may have edema and oliguria
Cerebrocortical function	Patient or family may report altered behavior patterns and evidence of diminished intellectual function; patient may exhibit asterixis, drowsiness, confusion, stupor, or coma
Clotting status	Patient may report prolonged bleeding with minor trauma (e.g., bleeding gums with toothbrushing), easy bruising, and tarry stools; bruising and petechiae may be evident

ASSESSMENT	OBSERVATIONS
Coping skills and support system	Patient may report difficulty dealing with stress, feelings of incompetence, feelings of inadequate support, and tendency to drink when overwhelmed; may report interpersonal conflict with significant others related to alcohol abuse; may report extreme anxiety and episodes of depression related to chronic illness and threat to health and life

2 DIAGNOSE

NURSING DIAGNOSIS	SUBJECTIVE FINDINGS	OBJECTIVE FINDINGS
Altered nutrition: less than body requirements related to anorexia, nausea, and vomiting	Reports anorexia, nausea, and vomiting; may report recent weight loss	Weight less than 85%-90% of usual weight (this finding may be absent in patient with ascites and edema); nutrient intake less than 75% of prescribed diet; signs of malnutrition (e.g., dry, thin skin; muscle wasting; fissures in corners of mouth)
Fluid volume excess related to ascites and edema or hepatorenal syndrome	Reports swelling in abdomen and legs; may complain of shortness of breath	Dependent edema; evidence of ascites (generalized abdominal distention, increasing abdominal girth, dilated abdominal veins, shifting dullness on percussion); may be oliguric and dyspneic
Altered renal, cerebral, cardiopulmonary, gastrointestinal, and peripheral tissue perfusion related to gastrointestinal bleeding (e.g., severe gastritis or bleeding varices)	Reports vomiting blood or having bloody or tarry stools; may report feeling faint, dizzy, or short of breath; may report feelings of anxiety and abdominal pain	Hematemesis (may be massive); melena or hematochezia; hypotension, tachycardia, tachypnea; may have diaphoresis, and oliguria
Altered thought processes related to hepatic encephalopathy	Patient or family reports altered behavior and diminished intellectual function; may report unusual lethargy or confusion	Asterixis; drowsiness; varying levels of confusion; stupor; coma
High risk for impaired skin integrity related to diarrhea or to pressure, shear, or friction	May report multiple watery stools	Multiple loose stools *or* thin, dry skin in patient who is bedbound *or* has limited mobility, reduced sensory awareness, and edema
High risk for injury related to thrombocytopenia and diminished clotting factors	Reports prolonged bleeding with minor trauma; may report tarry stools	Bruises; petechiae; prolonged bleeding following venipuncture or other minor trauma; tarry stools
Ineffective individual coping related to alcohol abuse or chronic illness	Reports feelings of stress and anxiety; may report continued alcohol ingestion or may deny alcohol abuse despite evidence	Inappropriate response to issues and situation; fails to follow treatment plan

→ › ›

NURSING DIAGNOSIS	SUBJECTIVE FINDINGS	OBJECTIVE FINDINGS
Ineffective family coping related to chronic illness, alcohol abuse, or both	Patient and family members verbalize feelings of anxiety, difficulty handling issues related to diagnosis and treatment, feeling overwhelmed, and inability to share feelings	Interactions between patient and family members marked by conflict; family members fail to support treatment plan; family members express anger with patient over alcohol abuse and subsequent illness

3   PLAN

Patient goals

1. The patient will attain and maintain his usual body weight and will ingest adequate nutrients daily.
2. The patient will maintain normal intravascular and interstitial fluid volumes.
3. The patient will maintain normal perfusion of renal, cerebral, cardiopulmonary, gastrointestinal, and peripheral tissues.
4. The patient will maintain normal thought processes and cerebrocortical function.
5. The patient will maintain normal skin integrity.
6. The patient will have no abnormal bleeding.
7. The patient will demonstrate effective coping strategies and will make appropriate decisions about treatment.
8. The family members will demonstrate effective coping strategies and healthy interpersonal interactions.

4   IMPLEMENT

NURSING DIAGNOSIS	NURSING INTERVENTIONS	RATIONALE
Altered nutrition: less than body requirements related to anorexia, nausea, and vomiting	Monitor patient's nutrient intake and nutrient losses (e.g., vomiting), as well as indicators of compromised nutritional status (e.g., muscle wasting, joint edema).	Prompt recognition of nutritional deficits permits early intervention; correcting nutritional deficits supports liver regeneration and improves the patient's general status.
	Collaborate with patient and dietitian to provide a high-protein, high-calorie diet based on patient's preferences.	Maintaining body weight and positive nitrogen balance reduces morbidity and helps maximize health.
	For patient with jaundice, provide low-fat diet.	Jaundice is an indicator of compromised bile production or transport; biliary insufficiency reduces the ability to digest and absorb fats.
	For patient with preclinical or mild encephalopathy: modify diet to limit protein load (i.e., 15-20 g daily of all-vegetable or low-ammonia protein initially; gradually increase to 35-50 g daily as tolerated); administer branched chain–enriched amino acid solution (e.g., HepatAmine).	Encephalopathy results from altered protein metabolism and increased levels of protein by-products such as ammonia; intake of dietary protein must be titrated to patient's tolerance; administration of branched chain–enriched supplements improves protein tolerance.
	Monitor glucose levels, and administer insulin as needed.	Patients with compromised liver function frequently are glucose intolerant.
	Administer vitamin and mineral supplements as ordered.	Patients with compromised nutritional status frequently are deficient in vitamins and minerals.

NURSING DIAGNOSIS	NURSING INTERVENTIONS	RATIONALE
	For patient who cannot tolerate oral or enteral feedings: collaborate with physician and nutritional support team to provide TPN.	TPN corrects nutritional deficits and prevents complications associated with malnutrition.
Fluid volume excess related to ascites and edema or hepatorenal syndrome	Monitor patient for intake exceeding output, increasing edema, increasing abdominal girth, shortness of breath, and weight gain.	Prompt recognition of fluid volume excess permits early intervention and correction of intravascular volume.
	Restrict sodium intake to 250-500 mg daily.	Patients with edema and ascites aggressively retain sodium because of altered renal function.
	For patient with serum sodium <130 mEq/L: restrict fluid intake to 1,000 ml daily.	Low serum sodium in a patient with edema and ascites indicates aggressive fluid retention and dilutional hyponatremia.
	Limit physical activity (bed rest or light activity spaced with frequent rest periods).	Adequate rest and reduced activity support diuresis.
	Administer diuretics as ordered (e.g., spironolactone or spironolactone plus hydrochlorothiazide, or spironolactone plus furosemide).	Diuretics reduce sodium and water reabsorption in the renal tubules and thus increase urine output.
	Administer salt-poor albumin per IV infusion as ordered; monitor patient for signs of fluid overload.	Salt-poor albumin increases intravascular oncotic pressure, which causes an interstitial-to-plasma fluid shift; the increased intravascular volume increases glomerular filtration and urinary output.
	For patient with hepatorenal syndrome: administer levodopa as ordered (preceded by antacid).	Levodopa is the precursor to the neurotransmitters dopamine and norepinephrine, which increase peripheral vascular resistance and improve renal perfusion.
	For patient with shortness of breath or dyspnea: elevate the head of the bed, and gatch the knees.	Elevating the head of the bed lowers the diaphragm and improves lung expansion and ventilatory function.
	For patient with resistant or severe ascites: prepare patient for paracentesis as ordered.	Paracentesis provides immediate temporary relief of ascites.
	For patient with persistent, severe ascites unresponsive to therapy: prepare patient for placement of peritoneovenous shunt as ordered.	A shunt provides for continuous reinfusion of ascitic fluid.
	For patient with hemodynamic instability: assist with insertion of Swan-Ganz or central venous catheter (as ordered), and monitor pressures.	Accurate monitoring of CVP permits appropriate adjustments in fluid and diuretic therapy.

→ > >

NURSING DIAGNOSIS	NURSING INTERVENTIONS	RATIONALE
Altered renal, cerebral, cardiopulmonary, gastrointestinal, and peripheral tissue perfusion related to gastrointestinal bleeding (e.g., severe gastritis or bleeding varices)	Monitor stools, emesis, and gastric aspirate (if applicable) for frank or occult blood; measure amount of bloody stools, emesis, or aspirate.	Bleeding may occur as a result of gastritis, peptic ulcer disease, or esophageal or gastric varices; measuring stool/emesis/aspirate helps quantify blood loss.
	Monitor vital signs for evidence of hypovolemia (tachycardia, tachypnea, hypotension).	Hypovolemia is reflected by changes in BP; compensatory responses to hypovolemia produce tachycardia and tachypnea.
	During bleeding episodes: keep patient NPO, and place an N/G tube as ordered (or assist with placement).	An N/G tube allows monitoring of gastric aspirate and provides access for gastric lavage; N/G intubation and NPO status provide gastric decompression and reduce vomiting.
	For patient with bleeding varices: assist with insertion of triple- or quadruple-lumen N/G tube for compression of bleeding esophageal or gastric varices.	Balloon tamponade provides initial control of bleeding varices in 76%-90% of patients and long-term control in about 46% of patients.
	Lubricate nasal passages and nasopharynx with topical anesthetic.	Topical anesthesia reduces the discomfort of tube insertion.
	Ascertain correct placement of tube (by x-ray), and inflate gastric balloon with 250-450 ml of air, and pull tube taut against gastroesophageal junction.	Tube placement must be confirmed to prevent complications; balloon inflation compresses the bleeding varices.
	For continued bleeding: inflate esophageal balloon (of double-balloon tube) to pressure of about 35 mm Hg.	Distal esophageal compression may be needed for control of esophageal varices.
	Maintain correct position of tube by taping tube to mask of football helmet that patient wears (or by taping a split tennis ball to the patient's nose).	Accurate positioning of the tube must be maintained to compress the bleeding varices and prevent complications of balloon displacement (e.g., asphyxiation and esophageal tears or rupture).
	Pass catheter for esophageal aspiration through opposite nostril, and connect to suction (or connect esophageal aspiration lumen of four-lumen tube to suction).	The most common complication of balloon tamponade is aspiration pneumonia, because the patient cannot swallow with the balloon or balloons inflated.
	Carry out iced saline or tap water lavage as ordered through N/G or special "balloon tamponade" tube.	Iced solutions promote mucosal vasoconstriction, which helps stop the bleeding; however, iced solutions can inhibit platelet function and prolong bleeding; water breaks up blood clots more readily but is hypotonic; saline is isotonic but can contribute to sodium and water retention.
	Administer IV fluids and blood replacement as ordered; if blood is administered, use fresh blood, and observe for transfusion reactions.	IV fluids are administered to maintain plasma volume; blood may be required for replacement of RBCs and platelets during massive bleeding; fresh blood contains clotting factors.

NURSING DIAGNOSIS	NURSING INTERVENTIONS	RATIONALE
	Prepare patient for endoscopy with laser coagulation (for gastritis or peptic ulcer) or sclerotherapy (for esophageal varices) as ordered.	Endoscopy and laser coagulation are commonly used for control of gastric and duodenal bleeding caused by erosive gastritis or ulcer disease; sclerotherapy is a safe and effective technique for control of bleeding varices.
	Administer vasopressin IV as ordered; administer nitroglycerin as ordered to help reduce adverse cardiovascular responses to vasopressin.	Vasopressin significantly reduces mesenteric blood flow and also reduces gastric acid secretion; it may be used to provide short-term control of variceal bleeding; vasopressin may cause hypertension, cardiac dysrhythmias, and myocardial infarction; nitroglycerin dilates cardiac vessels and helps prevent these complications.
	Administer propranolol as ordered for patient with mild and self-limiting variceal bleeding.	Propranolol has been used on a long-term basis to prevent bleeding in patients whose initial bleeding is too mild to justify sclerotherapy or surgical intervention.
	Administer H_2-receptor antagonists to patient with known varices, gastritis, or peptic ulcer disease.	Reducing gastric acidity helps to prevent reflux esophagitis (a possible causative factor in variceal bleeding) and to promote healing of gastric erosions and peptic ulcers.
	For patient with variceal bleeding that is unresponsive to tamponade, vasopressin, and sclerotherapy: prepare for surgery (portosystemic shunt).	Portosystemic shunts reduce portal hypertension and are effective in preventing recurrent variceal bleeding.
Altered thought processes related to hepatic encephalopathy	Monitor patient for evidence of developing or worsening encephalopathy (altered behavior patterns or diminished intellectual function, asterixis, agitation, drowsiness, confusion, stupor, coma, and decerebrate-decorticate posturing).	Early signs of encephalopathy include altered behavior patterns and diminished intellectual function; later signs include asterixis, agitation, confusion, and drowsiness; severe encephalopathy is evidenced by stupor, coma, and decerebrate-decorticate posturing.
	For patient with gastrointestinal bleeding: once bleeding has been controlled, administer saline enemas to "purge" the colon of blood.	GI bleeding increases the protein load within the gut and contributes to development of encephalopathy.
	Restrict dietary protein intake based on patient's tolerance: low-protein, high-carbohydrate diet (15-20 g low-ammonia or all-vegetable protein) until all signs of encephalopathy have resolved; gradually increase dietary protein 5-10 g daily until patient can tolerate 35-50 g a day.	Encephalopathy is a result of altered protein metabolism; treatment involves reducing protein intake to a level tolerated by the patient.
	Administer tap water enemas until clear as ordered.	Enemas are given to purge the colon of ammonia sources (e.g., blood and stool) and ammonia-producing bacteria.

→ > >

NURSING DIAGNOSIS	NURSING INTERVENTIONS	RATIONALE
	Administer neomycin as ordered (usually 1-1.5 g PO qid until encephalopathy has resolved; then 2-3 g PO daily until patient can tolerate protein without becoming encephalopathic; may give up to 12 g daily in acute encephalopathic states; can also be given rectally).	Neomycin reduces the ammonia-producing bacteria in the colon.
	Administer lactulose as ordered (usually 20-30 g tid or qid to maintain soft stools, or 30-45 ml in 100 ml of fluid as retention enema).	Lactulose is not metabolized in the small intestine and is broken down in the colon by bacteria; it lowers the pH of the stool, which creates a gradient between the acidified stool and the interstitial fluid that causes ammonia to diffuse out of the interstitial fluid and into the colon; the net result is increased elimination of ammonia through the stool.
	Collaborate with physician to modify dosage or to avoid administration of sedatives, tranquilizers, or narcotic analgesics.	The damaged liver is less able to detoxify drugs; sedative drugs may precipitate encephalopathy.
	For patient with severe encephalopathy and altered level of consciousness: keep patient NPO, and insert N/G tube to suction as ordered; irrigate tube as needed to maintain patency.	NPO status and N/G suction provide gastric decompression and help prevent vomiting and aspiration in patient with altered level of consciousness.
	For patient with severe encephalopathy producing coma: protect patient's airway by oral and endotracheal suction or endotracheal intubation as needed.	A comatose patient cannot protect his airway or clear secretions.
High risk for impaired skin integrity related to diarrhea or to pressure, shear, or friction	For patient with diarrhea: cleanse perianal skin gently after each bowel movement; protect perianal skin with sealants (e.g., skin wipes or incontinent spray), moisture barrier ointment, or both (if both are used, apply sealant and allow to dry before applying ointment); for severe diarrhea, consider fecal incontinence collector.	Diarrhea causes maceration and denudation of perianal skin; gentle skin care prevents additional trauma; sealants provide a copolymer film on the skin, and moisture barrier ointment repels liquid stool; a fecal incontinence collector contains the stool and protects the skin.
	Implement measures to protect fragile skin from friction and shear (use lift sheets, limit head of bed elevation, use knee gatch when head of bed is elevated, use foam overlay or other low-shear surface).	Friction causes mechanical damage to skin from "rubbing"; shear occurs when the patient slides down, which causes tissue layers to slide against each other, disrupting blood vessels.
	For patient with altered level of consciousness or reduced mobility: initiate routine turning schedule (q 1-2 h) based on patient's tolerance, and consider using pressure reduction device (e.g., mattress overlay or replacement mattress).	Pressure ulcers occur when the patient is allowed to remain in one position for prolonged periods; frequency of repositioning is titrated for each patient (ideal interval is one that provides for prompt resolution of reactive hyperemia [i.e., complete resolution of reddened areas within 20 min of repositioning]); may lengthen interval if pressure-reducing device is used.

NURSING DIAGNOSIS	NURSING INTERVENTIONS	RATIONALE
	Monitor patient for evidence of impending breakdown, and adjust care plan appropriately (e.g., modify turning schedule to eliminate pressure on erythematous area).	Erythema that does not resolve is the first sign of impending damage; it is critical to identify causative factors and take corrective action to prevent breakdown.
High risk for injury related to thrombocytopenia and diminished clotting factors	Monitor patient for evidence of clotting abnormalities (bruising with minimal trauma, hematuria, melena, and epistaxis).	Prompt recognition of clotting deficiencies permits appropriate intervention.
	Administer vitamin K as ordered to patient with loss of bile flow to intestine.	Loss of bile flow to intestine reduces absorption of fat-soluble vitamins; vitamin K is essential for synthesis of a number of clotting factors.
	Instruct patient with clotting abnormalities to avoid using straight razors and hard toothbrushes.	Minor trauma can result in prolonged bleeding.
	For patient with severe or persistent bleeding: administer whole blood or fresh frozen plasma.	Bank blood replaces all clotting factors except factor V, which is found only in fresh frozen plasma or fresh whole blood.
Ineffective individual coping related to alcohol abuse or chronic illness	Provide information about the relationship between excessive alcohol intake and the development of cirrhosis (if applicable) and between alcohol ingestion and worsening of liver status.	The patient must be informed about factors that contribute to his disease to make informed decisions about continued alcohol intake.
	Provide supportive counseling (i.e., reflective listening with therapeutic confrontation as indicated).	Supportive counseling helps patient explore feelings, identify major issues, and consider options for dealing with them.
	Refer patient to local support groups as indicated (e.g., Alcoholics Anonymous or liver disease and transplant support groups).	Participation in support groups reduces the patient's sense of isolation, expands his support system, encourages development of new coping strategies, and has been demonstrated to be effective in modifying addictive behavior.
	Reassure patient that conflicting, confusing, and negative emotions are normal and that expressing these feelings is helpful in dealing with anxiety, anger, and grief (e.g., by talking, crying, yelling, thinking).	Recognizing that one's reactions are normal is reassuring and gives the patient "permission" to have and verbalize negative feelings.
	Offer professional counseling as an option.	Professional counseling helps the patient confront and deal with issues.
Ineffective family coping related to chronic illness, alcohol abuse, or both	Provide realistic information (about disease and effects of alcohol on liver function) to family members based on their readiness.	Information reduces anxiety and increases the ability to cope by relieving unfounded fears and clarifying issues.
	Provide opportunities for family members to discuss their feelings, concerns, and frustrations in private (away from the patient).	Family members must adapt to changes in patient's health status; if the disease resulted from alcohol abuse, family may have unresolved feelings of anger or guilt; family members need an opportunity to ventilate feelings and confront personal issues.

→ > >

NURSING DIAGNOSIS	NURSING INTERVENTIONS	RATIONALE
	Encourage family members to share their feelings and concerns with each other and the patient.	Open communication reduces resentment and misunderstandings and improves ability to cope with frustrations.
	If patient cannot carry out his usual family roles, help him and family to renegotiate tasks so that the patient contributes as much as possible.	Renegotiating tasks maintains patient's feelings of worth and reduces other members' overload and resentment.
	Acknowledge negative feelings as normal and "OK."	Acknowledging the normality of negative feelings reduces guilt and enhances coping ability.
	Suggest family counseling as an effective management approach.	Counseling supports family members in dealing effectively with the illness and their feelings.
	Encourage the patient and family to share recreational and pleasurable activities when possible.	Shared activities reduce stress and promote closeness, which improves the ability to cope.

5 EVALUATE

PATIENT OUTCOME	DATA INDICATING THAT OUTCOME IS REACHED
Patient has attained and maintains usual weight and ingests adequate nutrients daily.	Weight is within 90% of usual weight; patient consumes at least 75% of prescribed diet or receives enteral or parenteral support; patient has no signs of malnutrition (e.g., dry, pluckable hair; muscle wasting; joint edema).
Patient maintains normal intravascular and interstitial fluid volumes.	Intake and output are balanced; abdominal girth remains stable; ascites has resolved or is stable; edema is minimal or absent; patient has no shortness of breath; BP and pulse are within normal limits.
Patient maintains normal perfusion of renal, cerebral, cardiopulmonary, gastrointestinal, and peripheral tissues.	BP, pulse, and respiratory rates are within normal limits; urine output is within normal limits; patient has no hematemesis, melena, or hematochezia.
Patient maintains normal thought processes and cerebrocortical function.	Patient is alert and oriented; patient and family state that behavior patterns and intellectual acuity are normal; no asterixis, agitation, or confusion is observed.
Patient maintains normal skin integrity.	Skin remains intact over entire body surface; there are no areas of erythema persisting longer than 20 min after pressure relief; there are no areas of induration over bony prominences.

PATIENT OUTCOME	DATA INDICATING THAT OUTCOME IS REACHED
Patient has no abnormal bleeding.	Inspection reveals no unexplained bruises, petechiae, or epistaxis; patient has no melena, hematuria, or episodes of prolonged bleeding.
Patient demonstrates effective coping strategies and healthy interpersonal interactions.	Patient acknowledges relationship between excessive alcohol ingestion and disease (if applicable); he verbalizes need to omit alcohol; he has identified an effective support system and appropriate strategies for dealing with stress; he can discuss his feelings openly.
Patient and family demonstrate effective coping and healthy interpersonal interactions.	Patient and family members share their feelings with health team members and each other; they are able to acknowledge negative feelings such as anger and resentment and are able to negotiate issues and concerns; they are able to share pleasurable experiences; they report reduced conflict and increased ability to deal with issues; they deal appropriately and realistically with treatment decisions.

PATIENT TEACHING

1. Explain the causative factors for the patient's cirrhosis, if known, and explain measures he can take to reduce the risk of further liver damage (e.g., forgo alcohol, follow the prescribed diet, adopt a healthy life-style with balance between rest and activity).
2. Explain the rationale for the prescribed diet (i.e., the need to balance protein to meet bodily needs without exceeding the liver's ability to convert ammonia into urea, and restricting sodium to reduce fluid accumulation, edema, and ascites). Instruct the patient in the specifics of the prescribed diet (i.e., foods allowed, foods prohibited, foods restricted).
3. Explain the rationale for medications, and teach the patient the schedule, dosage, and potential adverse reactions.
4. Instruct the patient to inform all physicians and dentists he sees about his cirrhotic liver disease and reduced ability to tolerate sedative and analgesic medications. Encourage the patient to acquire Medic-Alert identification.
5. Teach the patient the signs and symptoms of complications that he must report to his physician immediately (increasing ascites, edema, and shortness of breath; gastrointestinal bleeding; a change in behavior pattern or intellectual functioning, and asterixis).
6. Explain the treatment options (life-style changes, medications, and surgical options), and give the patient and family a chance to ask questions and clarify their concerns.

CHAPTER 6

Disorders of Nutrient Intake and Absorption

Short Bowel Syndrome

Short bowel syndrome results when the length of functional small bowel is insufficient to provide adequate absorption of nutrients, vitamins, minerals, fluids, and electrolytes. The condition is characterized by steatorrhea, weight loss, malabsorption, malnutrition, and fluid-electrolyte derangements.

EPIDEMIOLOGY

Short bowel syndrome most commonly results from massive small bowel resection, which may be necessitated by ischemic processes affecting the intestinal wall. Intestinal ischemia may be caused by mesenteric vascular disease, volvulus, strangulated hernias, or massive abdominal trauma that causes transection or avulsion of the mesenteric vasculature. Severe or recurrent inflammatory processes involving the small bowel may also precipitate short bowel syndrome because (1) massive or repetitive surgical resections may be required to control the disease or its complications; (2) mucosal damage may compromise absorptive capacity in the remaining small bowel; and (3) internal fistulas may form between proximal and distal loops of small bowel, causing nutrients to "bypass" a significant amount of the absorptive surface. A less common cause of short bowel syndrome is surgical resection of a retroperitoneal malignancy involving the superior mesenteric vessels; curative resection for such a lesion must include the superior mesenteric artery and the bowel it supplies.

There has been much controversy over the length of intact bowel that defines "short bowel syndrome." This inability to define precisely the length of bowel required for adequate absorptive capacity is due in part to inconsistencies in measurement; the measurable length of the intact small bowel varies from about 260 to 800 cm (depending on the state of contraction), which means that intraoperative evaluations of the length of remaining small bowel vary also. The difficulty in defining the length of small bowel required for adequate nutrient absorption is also a reflection of the many variables affecting bowel function and nutrient absorption; for example, distal resections may cause greater compromise than proximal resections, and removal of the duodenum is not well tolerated. It is now recognized that the minimal amount of small bowel required to maintain life without long-term parenteral nutritional support varies from patient to patient. Most patients can tolerate the loss of 40% or more of the small bowel so long as the duodenum, distal ileum, and ileocecal valve remain intact. Factors that increase the risk of short bowel syndrome include resection of 75% or more of the small bowel (with residual length of less than 100 cm) and resection of the terminal ileum and ileocecal valve. Retention of the ileocecal valve may enable the patient undergoing massive intestinal resection to regain adequate absorptive function; when the ileocecal valve is retained, intestinal motility is slowed, which promotes absorption, and bacterial contamination of the small bowel is prevented, which promotes fat absorption by preventing deconjugation of bile salts.

PATHOPHYSIOLOGY

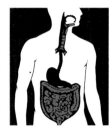

Malabsorption of nutrients, vitamins, minerals, fluids, and electrolytes is the primary pathologic effect of short bowel syndrome; secondary derangements include gastric hypersecretion, hyperbilirubinemia, increased intestinal motility, intractable diarrhea, and development of oxalate renal stones. The specific manifestations depend on the length and specific segments of bowel resected.

The macronutrients (proteins, fats, and carbohydrates) normally are digested and absorbed in the proximal 150 cm of jejunum; however, these nutrients can also be absorbed by the distal jejunum or by the ileum. Carbohydrates and proteins are more readily digested and absorbed than fats; this explains why fat intolerance is a common problem in short bowel syndrome, whereas carbohydrate and protein malabsorption is uncommon even after massive small bowel resection. (However, lactose may be poorly tolerated, because massive small bowel resection creates a lactase deficiency.) Fat malabsorption creates significant secondary problems such as deficiencies of fat-soluble vitamins, weight loss, and steatorrhea.

Vitamin and mineral deficiencies may also occur in the patient with short bowel syndrome, depending on the segments of bowel resected and on the severity of fat intolerance. Resection of the terminal ileum causes vitamin B_{12} deficiency, which becomes manifest once the liver stores of the vitamin have been depleted; vitamin B_{12} malabsorption requires lifelong parenteral replacement to prevent anemia and peripheral neuropathy. Massive small bowel resection resulting in fat intolerance also causes malabsorption of the fat-soluble vitamins (A, D, E, and K); parenteral administration of vitamin K may be required to prevent coagulopathies until oral vitamin supplements can be tolerated. Deficiencies of water-soluble vitamins also can occur, although water-soluble vitamins are absorbed much more readily than fat-soluble vitamins; most patients can maintain adequate levels of water-soluble vitamins with liquid supplements. Uncorrected vitamin deficiencies cause a wide variety of clinical signs and symptoms (Table 6-1). Deficiencies of minerals, such as iron, folic acid, and calcium, are also common in the patient with short bowel syndrome, especially in patients undergoing partial or total duodenectomy. These deficiencies must be corrected by means of oral or parenteral supplements to prevent sequelae such as anemia and osteoporosis.

In addition to malabsorption of macronutrients and micronutrients, short bowel syndrome can cause severe derangements in fluid and electrolyte balance. Normally the small bowel reabsorbs about 80% of the 8 to 10 L of fluid ingested and secreted daily into the small bowel. The patient with short bowel syndrome initially may lose as much as 5 L of fluid daily through the stool, with resultant hypovolemia, hypokalemia, hyponatremia, and metabolic acidosis. Proximal small bowel resections generally produce less long-term imbalance than distal small bowel resections; this is because the distal ileum and colon have tremendous reserve capacity for absorption of fluid and electrolytes, whereas loss of the distal ileum not only presents a large fluid load to the colon but also results in malabsorption of bile salts, which causes a bile salt–induced diarrhea.

Gastric hypersecretion is a common secondary effect of short bowel syndrome; the degree of hypersecretion is directly related to the extent of the small bowel resection, with a 75% resection more than doubling the usual amount of acid secreted. The massive secretion of acid overwhelms the buffering mechanisms of the small bowel, producing a low intraluminal pH that inactivates pancreatic enzymes and damages the small bowel mucosa, possibly causing ulceration. Inactivation of the pancreatic enzymes further compromises digestion and absorption of fats and proteins, and the increase in intraluminal acid exacerbates the diarrhea by causing an increased solute load. The cause of the hypersecretion is not known but is hypothesized to be loss of an inhibitor (to gastric acid secretion) normally produced by the intact small bowel.

Many patients with short bowel syndrome also have transient changes in liver function, and hyperbilirubinemia and jaundice are common developments during the initial period following massive small bowel resection. The causative mechanism is not well understood but is thought to be due either to bacteria arising from the ischemic bowel and passing through the portal circulation into the liver or to the sudden reduction in portal blood flow caused by massive small bowel resection.

Cholelithiasis is another complication of short bowel syndrome; studies have shown that most patients with short bowel syndrome eventually develop gallstones, and many require surgical intervention within the 2 years following massive small bowel resection. Gallstones develop because resection of the terminal ileum leads to loss of bile salt reabsorption. The liver's ability to increase bile salt synthesis is relatively fixed, and bile salt depletion results in a more lithogenic bile.

Calcium oxalate renal stones also are more common among patients with short bowel syndrome and an intact colon. These stones occur because absorption of dietary oxalate is increased. Oxalate normally is bound to

Table 6-1

SYMPTOMS OF WATER-SOLUBLE VITAMIN DEFICIENCIES

Vitamin	Function	Signs of deficiency
B_1 (thiamine)	Supports carbohydrate and amino acid metabolism; required for growth	Muscle weakness, paralysis, neuritis
B_2 (riboflavin)	Involved in citric acid cycle	Fissures at corners of mouth, eye disorders
Pantothenic acid (component of B_2 complex)	Promotes gluconeogenesis and synthesis of steroid hormones; constituent of coenzyme A	Fatigue, neuromuscular dysfunction
B_3 (niacin)	Supports metabolic processes (glycolysis and citric acid cycle)	Diarrhea, dermatitis, mental confusion
B_6 (pyridoxine)	Amino acid metabolism	Dermatitis, growth retardation, nausea
Folic acid	Hematopoiesis and nucleic acid synthesis	Macrocytic anemia
B_{12} (cobalamin)	Erythrocyte production; nucleic acid and amino acid metabolism	Pernicious anemia, nervous system disorders (e.g., peripheral neuropathy)
C (ascorbic acid)	Collagen synthesis; protein metabolism	Delayed wound healing, capillary fragility, defective bone formation
H (biotin)	Fatty acid and purine synthesis; citric acid cycle	Fatigue, nausea, mental and muscle dysfunction

calcium in the bowel lumen and therefore is unabsorbable; however, in the presence of steatorrhea, the calcium binds to the unabsorbed fatty acids, leaving the oxalate in an absorbable state.

One of the most debilitating effects of short bowel syndrome is the intractable diarrhea. Diarrhea associated with short bowel syndrome involves a number of etiologic factors. Although the most obvious factors are the reduction in absorptive area and the increased fluid load presented to the colon, a number of additional factors exacerbate the diarrhea. One of these is the increased solute load created by the undigested nutrients, which causes an osmolar diarrhea. Another factor is the hypermotility that commonly accompanies short bowel syndrome; this is particularly significant when the small bowel resection includes the ileocecal valve. Resection of the ileocecal valve also permits bacterial contamination of the small bowel, which contributes to deconjugation of the bile salts, with resultant fat malabsorption and steatorrhea. Steatorrhea is also a factor when the terminal ileum is resected; the resulting depletion in bile salts further impairs fat absorption. Lactose ingestion in the presence of lactase deficiency contributes to diarrhea in two ways: (1) the undigested lactose causes an osmolar diarrhea in the small bowel, and (2) colonic bacterial action on the lactose produces lactic acid, which acts as a colonic irritant and causes further

diarrhea. Controlling diarrhea is a major challenge in the management of short bowel syndrome.

In terms of clinical presentation and management goals, short bowel syndrome commonly is divided into three phases. Phase 1 begins immediately after resection of the small bowel and continues for about 2 months; this phase is characterized by massive diarrhea, and the major challenge is to maintain fluid and electrolyte stability. Nutritional status is maintained through total parenteral nutrition, since any attempt at enteral feedings results in increased diarrhea and may also precipitate vomiting.

Phase 2 is the bowel adaptation phase; it begins about 2 months after surgery, when fecal output has stabilized at 2 L or less per day. Patients who have retained at least 10% of the small bowel usually progress to Phase 2. The reduction in diarrhea signals the beginning of bowel "adaptation," which involves hyperplasia of the small bowel mucosa and villi. The mechanisms mediating this adaptation response have not been clearly identified; it is hypothesized that the intraluminal presence of nutrient breakdown products somehow stimulates the hyperplastic mucosal response, and studies have shown that enteral feedings and the presence of pancreatobiliary secretions in the lumen of the bowel both serve to stimulate villous growth. This theory is supported by the fact that, in general, proximal resections generate a greater adaptive response than do distal resections; it is thought that this is because proximal resections result in increased amounts of intraluminal nutrients in the distal small bowel. Humoral and hormonal factors are also thought to play a role in the adaptation response. During Phase 2, enteral feedings are very gradually advanced, beginning with simple carbohydrates; parenteral nutrition is continued, and the volume and formula are adjusted as the patient's enteral tolerance increases. Phase 2 usually lasts until about 12 months after resection, although it may last longer.

Phase 3 is the stabilization and long-term management phase. By the end of 1 to 2 years, adaptation is maximized, and the patient is stabilized on an appropri-

ate management program. For most patients with at least 10% of the small bowel intact, nutritional needs can be met with oral feedings. Some patients will require supplemental enteral or parenteral support, and a few patients will require total parenteral nutrition (TPN).

COMPLICATIONS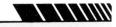

Fluid-electrolyte imbalance	Hypovolemia
Malabsorption syndromes	Malnutrition
Peptic ulcer disease	Intractable diarrhea
Calcium oxalate renal stones	Cholelithiasis

DIAGNOSTIC STUDIES AND FINDINGS

Diagnostic test	Findings
Serum electrolytes	May show decreased levels (e.g., hyponatremia, hypokalemia)
Arterial blood gases	May show metabolic acidosis (decreased levels of bicarbonate)
Liver studies	May show elevated bilirubin level, other alterations
Stool for fat	May show increased amount of fat in stool and decreased coefficient of fat absorption, indicating fat malabsorption (normal findings: <6 g of fat in stool per 24 h; coefficient of fat absorption >95%)
Hemoglobin and hematocrit	May be reduced
Serum albumin	May be reduced
Serum calcium, iron, magnesium, zinc, folic acid, vitamin B_{12}	May be reduced
Schilling test for vitamin B_{12} absorption	May show reduced urinary excretion of vitamin B_{12}
Prothrombin time (PT)	Prolonged PT may be seen with fat malabsorption and vitamin K deficiency
Hydrogen breath test	Elevated hydrogen level commonly seen in patient with lactose intolerance

MEDICAL MANAGEMENT

GENERAL MANAGEMENT

Phase 1 (postoperative phase)

NPO status to prevent exacerbation of diarrhea; nasogastric suction during initial postoperative period to prevent vomiting; IV fluids and TPN to supply needed nutrients, vitamins, minerals, fluids, and electrolytes; salt-poor albumin IV to correct hypoalbuminemia and maintain oncotic pressure. Hemodynamic monitoring (vital signs, intake and output, central venous pressure or Swan-Ganz readings).

Phase 2 (2 months to 1-2 years after surgery)

Gradual advancement in oral intake of nutrients and fluids, with corresponding decrease in volume of TPN feedings based on tolerance: initial oral feedings: simple electrolyte and carbohydrate solutions (e.g., flavored 5% dextrose in lactated Ringer's solution); gradual advancement to dilute solutions of chemically defined diets with short-chain peptides and simple amino acids; progressive advancement to high-carbohydrate, high-pro-

Continued.

MEDICAL MANAGEMENT—cont'd

tein, moderate-fat, low-lactose diet (initially solids should be given separately from liquids). Supplementation with short-chain and medium-chain triglycerides (e.g., coconut oil, 30 ml bid or tid) and essential fatty acids (e.g., safflower oil, 30 ml bid or tid) as needed; monitoring of nutritional status (weigh daily or weekly, serum determinations of nutritional indices).

Phase 3 (long-term management)

Oral feedings as tolerated (high carbohydrate, high protein, moderate fat, low lactose): Amount of oral intake should be greater than amount needed to compensate for malabsorbed nutrients. Enteral supplementation of oral intake as needed for patients unable to maintain weight with oral feedings (e.g., continuous-drip, lactose-free enteral feedings 8-12 h/day). Parenteral supplements as needed for patients unable to maintain weight with oral feedings and enteral supplements (e.g., cyclic infusion of TPN formula 12 h/day).

SURGERY

There are no definitive surgical procedures for managing short bowel syndrome, although surgery may be indicated to correct underlying disease processes exacerbating the syndrome (e.g., correction of loop-to-loop fistulas) or to manage complications (e.g., cholecystectomy). Surgical procedures that occasionally are performed for intractable short bowel syndrome include bowel-lengthening procedures (in which the bowel and its mesentery are divided longitudinally, producing two narrow intestinal tubes that are then anastomosed), intestinal interpositions (in which a bowel segment such as colon is surgically interposed, usually in an antiperistaltic position, to slow transit), or small bowel transplant (which is still experimental and has high morbidity and mortality rates).

DRUG THERAPY

Broad-spectrum antibiotics: IV first 5-7 days postoperatively.
Sodium bicarbonate: 8-12 g daily (powder, tablet, liquid, or wafer form) for patient with chronic metabolic acidosis; sodium bicarbonate IV for patient with acute metabolic acidosis (Phases 2 and 3).
Calcium gluconate: 6-8 g daily (powder, tablet, wafer, or liquid form) for patient with chronic hypocalcemia; calcium gluconate IV for patient with severe or recalcitrant hypocalcemia (Phases 2 and 3).
Multivitamin supplements in pediatric form: 1 ml bid (Phases 2 and 3) *or* multivitamin capsule or tablet 1 bid (if tolerated). Iron supplements (e.g., Fer-in-Sol, 1 ml 1-3 × daily) (Phases 2 and 3).
Vitamin B$_{12}$: 1 mg IM q 2-4 wk as needed (Phases 2 and 3).
Folic acid: 15 mg IM weekly as needed (Phases 2 and 3).
Vitamin K: 10 mg IM weekly as needed (Phases 2 and 3).
Antacids (e.g., Amphojel or Mylanta): 30-60 ml q 2 h to counteract gastric hypersecretion (Phase 1; Phases 2 and 3 as needed).
Sucralfate (e.g., Carafate): 1 g PO q 6 h to protect gastric and duodenal mucosa from gastric acid (Phase 1; Phases 2 and 3 as needed)
Cimetidine (Tagamet): 300-600 mg q 6 h (IV or PO); *or* ranitidine (Zantac): 150 mg q 12 h (IV or PO); *or* famotidine (Pepcid): 20 mg bid (IV or PO) to reduce gastric hypersecretion and prevent ulceration (Phase 1; Phases 2 and 3 as needed).
Somatostatin (Sandostatin): 50-150 µg IV or SQ to reduce intestinal secretions and fecal output (Phase 1).
Cholestyramine (Questran): 4 g PO q 8 h to bind bile acids and reduce bile salt–induced diarrhea (Phase 1; Phases 2 and 3 as needed).
Loperamide (Imodium): 4-16 mg PO daily; *or* diphenoxylate (Lomotil): 20 mg PO q 6 h to control diarrhea (Phases 1 and 2; Phase 3 as needed).
Codeine: 60 mg IM q 4 h *or* acetaminophen with codeine: 30-60 mg PO q 4 h as needed to control diarrhea (Phases 1 and 2; Phase 3 as needed).
Propantheline (Pro-Banthine): 15 mg PO q 4-6 h for intractable diarrhea (Phase 2; Phase 3 as needed).
Omeprazole (Prilosec): 20 mg PO daily for intractable diarrhea (Phase 2; Phase 3 as needed).
Dicyclomine (Bentyl): 20-40 mg PO q 6 h for intractable diarrhea (Phase 2; Phase 3 as needed).
Deodorized tincture of opium: 10-30 drops q 4 h for intractable diarrhea (Phase 2; Phase 3 as needed).
Insulin: as needed for patient who is glucose intolerant and receiving TPN.

_1_ ASSESS

ASSESSMENT	OBSERVATIONS
Surgical history	May report massive or repetitive small bowel resections for management of inflammatory or ischemic disease
Fluid and electrolyte balance	May report frequent large-volume diarrheal stools; may report reduced frequency of urination and increased urine concentration; may report signs and symptoms of fluid-electrolyte imbalance (e.g., dry mouth and skin, feeling dizzy or weak when standing; extreme fatigue; muscle weakness); may have postural hypotension, diminished skin turgor, diminished muscle tone and reflexes, cardiac dysrhythmias, and altered level of consciousness
Gastrointestinal function and symptoms	May report frequent diarrheal stools; may report large amounts of flatus and explosive diarrhea after ingesting milk or milk products (lactose intolerance); may report greasy, foul-smelling stools (fat malabsorption)
Nutritional status	Weight may be less than 85%-90% of usual weight; may have signs and symptoms of nutrient, vitamin, and mineral depletion (e.g., skin rashes; sore tongue; fissures at corners of mouth; fatigability; joint edema; dry, pluckable hair; easy bruising; diminished night vision; hip pain or pain on walking; tingling in fingers or toes; numbness or burning sensation in legs and feet); may report persistent weight loss despite increased oral intake of nutrients
Perianal skin	May report perianal burning, itching, or soreness; perianal area may appear erythematous and denuded

_2_ DIAGNOSE

NURSING DIAGNOSIS	SUBJECTIVE FINDINGS	OBJECTIVE FINDINGS
Diarrhea related to malabsorption of nutrients and fluids	Reports frequent loose stools; describes stools as watery or "greasy and malodorous"; may describe stools as "explosive"	Watery or fatty stools that may be malodorous; increased frequency of stools
Altered nutrition: less than body requirements related to malabsorption of nutrients.	Reports unplanned and persistent weight loss despite increased oral intake; may report persistent diarrhea; may report signs of nutrient, vitamin, and mineral deficiencies (e.g., skin rashes, sore tongue, fatigability, hip pain or pain on walking, tingling in fingers or toes, numbness or burning sensation in legs and feet).	Weight less than 90% of usual weight; may exhibit signs of nutrient, vitamin, and mineral deficiencies (e.g., skin rashes, fissures at corners of mouth, joint edema, dry, pluckable hair, bruising).
Fluid volume deficit related to diarrhea	Reports diarrhea and signs and symptoms of fluid volume deficit (e.g., dry mouth, dizziness when standing, extreme fatigue, tingling in hands or feet)	Frequent, large-volume, watery stools; signs of fluid volume deficit (e.g., oliguria, increased concentration of urine, diminished skin turgor, tachycardia, hypotension, decreased central venous pressure or Swan-Ganz readings, diaphoresis)

_3_ PLAN

Patient goals

1. The patient's diarrhea will be controlled.
2. The patient will regain and maintain his usual weight and will have no signs or symptoms of nutrient, vitamin, or mineral deficiencies.
3. The patient will maintain normal levels of intravascular, interstitial, and intracellular fluids and electrolytes.

→ > >

4 IMPLEMENT

NURSING DIAGNOSIS	NURSING INTERVENTIONS	RATIONALE
Diarrhea related to malabsorption of nutrients and fluids	Monitor stools for frequency, volume, and consistency.	Diarrhea is a common clinical indicator of nutrient malabsorption; volume, frequency, and consistency of stools reflect GI tract's ability to digest and absorb nutrients.
	Keep patient NPO until fecal losses are less than 2 L/day.	Fecal losses greater than 2 L/day indicate that bowel adaptation has not yet begun; oral feedings initiated before bowel adaptation has begun increase the fluid load in the gut and exacerbate diarrhea.
	Initiate oral or enteral feedings with balanced solutions containing simple carbohydrates and electrolytes.	Balanced solutions containing salt and simple sugars are readily absorbed and thus less likely to increase diarrhea.
	Collaborate with physician and dietitian to advance oral and enteral feedings very slowly according to patient's tolerance.	Gradual advancement of oral and enteral feedings stimulates bowel adaptation without exacerbating malabsorption and diarrhea.
	Administer antisecretory medications as ordered (e.g., cimetidine, ranitidine, famotidine, somatostatin).	Antisecretory medications reduce intestinal secretion and thus help reduce fecal losses.
	Administer antimotility agents as ordered (e.g., loperamide, diphenoxylate, codeine, deodorized tincture of opium).	Antimotility agents reduce peristalsis and thus increase intestinal transit time and nutrient contact with the intestinal mucosa.
	Administer cholestyramine as ordered for patient with bile salt–induced diarrhea caused by resection of the terminal ileum and failure to reabsorb bile salts.	Failure to reabsorb bile salts in the terminal ileum results in bile salts being delivered to the colon, which causes colonic irritation and diarrhea; cholestyramine prevents this by binding with unabsorbed bile acids.
	Provide appropriate perianal skin care: gentle cleansing with tap water or mineral oil; protection of intact skin with copolymer film (e.g., Bard Incontinent Spray or Skin Prep); treatment of denuded skin with pectin-based powder (e.g., Stomahesive Powder) and a moisture-barrier cream or ointment (e.g., Critic-Aid or Calmoseptine).	Diarrhea associated with short bowel syndrome contains proteolytic enzymes and may be acidic; scrupulous skin care is essential to prevent massive skin breakdown.
Altered nutrition: less than body requirements related to malabsorption of nutrients	Monitor indicators of nutritional status: body weight, fecal losses, signs of malnutrition (e.g., skin rashes, joint edema, easy bruising, hip pain or pain on walking, diminished muscle mass, cheilosis, pluckable hair).	Continuing assessment provides the basis for appropriate intervention.

NURSING DIAGNOSIS	NURSING INTERVENTIONS	RATIONALE
	Keep patient NPO, and collaborate with physician and nutritional support team to provide TPN during initial postoperative phase and until fecal losses have stabilized at less than 2 L/day.	All nutrient needs must be met through the parenteral route until initial bowel adaptation occurs; oral feedings given before this will exacerbate the diarrhea.
	Initiate oral or enteral feedings with a balanced solution of electrolytes and simple carbohydrates (e.g., flavored D_5 lactated Ringer's solution).	Once initial bowel adaptation has begun, oral or enteral feedings stimulate mucosal hyperplasia and help stimulate pancreatic secretions, which also promote bowel adaptation; balanced solutions of electrolytes and simple carbohydrates are the most readily absorbed enteral nutrient.
	Collaborate with physician and nutritional support team to gradually advance enteral feedings to dilute formulas with short peptide chains, to high-protein, high-carbohydrate, low-fat, low-lactose diet, to near-normal diet, with rate of advancement determined by patient's tolerance.	Gradual advancement of enteral nutrients stimulates the adaptation response while minimizing malabsorption and diarrhea.
	Taper parenteral nutrients as patient is able to increase oral and enteral intake.	Nutrient intake should be gradually shifted to the oral or enteral route.
	Provide supplemental intake of vitamins and minerals as indicated (e.g., general multivitamin and mineral supplements, folic acid, vitamin B_{12}, vitamin K); administer orally (e.g., in liquid or chewable form) if tolerated; administer parenterally if needed to maintain normal levels.	Vitamins and minerals are essential for many bodily functions, and normal levels must be maintained; liquid or chewable forms may be more readily absorbed.
	Administer medium-chain triglycerides and short-chain triglycerides as indicated (coconut oil and safflower oil) for patient with fat malabsorption.	Medium-chain and short-chain triglycerides do not require bile for absorption; they provide essential fatty acids and support absorption of fat-soluble vitamins.
	For patient unable to maintain weight and nutritional status with oral feedings: collaborate with physician and nutritional support team to provide cyclic administration of enteral feedings by continuous-drip infusion.	Continuous-drip enteral feedings on a cyclic basis provide for increased absorption of nutrients without exacerbating diarrhea and may enable a patient to maintain nutritional status without parenteral support.
	For patient unable to maintain weight on a combination of oral and enteral feedings: collaborate with physician and nutritional support team to provide parenteral nutritional support on either a cyclic or continuous basis.	Long-term parenteral nutritional support may be required for patients with severe short bowel syndrome.
Fluid volume deficit related to diarrhea	Maintain accurate records of fluid intake and fluid loss (urine output, N/G suction or emesis, liquid stools).	Accurate records permit early recognition of fluid deficits and also provide the basis for accurate fluid replacement.

→ > >

NURSING DIAGNOSIS	NURSING INTERVENTIONS	RATIONALE
	Monitor indicators of intravascular volume depletion (BP, CVP, or Swan-Ganz pressure readings, urine output, diaphoresis, skin turgor, pulse).	Prompt recognition of fluid volume deficit permits early intervention; hypovolemia causes hypotension and oliguria, and compensatory responses cause tachycardia, diaphoresis, and reduced skin turgor.
	Administer IV fluids and electrolytes as ordered.	IV fluids and electrolytes restore plasma volume and correct fluid volume deficits.
	Administer salt-poor albumin IV as ordered.	Hypoalbuminemia contributes to intravascular depletion by reducing intravascular oncotic pressure.
	Administer calcium gluconate and sodium bicarbonate PO or IV (as ordered) for patient with chronic or acute hypocalcemia or metabolic acidosis.	Hypocalcemia and metabolic acidosis are common electrolyte imbalances in patients with short bowel syndrome; hypocalcemia affects neuromuscular function adversely, and acidosis causes multiple derangements in body functions and level of consciousness.

5 EVALUATE

PATIENT OUTCOME	DATA INDICATING THAT OUTCOME IS REACHED
Patient's diarrhea has been controlled.	Patient reports fewer than five loose stools per day; he states that perianal skin is not painful, and inspection reveals intact perianal skin.
Patient has regained and maintains usual weight and has no signs or symptoms of nutrient, vitamin, or mineral deficiencies.	Patient's weight is within 90% of his usual or desired weight; patient has no signs or symptoms of nutrient deficiencies (e.g., joint edema, dry skin, skin rashes, cheilosis, easy bruising, fatigability, diminished night vision, numbness and burning in feet and legs, tingling in hands and feet, hip pain or pain on walking).
Patient maintains normal levels of intravascular, interstitial, and intracellular fluids and electrolytes.	BP and pulse are within normal limits; urine output is normal; fluid intake and fluid losses are balanced; skin turgor is normal; patient has no symptoms of electrolyte imbalance (e.g., extreme muscle weakness, muscle cramping, dizziness when standing, tingling in hands and feet, altered level of consciousness).

PATIENT TEACHING

1. Explain what is meant by short bowel syndrome, and explain the effects of the disorder on nutritional status, gastrointestinal functioning, and fluid and electrolyte balance.
2. Explain the treatment plan, including the rationale and general guidelines for a staged management approach.
3. Instruct the patient in the specifics of his individualized treatment plan (e.g., prescribed diet, enteral feedings, oral or parenteral supplements of vitamins

and minerals, parenteral support). Teach the patient or family member the procedures for (1) administering enteral or parenteral feedings and (2) caring for the enteral feeding tube and setup or the TPN venous access device and site. Instruct the patient in possible adverse reactions or complications and appropriate management (e.g., how to manage an obstructed feeding tube; how to manage a cracked or broken venous access line).

4. Explain the rationale and administration guidelines for prescribed medications.
5. Teach the patient the signs and symptoms of fluid and electrolyte imbalance, and instruct him to notify his physician if he develops any of them; explain that minor viral illnesses must be treated promptly because they may cause severe fluid-electrolyte disturbances in an individual with short bowel syndrome.

Malnutrition

Malnutrition occurs when the amount of nutrients ingested and absorbed is insufficient to maintain normal body structure and function.

Malnutrition is classified according to the body compartment affected by the deficiency: marasmus involves loss of fat stores and skeletal muscle, but visceral proteins usually are maintained within the low normal range; kwashiorkor involves loss of visceral proteins, but body fat stores and skeletal muscle mass are maintained; mixed marasmus-kwashiorkor (protein-calorie malnutrition) involves loss of body fat, skeletal muscle wasting, and depletion of visceral proteins (Figure 6-1).

EPIDEMIOLOGY

Malnutrition long has been recognized as a serious health problem in underdeveloped countries, where famine is a constant threat. More recently it has been identified as an important and treatable complication of many chronic illnesses and as a major contributor to morbidity and mortality among hospitalized patients. Malnutrition continues to be a serious problem among hospitalized patients, despite the proliferation of information on the causes, effects, prevention, and treatment of nutritional deficiencies. Factors contributing to malnutrition in hospitalized patients are listed on p. 238.

Malnutrition commonly results from inadequate nutrient intake; causative factors include anorexia (from either psychologic or physical causes), chewing or swallowing disorders, fad diets, dietary restrictions necessitated by chronic medical conditions, and socioeconomic factors restricting access to appropriate foods.

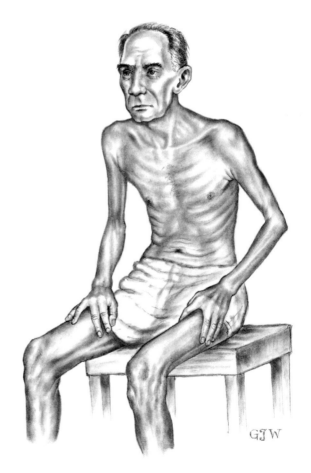

FIGURE 6-1
Celiac sprue (primary malabsorption).

Malnutrition may also result from impaired nutrient absorption; this is the basis for nutritional compromise in patients with short gut syndrome, malabsorption syndromes, and high-output small bowel fistulas. Hypermetabolic conditions such as sepsis can contribute to malnutrition by increasing nutrient demands.

MARASMUS

Marasmus results from prolonged periods of inadequate nutrient intake or compromised nutrient absorption, as occurs with starvation, chronic anorexia, or chronic illness. Nutrient intake is balanced in that the ratio of calories to protein is appropriate, but overall nutrient intake is insufficient to provide the calories needed to support bodily functions. As a result, the body begins to break down its own tissues to meet its energy needs. The immediate effect of inadequate caloric intake is a reduction in blood glucose levels; this causes a reduction in insulin production and an increase in glucagon production. Glucagon mediates the breakdown of stored glycogen, which provides a temporary source of glucose. Since glycogen reserves are limited, this alternative fuel source is exhausted fairly quickly. If the deficit state continues, the body turns to its fat and muscle stores as alternative sources of energy. Fat, which is stored in the body as triglycerides, is degraded into fatty acids and glycerol; fatty acids are metabolized to produce ketones, which become the body's major source of energy. Although most of the body's energy demands can be met by ketones, some tissues require glucose (e.g., the renal medulla, the white blood cells, and part of the brain). This glucose is provided through neoangiogenesis, the process by which the liver synthesizes glucose from amino acids (derived from lean body mass) and glycerol (derived from triglycerides). The major source of energy in the patient with marasmus is breakdown of fat, which causes loss of adipose tissue and progressive weight loss. Gradual muscle wasting may also be seen, because skeletal muscle mass serves as a secondary fuel source. Because protein intake is sufficient to support production of visceral proteins by the liver, the visceral protein compartment is spared.

KWASHIORKOR

Kwashiorkor is a protein deficiency that results when caloric intake is maintained but protein intake is very deficient; this may be seen in individuals on fad diets. Failure to maintain an adequate protein intake results in loss of visceral proteins, because there is insufficient protein to support production of visceral proteins by the liver. Loss of visceral proteins (e.g., albumin, transferrin, fibronectin) results in loss of intravascular oncotic pressure and compromised immune function. Because the caloric intake is sufficient to meet the body's energy needs, there is no breakdown of adipose tissue

---

FACTORS CONTRIBUTING TO MALNUTRITION IN HOSPITALIZED PATIENTS

Failure to accurately assess height and weight
Failure to assess nutritional status before major surgical procedures
Failure to record patient's nutrient intake and to perform calorie counts
Elimination of nutrients as preparation for diagnostic studies
Prolonged NPO status without nutritional replacement (IV fluids only form of intervention)
Failure to provide nutritional support until malnutrition advanced
Lack of knowledge about metabolic response to injury and illness
Lack of knowledge about options for nutritional support and appropriate use of nutritional products
Lack of knowledge about effects of malnutrition on immunocompetence

---

or skeletal muscle to provide ketones or glucose; the patient does not lose weight and does not appear malnourished.

MIXED MARASMUS-KWASHIORKOR

Mixed marasmus-kwashiorkor (protein-calorie malnutrition) involves acute deficiency of both calories and protein, as may occur in a hospitalized patient who is maintained on intravenous fluids. In this situation the acute protein deficiency results in visceral protein depletion, as is seen in kwashiorkor. The calorie deficiency triggers breakdown of fats and skeletal muscle to provide ketones and glucose for energy; this produces the weight loss and skeletal muscle wasting commonly associated with marasmus. However, protein-calorie malnutrition in an individual who is acutely ill or injured precipitates greater loss of skeletal muscle mass and less breakdown of body fats than occur in the chronic deficit state known as marasmus. This is explained by the metabolic changes induced by acute physiologic stress. Acute stress causes stimulation of the sympathetic nervous system and increased production of corticosteroids, which results in an increased metabolic rate and increased mobilization of amino acids from the skeletal muscles. Because glucose remains the preferred fuel source, continuous breakdown of skeletal muscles occurs to provide the amino acids required for gluconeogenesis. (In chronic deficit states, ketones derived from fat breakdown become the primary energy source.) The result is significant loss of muscle mass and depletion of visceral proteins, and gradual loss of body fat. Protein-calorie malnutrition in an acutely ill or injured individual is associated with significant morbidity and mortality.

PATHOPHYSIOLOGY

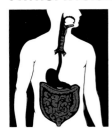

The pathologic results of malnutrition vary, depending on the body compartment affected and the severity of the deficiency. When the primary deficit is calories (as is seen in marasmus), the effect is loss of body fat and gradual loss of skeletal muscle mass. The patient loses weight, and he may also note loss of endurance related to loss of muscle mass and reduced energy production. Serious morbidity does not usually occur unless the deficit state is prolonged enough to exhaust the body's fat stores; at this point the body must use its muscle mass to produce energy, and the patient experiences the signs and symptoms of protein depletion (e.g., edema, delayed wound healing). Patients with a primary calorie deficiency (marasmus) retain the ability to fight infection and to respond to stress, because the visceral protein compartment is relatively unaffected.

Protein deficiency, as is seen in kwashiorkor and mixed protein-calorie malnutrition, has serious pathologic consequences. Protein is the structural component for all lean body mass, including organ mass and muscle mass, and is required for production of visceral proteins such as albumin, antibodies, hormones, enzymes, and carrier substances such as transferrin. Normally the body's protein structures undergo a continual "turnover" process, which involves breaking down existing proteins and replacing them with newly synthesized proteins; this "new" protein is composed primarily of "recycled" amino acids derived from the breakdown of old proteins. However, during each turnover cycle, some protein is degraded and excreted; therefore a constant supply of exogenous protein is needed to maintain muscle mass and organ function and to support production of visceral proteins by the liver.

Protein deficiency alone, as is seen in kwashiorkor, primarily affects the visceral protein compartment; loss of muscle mass is gradual, since most of the amino acids required for protein turnover are derived from breakdown of endogenous protein. Visceral protein deficiency causes serious adverse effects, however. Loss of albumin causes reduced intravascular oncotic pressure, which results in edema and ascites; edema of the bowel wall reduces nutrient absorption and causes diarrhea.

Loss of carrier proteins such as transferrin, prealbumin, and retinol-binding protein causes reduced transport of iron, thyroxin, and vitamin A in the bloodstream. Loss of antibodies, lymphocytes, and fibronectin impairs the immune response. In addition, wound healing and tissue repair are severely compromised, since these processes are protein dependent; wound dehiscence is common. The patient with kwashiorkor, therefore, is at greater risk for infection and is less able to heal than the patient with marasmus, although the patient with marasmus *appears* to be more compromised.

The patient with combined protein and calorie deficits is at the greatest risk for morbidity and even mortality. In addition to the adverse effects associated with loss of visceral proteins, this patient experiences progressive loss of lean body mass as the body cannibalizes its own protein structures to obtain the amino acids required for gluconeogenesis and energy production. Loss of skeletal muscle mass results in generalized muscle wasting and diminished activity tolerance; wasting of intercostal and diaphragmatic muscles compromises ventilatory function and renders the patient more susceptible to respiratory complications such as pneumonia. Loss of smooth muscle in the gastrointestinal tract reduces peristalsis and increases the risk of constipation and ileus. Loss of cardiac muscle results in reduced cardiac output. Organ mass is also diminished, resulting in progressive organ failure; the kidneys and liver are particularly susceptible. Renal and hepatic failure increase the risk of secondary metabolic complications, since breakdown of proteins requires deamination and conversion to urea within the liver and excretion of urea by the kidneys.

Micronutrient deficiencies frequently accompany malnutrition states, since the nutrients that provide calories and protein also provide vitamins and minerals. Signs and symptoms of vitamin and mineral deficiencies are listed in Tables 6-1 and 6-2; assessment of nutritional status should include observation and questioning about these indicators, and nutritional repletion must always include micronutrients as well as macronutrients.

COMPLICATIONS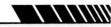

Infection/sepsis
Delayed healing/wound breakdown
Pulmonary complications (pneumonia, ventilator
   dependence)
Cardiac failure
Renal failure
Hepatic failure
Malabsorption/diarrhea

Table 6-2

SIGNS OF MINERAL DEFICIENCY

Mineral	Function	Signs of deficiency
Calcium	Formation of bones and teeth; neuro-muscular function; clotting	Neuromuscular irritability and tetany
Chromium	Glucose metabolism	Resistant hyperglycemia
Copper	Hemoglobin and melanin production; electron transport	Anemia, activity intolerance
Iodine	Production of thyroid hormone; metabolism	Reduced metabolic rate
Iron	Component of hemoglobin; energy production in electron-transport system	Anemia, reduced oxygen transport, loss of energy
Magnesium	Bone formation; nerve and muscle function	Neuromuscular irritability, vasodilation, dysrhythmias
Manganese	Hemoglobin synthesis; growth; enzyme activation	Tremors and convulsions
Molybdenum	Component of enzymes	Unknown
Phosphorus	Formation of bones and teeth; energy transfer; component of nucleic acids	Loss of energy and cellular function
Selenium	Component of enzymes	Unknown
Zinc	Protein metabolism; carbon dioxide transport and metabolism; component of enzymes	Deficient protein metabolism and delayed wound healing, deficient carbon dioxide transport

DIAGNOSTIC STUDIES AND FINDINGS

Diagnostic test	Findings
Triceps skin fold measurement	Used to estimate body's fat stores; may be below normal in patient with marasmus or protein-calorie malnutrition
Midarm muscle circumference or midarm muscle area	Used to estimate skeletal muscle mass; calculation requires measurement of triceps skin fold thickness also; may be below normal in patient with marasmus or protein-calorie malnutrition
Creatinine-height index	May be below normal in patient with skeletal muscle depletion; considered unreliable because results can be altered significantly by small errors in urine collection
Serum albumin	May be below normal in patients with kwashiorkor or protein-calorie malnutrition; <2.4 g/dl indicates severe deficiency; considered a poor indicator of nutritional status because of its long half-life (20 days), because hydration significantly affects values, and because of the large total body pool of albumin
Serum transferrin	Low level commonly seen in patients with protein deficiencies; preferred over albumin test because transferrin's shorter half-life (8 days) means that it more rapidly reflects changes in protein status; <100 mg/dl indicates severe protein deficiency
Prealbumin	Low level commonly seen in patients with protein deficiency; prealbumin's extremely short half-life (2 days) makes it valuable for monitoring changes in protein status; <5 mg/dl indicates severe protein deficiency
Retinol-binding protein	Low level may be seen in patients with protein deficiency; because half-life is 12 hours, values reflect current protein status
Total lymphocyte count	Low level may be seen in patient with visceral protein deficiency resulting in immunocompromise; results must be correlated with other indicators of malnutrition, since other factors can affect total lymphocyte count
Delayed cutaneous hypersensitivity (skin testing for antigens such as *Candida* organisms, mumps, coccidioidin, histoplasmosis, and *Trichophyton* sp.)	Failure to demonstrate positive response at 24 and 48 hours indicates reduced cell-mediated immunity and may be seen in cases of severe malnutrition

DIAGNOSTIC STUDIES AND FINDINGS—cont'd

Diagnostic test	Findings
24-hour urine for urea nitrogen	Used to calculate nitrogen balance; negative nitrogen balance exists when nitrogen excretion (measured by 24-hour urine for urea nitrogen plus a correction factor for other sources of nitrogen loss) exceeds nitrogen intake (calculated by a formula converting ingested or infused protein into nitrogen)

MEDICAL MANAGEMENT

GENERAL MANAGEMENT

Nutritional assessment to determine nutrient needs and nutrient intake. Collaboration with nutritional support team to provide appropriate nutritional replacement:

Dietary modifications and/or use of oral nutritional supplements for patient who can ingest adequate nutrients orally and who has normal gut function (specific dietary modifications and selection of supplements are determined by nutrient needs and type of deficiency).

Placement of enteral feeding tube and administration of selected formula at appropriate rate for patient who is unable or unwilling to ingest adequate nutrients orally but whose gut function is within normal limits (specific formula and rate of administration depend on length and function of distal bowel, site of enteral feeding tube, and type and amount of nutrients to be provided).

Insertion of peripheral intravenous catheter and administration of amino acid formulas and lipids to supplement protein and calorie intake in patient who can partially meet nutrient requirements through oral or enteral feedings (e.g., patient who has impaired nutrient absorption due to hypoalbuminemia and bowel wall edema may benefit from peripheral parenteral protein administration to help correct hypoalbuminemia).

Note: Peripheral parenteral nutrition cannot be used for total nutritional support and is appropriate only on a short-term basis.

Placement of a central venous catheter and administration of TPN for patient who cannot meet nutrient needs through oral, enteral, or peripheral parenteral routes (e.g., patient with multiple small bowel fistulas in proximal and mid ileum).

SURGERY

Surgical placement of an enteral feeding tube (e.g., gastrostomy or jejunostomy) may be indicated for a patient with conditions requiring long-term enteral feeding support (e.g., patient with neurologic or mentation deficit that interferes with oral intake of nutrients).

Surgical placement of a central venous catheter is indicated for a patient requiring TPN.

DRUG THERAPY

Vitamin and mineral supplements for patient being managed with oral or enteral feedings.

Salt-poor albumin IV for patient with edema and ascites secondary to hypoalbuminemia.

Insulin as needed to control hyperglycemia in patient receiving TPN.

Antidiarrheal agents may be required to control diarrhea in patient receiving enteral feedings. (*Note:* Antiperistaltic agents such as loperamide should not be administered until infection with *Clostridium difficile* has been ruled out.)

1 ASSESS

ASSESSMENT	OBSERVATIONS
Weight history	May report recent nonvolitional weight loss; current weight may be < 85%-90% of usual
Nutrient intake and absorption	May report difficulty chewing or swallowing foods; may report anorexia and nausea that interfere with nutrient intake; may report frequent vomiting; may report diarrhea or fistulous drainage; may report socioeconomic factors limiting food choices and nutrient intake; nutritional history and documentation of nutrient intake may reveal inadequate intake of calories or protein or both; may have history of small bowel resections
Indicators of nutritional deficits	Triceps skin fold thickness and midarm muscle circumference may be below normal range; muscle wasting may be evident; patient may report diminished activity tolerance and generalized weakness; reflexes may be hypoactive; hair may be sparse, dull, dry, and easily pluckable; skin may be dry and have petechiae, rashes, or follicular hyperkeratosis; gums may be spongy and may bleed easily; oral ulcers and fissures at corners of mouth may be seen; conjunctivae may be pale; seborrheic dermatitis may be seen on face and in nasolabial folds; generalized edema and joint edema may be evident; delayed healing or wound and tissue breakdown may be seen; palpation may reveal enlargement of thyroid and parotid glands and liver

2 DIAGNOSE

NURSING DIAGNOSIS	SUBJECTIVE FINDINGS	OBJECTIVE FINDINGS
Altered nutrition: less than body requirements related to inadequate nutrient intake, compromised nutrient absorption, or excessive nutrient losses	Reports recent nonvolitional weight loss; may report reduced nutrient intake related to anorexia, nausea, chewing or swallowing difficulties, or inadequate food availability; may report chronic diarrhea or large-volume fistulous drainage; may report reduced activity tolerance	Present weight less than 85%-90% of usual weight; signs of nutritional compromise (e.g., muscle wasting; loss of muscle tone; hypoactive reflexes; tissue and joint edema; sparse, pluckable hair; dry skin; rashes; fissures at corners of mouth); palpation may reveal enlargement of thyroid and parotid glands and hepatomegaly

3 PLAN

Patient goal
1. The patient will regain and maintain usual weight and have no signs or symptoms of nutritional deficiencies.

4 IMPLEMENT

NURSING DIAGNOSIS	NURSING INTERVENTIONS	RATIONALE
Altered nutrition: less than body requirements related to inadequate intake, poor absorption, or excessive nutrient losses	Monitor patient's weight, nutrient intake, and indicators of compromised nutritional status (e.g., muscle wasting, tissue and joint edema, hypoalbuminemia).	Prompt recognition of nutritional deficits permits early intervention; correction of nutritional deficits helps prevent complications.

NURSING DIAGNOSIS	NURSING INTERVENTIONS	RATIONALE
	Collaborate with nutritional support team to accurately assess nutritional status, nutrient intake, nutrient needs, ability to ingest nutrients orally, and length and function of small bowel.	Accurate assessment provides the basis for intervention; nutritional support plan must address the gap between nutrient needs and intake and must use appropriate routes for nutritional replacement.
	For patient who can ingest nutrients orally and who has adequate small bowel function: provide diet that supplies the needed proteins, calories, and micronutrients; document nutrient intake at each feeding.	The oral route is preferred for nutritional support because it is the most physiologic, the safest, and the least expensive.
	For patient who can ingest nutrients orally but has difficulty consuming the needed volume of food: collaborate with dietitian to supplement dietary intake with appropriate liquid formulas.	Oral supplements are an alternative to dietary intake of nutrients; liquid supplements require less energy to ingest and are more rapidly emptied from the stomach.
	For patient with adequate small bowel function who is unable or unwilling to ingest adequate nutrients orally: collaborate with physician and nutritional support team to insert an appropriate tube for enteral feedings and to select an appropriate formula for enteral feedings.	The enteral route for nutritional support is preferred to the parenteral route because it is safer, less expensive, and maintains the integrity and function of the small bowel (i.e., absorptive capacity and immune functions).
	For patient with gastric tube: administer bolus feedings at regular intervals; check for gastric residuals before each feeding, and hold feeding if residual exceeds 100 ml.	Because the stomach provides controlled emptying, continuous-drip administration is not necessary; feedings should not be given in the presence of high residuals because of the risk of vomiting and aspiration.
	For patient with jejunostomy tube: administer formula by continuous drip; begin with isotonic solutions at a slow rate (e.g., 30-50 ml/h); gradually increase the rate (and concentration, if applicable) until the desired volume of nutrients is being administered without adverse reactions.	Continuous-drip feeding is required because the gastric reservoir has been bypassed; isotonic solutions given slowly are more readily absorbed and less likely to cause osmotic diarrhea; as absorption improves, administration rate can be increased without adverse effects.
	For patient receiving oral or enteral feedings: give vitamin and mineral supplements as ordered.	Micronutrient deficiencies are common in patients with compromised nutrient intake; micronutrients are essential to health.
	For patient who cannot meet all nutrient needs by oral or enteral route, and for patient with bowel wall edema secondary to hypoproteinemia and resultant poor absorption of enteral formulas: collaborate with physician and nutritional support team to establish peripheral IV access and to administer amino acids and lipid solutions.	Peripheral parenteral alimentation can be used on a short-term basis to help correct hypoproteinemia and to provide supplemental calories through lipid administration; TPN cannot be provided through a peripheral line because of the hypertonicity of the required solutions and resultant severe phlebitis.
	Administer salt-poor albumin IV as ordered for patient with hypoproteinemia and generalized edema.	Salt-poor albumin restores intravascular oncotic pressure and acts as an osmotic diuretic.

→ › ›

NURSING DIAGNOSIS	NURSING INTERVENTIONS	RATIONALE
	For patient who cannot meet nutrient needs through oral, enteral, or peripheral parenteral routes: collaborate with physician and nutritional support team to insert central venous line and to initiate TPN.	TPN provides all needed nutrients and is indicated for any patient who cannot meet nutrient needs through alternate routes; TPN must be administered through a large-volume central vein to provide dilution of the hypertonic solution.
	For patient receiving TPN: monitor blood glucose levels, and administer insulin as ordered and indicated.	Hyperglycemia is a common complication of TPN due to the high concentration of glucose.
	Supplement TPN with enteral feedings of isotonic solutions at a slow rate when patient can tolerate them; gradually increase enteral feedings as tolerance increases, and taper TPN accordingly.	Enteral feedings are indicated for maintaining bowel wall integrity and function (i.e., absorption and immune functions); the long-term goal is to maintain nutritional status with oral and enteral feedings.
	For patient receiving enteral feedings who develops diarrhea: administer antidiarrheal agents as ordered and needed; **do not** administer antiperistaltic agents until infection with *C. difficile* and impaction have been ruled out as causative factors.	Antidiarrheal agents slow intestinal motility and therefore promote absorption; antiperistaltic agents delay intestinal transit, which increases the risk of impaction and mucosal damage from bacterial toxins.
	For patient discharged home while still receiving parenteral or enteral nutrition: initiate home health care referral.	Follow-up care is essential to prevent complications.

5 EVALUATE

PATIENT OUTCOME	DATA INDICATING THAT OUTCOME IS REACHED
Patient has regained and maintains usual weight and has no signs or symptoms of nutritional deficits.	Patient's current weight is within 90% of usual weight; patient has no signs or symptoms of nutritional deficits (e.g., muscle wasting; diminished muscle tone; hypoactive reflexes; sparse, dry, pluckable hair; pale conjunctivae; dry skin with rashes, petechiae, keratosis, facial and nasolabial seborrheic dermatitis; activity intolerance; thyroid and parotid gland enlargement; hepatomegaly); wounds are healing or have healed.

PATIENT TEACHING

1. Explain the importance of nutrition to health and recovery; explain that wound healing, infection control, and normal bodily functions depend on an adequate intake of calories, proteins, fats, vitamins, and minerals.
2. Discuss the factors leading to the patient's compromised nutritional status (e.g., anorexia, nausea, diarrhea, fad diet, fistulous drainage, inability to chew or swallow).
3. Explain the treatment plan for correcting nutritional deficits (dietary modifications, oral supplements, enteral feedings, peripheral parenteral nutrition, total parenteral nutrition, vitamin and mineral supplements).
4. Instruct the patient in the specifics of his individualized treatment plan. Teach the patient or family member the procedures for administering enteral or parenteral feedings and for caring for the enteral feeding tube and setup or the TPN venous access device and site. Instruct the patient in possible adverse reactions or complications and their appropriate management (e.g., how to manage an obstructed feeding tube or a cracked or broken venous access line).

Intestinal Fistulas

A fistula is an abnormal communication between two body structures. They may be categorized as internal or external and as high output or low output. Internal fistulas are those between two internal organs, with no external drainage (e.g., a fistula between two loops of small intestine). An external fistula is one that drains to the outside of the body; a fistula between the small bowel and the skin is an external fistula. High-output fistulas are those with more than 500 ml of drainage per 24 hours; low-output fistulas are those with less than 500 ml of drainage per 24 hours.

Fistulas are named by the organ of origin and the organ of termination; for example, an enteroenteric fistula is one between two loops of small bowel, and an enterocutaneous fistula is one between the small bowel and the skin. The terms used to identify the organs involved in a fistula are:

Term	Organ	Term	Organ
Entero-	Small bowel	**Vesico-**	Bladder
Colo-	Colon	**Vaginal**	Vagina
Recto-	Rectum	**Cutaneous**	Skin

ETIOLOGY

Fistulas most commonly result from infectious or inflammatory processes that involve the bowel or from perforation of the bowel wall by trauma, surgical injury, or tumor invasion (Figure 6-2). Distal obstruction may be a contributing factor in fistula formation, and it is known to prevent spontaneous closure of a fistula.

Infectious processes such as abscesses may cause fistulas by direct erosion of the intestinal wall; inflammatory processes cause fistulas because the inflamed bowel becomes densely adherent to adjacent structures, and degeneration of the common wall results in fistula formation. Inflammatory processes that commonly cause fistulas include radiation damage, tumor-induced inflammation and adhesion, Crohn's disease, and diverticular disease. Crohn's disease is the most common cause of fistulas between adjacent loops of bowel (enteroenteric fistulas). Fistulas between the bowel and bladder or the bowel and vagina are most commonly caused by either Crohn's disease or diverticular disease; fortunately, such fistulas are not common.

The most common type of small bowel fistula is the enterocutaneous fistula, and most of these are precipitated by abdominal surgery. Fistulas may develop as a result of intraoperative trauma to the intestine or postoperative anastomotic breakdown. Although surgical technique plays a role in postoperative fistula forma-

tion, the condition of the bowel itself is an important contributing factor. For example, irradiated or ischemic bowel is more prone to fistula formation, and fistulas are also more common with intraabdominal sepsis. Enterocutaneous fistulas may also develop in a patient with Crohn's disease who has had abdominal surgery. Crohn's disease increases the potential for intestinal adherence to the abdominal wall, and fistulas may subsequently form, either early, as a result of anastomotic breakdown, or later, as a result of recurrent inflammation.

Blunt or penetrating trauma to the small bowel can cause perforation of the bowel and subsequent fistula formation, as can ingestion of perforating objects such as fishbones or toothpicks; however, these are infrequent causes. Another uncommon etiologic factor is intraoperative placement of tantalum or polypropylene mesh, which occasionally causes erosion of the bowel wall.

PATHOPHYSIOLOGY

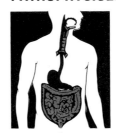

In the past fistulas were associated with significant morbidity and mortality, primarily because of the resultant fluid and electrolyte derangements and malnutrition. With the advent of hemodynamic monitoring, aggressive fluid and electrolyte replacement, and total parenteral nutrition, these complications can be managed more effectively. Today the mortality has been reduced from 54% to about 6%, and the major contributor to morbidity and mortality is intraabdominal sepsis.

The manifestations and complications associated with intestinal fistulas vary considerably, depending on the structures involved and whether the fistula is internal or external. This discussion differentiates among internal fistulas (fistulas between two loops of bowel), external fistulas between two hollow organs (e.g., the bowel and bladder or the bowel and vagina), and fistulas between the bowel and the skin.

Internal fistulas may involve two loops of small bowel (enteroenteric fistulas) or the small bowel and the colon (enterocolic fistulas). The most frequent location for internal fistulas is between the ileum and the cecum. Because external fluid loss does not occur and free intestinal perforation is unlikely, the manifestations of internal fistulas are frequently subtle and nonspecific; in many patients, the fistula is diagnosed incidentally at laparotomy. The clinical manifestations relate to nutritional compromise caused by nutrient "bypass" of absorptive surface (e.g., weight loss and diarrhea) and

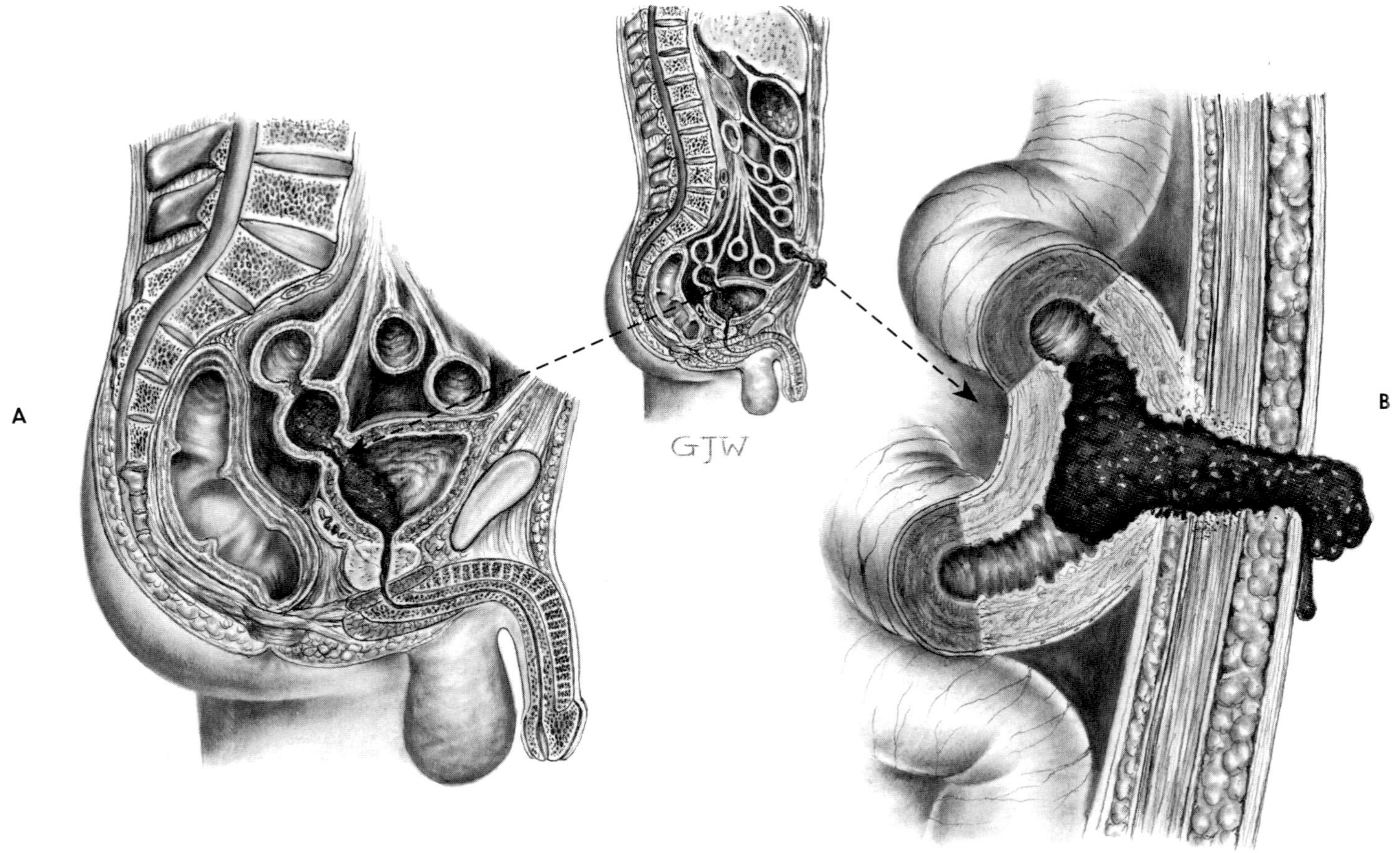

FIGURE 6-2
Fistula. **A,** Internal fistulas with communication between bowel and bladder. **B,** Enterocutaneous fistula with communication between small bowel and abdominal wall.

to possible abscess formation in the area of the fistula (e.g., abdominal tenderness and fever). Because internal fistulas usually are caused by chronic inflammatory conditions, it may be difficult to differentiate between manifestations of the fistula and manifestations of the underlying disease. Management usually involves resection of the involved bowel along with the fistulous tract; a staged procedure with temporary diversion may be required with significant inflammation or abscess formation. Recently controversy has developed over management of internal fistulas (i.e., resection versus conservative management); however, current studies indicate that resection eventually is required in most of these cases.

Fistulas between the bowel and a hollow organ include enterovesical and colovesical fistulas and, in women, enterovaginal and colovaginal fistulas. These fistulas are not common, but they are associated with significant morbidity. Fistulas between the bowel and the bladder usually are manifested by recurrent urinary tract infections and by complaints of frequency, dysuria, and elimination of flatus via the urethra; some patients may have acute sepsis. Management includes infection control measures followed by resection of the

involved section of bowel and bladder. If there is significant inflammation, a staged procedure with temporary fecal diversion may be required. Fistulas between the bowel and the vagina usually cause a purulent or feculent vaginal discharge; the patient may also report passage of gas through the vagina and may complain of fever, chills, and abdominal pain and tenderness. Patients with enterovaginal fistulas may have copious volumes of vaginal drainage, resulting in severe perineal skin damage and in serious fluid and electrolyte abnormalities. Initial management involves control of infection, correction of fluid and electrolyte imbalances, nutritional support, and control of fistula output through appropriate drainage systems. If the fistula fails to close with this conservative approach, surgical resection of the fistulous tract usually is curative. If resection is not feasible, a fecal diversion may be constructed to promote healing of the fistula.

Fistulas between the small bowel and the skin (enterocutaneous fistulas) are the most common type of intestinal fistula; they can originate anywhere in the small bowel but most commonly originate from the ileum. Clinical manifestations include persistent purulent drainage or identifiable intestinal drainage through an

MANAGEMENT OF A VAGINAL FISTULA

1. Obtain a soft rubber nipple shield (e.g., Curity) and a Malecot or mushroom catheter.
2. Cut a small hole in the tip of the nipple shield, and thread the catheter through so that the mushroom tip is resting within the nipple shield.
3. Fold the nipple shield down around the catheter tubing; lubricate the nipple shield generously with a water-soluble lubricant,* and gently insert it into the vagina until the entire shield is past the vaginal orifice; gently pull back on the catheter until the nipple shield is positioned in the vaginal vault.
4. Connect the open end of the catheter to the bedside drainage unit; irrigate as needed to maintain patency.

Note: For a patient with vaginal stenosis, a soft baby nipple may be substituted for a nipple shield.

*Check with the physician about using Xylocaine jelly as a lubricant for a patient with pelvic pain or vaginal tenderness.

CLOSED SUCTION MANAGEMENT OF FISTULOUS DRAINAGE*

1. Apply overlapping strips of a solid skin barrier around the wound edges to provide protection from drainage; apply a skin barrier paste to "caulk" the seams between the overlapping strips.
   Note: The inferior aspect of the wound should be bordered with a solid piece of barrier instead of overlapping strips to prevent leakage.
2. Place one layer of damp gauze in the wound bed (to protect the friable wound bed from damage caused by suction).
3. Position suction catheters in the base of the wound bed inferior to the fistula opening or openings; suction catheters are positioned *on top of* the gauze.
4. Cut strips of transparent dressing wide enough to cover the wound and surrounding barrier strips; apply the transparent dressing in overlapping strips to create a closed wound environment and to secure the suction catheters. Pectin-based paste may be applied to the exit site for suction catheters, if necessary, to prevent leakage.
5. Attach suction catheters to suction.

*This procedure is most appropriate for a fistula located in an open wound.

POUCHING AN ENTEROCUTANEOUS FISTULA

1. Preferred pouch: a drainable, odor-proof pouch with a solid barrier wafer attached.
2. Cut an opening in the pouch to "clear" the wound edges by about ⅛ to ¼ inch.
3. Treat any denuded skin by dusting on a light layer of pectin-based powder (e.g., Stomahesive by ConvaTec, Premium by Hollister); "seal" the powder by blotting lightly with water or skin sealant (e.g., Skin Prep by Smith and Nephew United).
4. Fill any irregular areas or crevices with pectin-based paste to create a smooth pouching surface (e.g., Stomahesive by ConvaTec or Premium by Hollister). Apply a thin layer of paste around the wound edges. (*Note:* If using a wound pouch with an access cap, a two-piece pouching system, or a drainable pouch with a wide bottom opening, application of paste to wound edges may be delayed until *after* the pouch has been applied to the skin.)
5. Be sure the skin surface is dry, and press pouch firmly into place.
6. Apply a thin layer of skin barrier paste to the junction between the skin and the solid barrier wafer (if possible); this helps prevent undermining of the fistulous drainage. *Note:* This step is easier with a wound pouch with an access cap, a two-piece pouching system, or a drainable pouch with a wide bottom opening.
7. Apply closure, or connect the spout of the pouch to the bedside drainage system.
8. Tape pouch edges.

Note: Suction can be added to the system by inserting a suction catheter and a "vent" catheter through a small **X** cut in the anterior surface of the pouch; paste is applied around the catheter exit site to prevent leakage.

FACTORS INHIBITING SPONTANEOUS CLOSURE OF ENTEROCUTANEOUS FISTULAS

Obstruction of distal bowel
Foreign body in fistulous tract
Malignancy involving fistulous tract
Previous irradiation to the area
Epithelium-lined tract between skin and fistula
Eversion and granulation of bowel to skin (formation of "pseudostoma")
Complete disruption of GI tract continuity
Large abscess
Crohn's disease

incision, drain site, or skin defect. The volume of drainage varies. Fistulas originating from the proximal small bowel usually are high-output fistulas, meaning that the daily volume of output is greater than 500 ml. These fistulas are associated with significant derangements in fluid and electrolyte balance, and they may also cause more severe skin breakdown because of the increased volume of enzymatic drainage. In addition to causing fluid and electrolyte abnormalities and perifistular skin breakdown, enterocutaneous fistulas compromise nutritional status by interfering with digestion and absorption of nutrients. An additional concern is the potential for intraabdominal infection, which occurs when the intestinal disruption causes intraabdominal as well as extraabdominal spillage. Management of enterocutaneous fistulas initially is conservative and involves correcting any distal obstruction, draining any intraabdominal abscesses, restoring the fluid and electrolyte balance, providing ongoing nutritional support, and controlling drainage from the fistula. Although surgical intervention is indicated for draining abscesses and correcting

distal obstruction, definitive procedures involving anastomoses should not be undertaken until infection has been controlled and nutritional and fluid balances have been optimized; premature surgical intervention is associated with additional complications such as anastomotic breakdown and recurrent fistula formation. In addition, studies have shown that most enterocutaneous fistulas heal with conservative therapy and that 90% of the fistulas that will close spontaneously do so within 4 to 6 weeks. Thus most agree that a trial of conservative therapy is indicated before definitive surgical intervention is undertaken. However, some factors are recognized as inhibiting spontaneous closure of enterocutaneous fistulas; these are listed in the box on p. 247.

COMPLICATIONS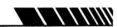

Intraabdominal, urinary tract, or pelvic sepsis
Fluid and electrolyte imbalance
Malnutrition
Perifistular skin breakdown

DIAGNOSTIC TESTS AND FINDINGS

Diagnostic test	Findings
Serum electrolytes	May show abnormalities, such as hypokalemia and hyponatremia
Oral administration of activated charcoal or indigo carmine	Appearance of charcoal or indigo carmine in wound drainage confirms presence of enterocutaneous fistula; appearance in urine confirms presence of enterovesical fistula
Fistulogram	Delineates anatomic location of fistulous tract; provides visualization of distal bowel to diagnose or rule out distal obstruction and to determine whether continuity exists between the fistulous tract and the distal bowel; may also reveal an undrained abscess adjacent to the fistulous tract
	Note: Water-soluble contrast agent usually is recommended for a fistulogram
Contrast study of entire bowel (small bowel series and colon study)	May reveal distal obstruction; provides information about fistula's location and underlying disease
	Note: Water-soluble contrast commonly is recommended with fistulous tract
Abdominal ultrasound study	May be used to define boundaries of abscess cavity
Abdominal computed tomography (CT) scan	May be done to evaluate intraabdominal abscess
Cystoscopy	Reveals presence of enterovesical or colovesical fistula
Vaginal examination with speculum	Fistulous orifice may be visualized; vaginal erosion may be seen
Urinalysis; urine culture	May reveal urinary tract infection with intestinal organisms (in patient with enterovesical fistula)

MEDICAL MANAGEMENT

GENERAL MANAGEMENT

NPO status for patient with proximal small bowel fistula; nasogastric intubation and suction may be required for high-output fistula from proximal small bowel.

IV fluids and electrolytes to restore fluid and electrolyte balance.

Accurate intake and output records; insertion of central venous pressure (CVP) or Swan-Ganz catheter for invasive monitoring in patient with hemodynamic instability.

MEDICAL MANAGEMENT—cont'd

Bowel rest and nutritional support:

NPO and TPN for patient with multiple small bowel fistulas, fistulas located in proximal ileum or midileum, or with known distal obstruction.

Low-residue diet (oral or enteral) for patient with fistula in distal ileum or colon (*Note:* must monitor impact of oral or enteral feedings on fistula's output).

NPO and enteral feedings through jejunostomy tube placed distal to fistula in patient with proximal jejunal fistula.

Note: Most patients require 3,000-5,000 nonprotein calories per day, in addition to 100-200 g of amino acids, to heal a fistulous tract.

Perifistular skin protection and containment of fistulous drainage (via wound pouch, suction, absorptive dressings, or combination therapy) for patient with enterocutaneous or colocutaneous fistula; perifistular skin protection and control of fistulous drainage (via vaginal diaphragm and drainage catheter) for patient with enterovaginal or colovaginal fistula.

Note: Consult ET nurse for assistance with fistula management. Home Health referral for patient discharged before fistula closes.

SURGERY

Percutaneous drainage of intraabdominal abscess (guided by CT or ultrasound).

Laparotomy may be required for open drainage of intraabdominal abscess or to correct distal obstruction.

Resection of fistulous tract with end-to-end anastomosis of remaining bowel for patient whose fistula fails to close with conservative therapy *and* who is free of intraabdominal infection.

Resection of fistulous tract with construction of proximal ostomy and distal mucous fistula for patient with intraabdominal infection in whom primary anastomosis is considered unsafe.

Intestinal anastomoses to bypass and exclude the fistulous tract for patient with unresectable fistula. The recommended procedure in this case is a bilateral exclusion procedure, which effectively defunctionalizes the fistulous tract. (The afferent and efferent loops of the fistulous tract are divided and anastomosed, which "excludes" the fistula. The ends of the tract can be oversewn and left in place, or they can be brought to the abdominal wall as mucous fistulas. The excluded segment of bowel can then be removed during a later procedure. Alternatively, the afferent loop to the fistulous tract is divided and anastomosed to the distal bowel, bypassing the fistula. The segment of bowel containing the fistulous tract is removed in a second procedure, if possible.)

Note: Simple suture closure of a fistula ("oversewing the defect") is not recommended, since there is a high rate of recurrence.

DRUG THERAPY

Broad-spectrum antibiotics (IV):   For management of infectious complications

Gentamicin (Garamycin) *or* **tobramycin (Nebcin):**   3-5 mg/kg daily IV in divided doses;

and

Clindamycin (Cleocin):   1.2-2.7 g daily IV in divided doses (may give up to 4.8 g daily for life-threatening infections) for severe intraabdominal infections.

Metronidazole (Flagyl):   15 mg/kg IV over 1 h as initial dose; then 7.5 mg/kg IV q6h, not to exceed 4 g daily.

Somatostatin analog (Sandostatin):   SQ bid or tid to reduce fistulous output by inhibiting intestinal secretions.

Insulin: As needed to control hyperglycemia in patient receiving TPN.

1 ASSESS

ASSESSMENT	OBSERVATIONS
Medical history	May report Crohn's disease, prior abdominal irradiation, diverticular disease, abdominal or pelvic malignancy, blunt or penetrating trauma, recent abdominal surgery
Fistula characteristics	Drainage may be reported and may be observed through the abdominal wall (incision, drain site, or skin defect), through the urethra, or through the vagina; drainage may appear purulent or may be frankly feculent; fistula may be high-output (>500 ml/24 h) or low output (<500 ml/24 h); fistulous tract may exhibit factors known to delay or prevent spontaneous closure (e.g., foreign body such as mesh or suture, epithelium-lined tract, or total disruption of intestinal tract continuity, as evidenced by mucosal eversion of fistulous opening)
Gastrointestinal function	May report absence of bowel movements and flatus per rectum (total diversion of fecal stream by fistula) or may report continued passage of stool and gas per rectum in addition to fistula drainage (partial diversion of fecal stream by fistula, with evidence of GI tract continuity and absence of distal obstruction)
Nutritional status	May report recent weight loss; weight may be less than 85%-90% of usual weight; may exhibit signs of nutritional compromise (e.g., muscle wasting; joint edema; dry, pluckable hair; fissures at corners of mouth; skin rashes; nonhealing wounds)
Fluid and electrolyte balance	May report reduced frequency of urination and increased urine concentration; output may exceed intake; may report symptoms of fluid-electrolyte imbalance (e.g., feeling dizzy or weak when standing, dry mouth and skin, extreme fatigue); may have signs of fluid volume deficit and electrolyte imbalance (e.g., postural hypotension, tachycardia, diminished skin turgor, flabby muscles, cardiac dysrhythmias)
Perifistular skin status	May report burning pain in skin around fistula; skin around fistula may appear erythematous and denuded
Evidence of intraabdominal infection	May have fever; may complain of acute abdominal pain; may have areas of marked tenderness to palpation

2 DIAGNOSE

NURSING DIAGNOSIS	SUBJECTIVE FINDINGS	OBJECTIVE FINDINGS
Altered nutrition: less than body requirements related to nutrient losses through fistulous tract	Reports recent weight loss; may report symptoms of nutritional compromise (e.g., delayed healing, easy fatigability)	Current weight less than 85%-90% of usual weight; exhibits signs of malnutrition (e.g., muscle wasting, nonhealing wounds, joint edema, skin rashes)
Fluid volume deficit related to losses through fistulous tract	Reports symptoms of fluid volume deficit (e.g., dry mouth, feeling weak or dizzy when standing, extreme fatigue)	Output exceeds intake; exhibits signs of fluid volume deficit (e.g., oliguria, increased urine concentration, diminished skin turgor, postural hypotension)
High risk for impaired skin integrity related to drainage from fistula	Reports drainage from fistula onto skin; may report burning and stinging of perifistular skin	Fistula between intestinal tract and skin; perifistular skin may appear erythematous or denuded

NURSING DIAGNOSIS	SUBJECTIVE FINDINGS	OBJECTIVE FINDINGS
High risk for infection related to drainage from fistula into abdominal cavity	May report abdominal pain or tenderness	May have fever; may show signs of intraabdominal infection (e.g., tenderness or pain)

3 PLAN

Patient goals

1. The patient will attain and maintain her usual weight and will have no signs or symptoms of nutritional compromise.
2. The patient will maintain a balance between intake and output and will have no signs or symptoms of fluid and electrolyte imbalance.

3. The patient will maintain intact perifistular skin.
4. The patient will be free of infection.

4 IMPLEMENT

NURSING DIAGNOSIS	NURSING INTERVENTIONS	RATIONALE
Altered nutrition: less than body requirements related to nutrient losses through fistulous tract	Monitor indicators of nutritional status: body weight, fistula output, signs of malnutrition (e.g., delayed healing, skin rashes, joint edema), laboratory data (if available).	Ongoing assessment provides the basis for appropriate intervention.
	Collaborate with physician and nutritional support team to provide nutritional support without increasing fistulous drainage: (1) low-residue oral or enteral feedings for distal small bowel or colonic fistulas; (2) distal jejunal feedings for proximal jejunal fistulas; (3) TPN for fistulas in distal jejunum or proximal ileum. Notify physician and nutritional support team if enteral feedings cause increased fistulous drainage.	Nutrient needs must be met and positive nitrogen balance must be maintained for fistula to heal; enteral route is preferred, because it is safer and less costly; enteral feedings are contraindicated in some patients because they increase drainage from the fistula and thus delay closure. Increased drainage in response to enteral feedings mandates modification of the nutritional support plan.
Fluid volume deficit related to losses through fistulous tract	Maintain accurate records of fluid intake and fluid loss (urine output, fistulous drainage, oral and IV fluid intake).	Accurate records permit early recognition of fluid deficits and also provide the basis for accurate fluid replacement.
	Monitor indicators of intravascular volume depletion (e.g., BP, CVP, or Swan-Ganz pressure readings, urine output, skin turgor, pulse) and electrolyte imbalance (e.g., cardiac dysrhythmias, muscle weakness).	Prompt recognition of fluid volume deficit permits early intervention. Hypovolemia causes hypotension and oliguria; compensatory responses cause tachycardia, diaphoresis, and diminished skin turgor. Electrolyte imbalance causes muscle weakness and cardiac dysrhythmias.
	Give IV fluids and electrolytes as ordered.	IV fluids and electrolytes restore plasma volume and correct fluid volume deficits and electrolyte imbalances.

→ > >

NURSING DIAGNOSIS	NURSING INTERVENTIONS	RATIONALE
	Give somatostatin analog (Sandostatin) as ordered.	Somatostatin reduces secretion of fluids in the GI tract and thus reduces fistulous drainage.
High risk for impaired skin integrity related to drainage from fistula	Monitor perifistular skin for erythema and denudation.	Intestinal secretions contain proteolytic enzymes that can cause severe skin damage.
	For patient with enterocutaneous or colocutaneous fistula: contain fistulous drainage by applying an odor-proof ostomy or wound pouch (apply pectin-based paste to protect any exposed skin edges; see p. 247 for pouching procedures).	Pouching provides an effective means of containing fistulous drainage and protecting the perifistular skin; all skin must be protected from the drainage.
	For patient with enterovaginal or colovaginal fistula: use a vaginal diaphragm and catheter to control drainage (see p. 247).	Fistulas between the intestine and the vagina can cause severe perineal skin damage.
	For patient with rectovaginal fistula: recommend measures for keeping stool formed, and instruct patient to douche after each bowel movement.	Rectovaginal fistulas usually can be managed by following measures to minimize fecal contamination of the vaginal vault.
	Treat denuded perifistular skin with pectin-based powder. If fistula is being pouched, "seal" powder by blotting with water or a skin sealant (e.g., Skin Prep or Bard Wipe). If fistula is being managed by alternate means (e.g., vaginal diaphragm and catheter), apply moisture barrier cream or ointment over the powder layer.	Pectin-based powder absorbs moisture from denuded skin and forms a protective coating. "Sealing" the powder with water or a skin sealant provides a nonpowdery pouching surface. Covering the powder with a moisture barrier cream or ointment provides an additional layer of protection from fistulous drainage.
High risk for infection related to drainage from fistula into abdominal cavity	Monitor patient for signs and symptoms of intraabdominal infection (e.g., fever, increasing abdominal tenderness), and report to physician.	Prompt recognition of intraabdominal infection permits early intervention.
	Administer antibiotics as ordered.	Antibiotics kill bacteria and help control infection and related complications.
	Prepare patient for diagnostic studies and possible drainage of intraabdominal abscesses.	Draining abscesses helps control infection.
	For patient who fails to respond to above measures: prepare patient for exploratory surgery and possible fecal diversion.	Emergency surgery is indicated to drain abscesses and control fistulous drainage; fecal diversion may be required to prevent further abdominal contamination, because resection of the fistula and primary anastomosis are contraindicated with intraabdominal infection.

5 EVALUATE

PATIENT OUTCOME	DATA INDICATING THAT OUTCOME IS REACHED
Patient has attained and maintains her usual weight and has no signs or symptoms of nutritional compromise.	Patient's weight is within 90% of her usual or desired weight; patient has no signs or symptoms of nutritional compromise (e.g., nonhealing wounds, joint edema, easy fatigability, skin rashes).
Patient maintains a balance between intake and output and has no signs of electrolyte imbalance.	Fluid intake and losses are balanced; skin turgor is normal; BP and pulse are normal; patient has no symptoms of electrolyte imbalance (e.g., muscle weakness, cardiac dysrhythmias, tingling or cramping in hands or feet).
Patient's perifistular skin remains intact.	Perifistular skin does not burn or sting, and inspection reveals no erythema or denudation.
Patient has no intraabdominal infection.	Patient's temperature is within normal limits; she has no abdominal pain, and palpation elicits no evidence of abdominal tenderness.

PATIENT TEACHING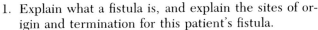

1. Explain what a fistula is, and explain the sites of origin and termination for this patient's fistula.
2. Explain the purpose and specifics of the treatment plan:
   - For the patient with distal obstruction: Explain the need for surgical intervention to correct the obstruction.
   - For the patient without distal obstruction: Explain that most fistulas close on their own as long as nutritional needs are met and the involved bowel is rested so that there is minimal drainage through the fistulous tract. Explain that this means that nutritional needs will be met through intravenous nutrition, tube feedings, or a low-residue diet (this is individualized on the basis of the patient's treatment plan). Explain that surgical closure usually is indicated if the fistula fails to close on its own within 4 to 6 weeks.
   - For the patient with severe intraabdominal inflammation: Explain that if surgical intervention is required, it may be delayed until the inflammatory process has subsided completely (to minimize complications).
   - Explain that drainage from the fistula is contained by means of pouching, suction, or drainage systems to protect the skin.
3. For the patient who is discharged before the fistula has closed: Teach the patient and family how to contain the fistulous drainage, and teach them home management of total parenteral nutrition or enteral feedings, if applicable.
4. Teach the patient to recognize the signs and symptoms of fluid and electrolyte imbalance, and instruct her to report them promptly to her physician if they develop.

CHAPTER 7

Interference with Fecal Elimination

Diarrhea

Diarrhea is defined as an increase in the volume, frequency, and fluid consistency of stools. It may be classified according to duration (acute or chronic) or type (secretory, osmotic, or mixed).

EPIDEMIOLOGY

Any pathologic condition that increases secretion into the bowel lumen, interferes with reabsorption from the bowel lumen, or significantly increases intestinal motility (thereby interfering with reabsorption) can cause diarrhea. The most common causative factors and the mechanisms by which they induce diarrhea are listed in Table 7-1.

Secretory diarrhea occurs when the normal mechanisms for production of intestinal fluid are stimulated so that excessive volumes of water and electrolytes are secreted into the intestinal lumen. If the rate of secretion is greater than the rate of reabsorption, diarrhea results. Secretory diarrhea usually is caused by infection with a toxin-producing organism such as *Vibrio cholerae* or enterotoxigenic *Escherichia coli*; hypersecretion can also be induced by a number of disorders that cause production of secretagogues, substances known to stimulate gastrointestinal secretion. Common secretagogues include deconjugated bile salts, which result from bacterial overgrowth in the small intestine, and hydroxy fatty acids, which are produced by bacterial action on undigested fats; these agents are thought to contribute to the diarrhea that is characteristic of bacterial overgrowth and fat malabsorption syndromes. Neoplastic

disorders may also cause production of secretagogues; for example, pancreatic cholera is characterized by the production of vasoactive intestinal peptide, and Zollinger-Ellison syndrome involves the production of excessive amounts of gastrin. Carcinoid syndrome, villous adenoma, and medullary carcinoma of the thyroid are also associated with secretory diarrheal syndromes.

Osmotic diarrhea is caused by osmotically active substances in the bowel lumen that prevent or retard reabsorption of water. This type of diarrhea is common in malabsorption syndromes; the malabsorbed nutrients are fermented to organic acids by the colonic bacteria, and the organic acids increase the osmotic load. (These organic acids may also stimulate colonic secretion.) Osmotic diarrhea may also follow ingestion of significant amounts of poorly absorbed substances; for example, the sorbitol in liquid medications frequently is a factor in the diarrhea commonly associated with enteral feedings.

The third category of diarrheal syndromes is the mixed type of diarrhea. This category includes diarrhea thought to result primarily from increased intestinal motility as well as that thought to result from a combination of increased secretion and decreased absorption. Increased motility contributes to diarrhea by reducing the contact time between the intraluminal contents and the intestinal mucosa, which compromises the reabsorption of water and electrolytes. In addition, increased motility may impair the normal digestive process and give rise to malabsorption of nutrients, which

Table 7-1 _____

CAUSATIVE FACTORS AND MECHANISMS OF ACTION IN DIARRHEAL DISORDERS

Causative factor	Mechanisms of action
Infectious agents	
V. cholerae, enterotoxigenic *E. coli, Salmonella* sp., *Shigella* sp., *Campylobacter* sp., *E. coli, Entamoeba histolytica, Giardia* sp., *Amoeba* sp.	Toxins cause secretory diarrhea. Organisms invade mucosa, reducing absorption and increasing motility
Clostridium difficile	Damages the mucosa and reduces absorption
Malabsorption syndromes	
Lactose intolerance, sorbitol intolerance, lactulose administration	Causes osmotic diarrhea secondary to nonabsorbable solutes; may increase secretion and motility
Celiac sprue	Damages the mucosa; causes increased secretion of fluid and electrolytes, malabsorption of nutrients with resulting osmotic diarrhea, and altered absorption
Fat malabsorption syndromes	Unabsorbed fatty acids act as secretagogues, causing secretory diarrhea
Inflammatory bowel disease	Damages the mucosa and reduces absorption; may increase motility
Short bowel syndrome	Reduces absorptive surface of bowel; unabsorbed substances may increase diarrhea by acting as secretagogues
Cholinergic drugs	Increase intestinal motility, reducing absorption
Malignant syndromes	
Zollinger-Ellison syndrome, pancreatic cholera syndrome, carcinoid syndrome, medullary carcinoma thyroid, villous adenoma	Produce substances that increase intestinal secretion (secretory diarrhea)
Saline cathartics	Produce osmotic diarrhea
Laxative abuse	Causes osmotic diarrhea and produces chronic changes in intestinal motility
Irritable bowel syndrome	Associated with changes in intestinal motility

in turn creates an osmotic effect. The breakdown of these malabsorbed nutrients by colonic bacteria may then produce substances that act as secretagogues, adding a secretory component to the diarrhea. In patients with mixed-type diarrhea, it may be difficult to determine the primary mechanism causing the diarrhea.

PATHOPHYSIOLOGY

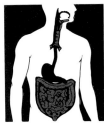

The pathologic effects of diarrhea vary depending on the causative mechanism and the severity of the diarrhea (volume of output). General effects include fluid and electrolyte derangements, possible damage to perianal skin, and potential fecal incontinence.

Secretory diarrhea occurs when secretory stimuli cause overproduction of intestinal fluid; the increased volume of intestinal secretions overwhelms the absorptive capacity of the small bowel and colon and causes diarrhea. Secretory diarrhea typically is high volume (more than 1 L per day) and is relatively unaffected by fasting, since the cause of the diarrhea is intestinal secretion rather than malabsorption of ingested substances. Secretory diarrhea is commonly associated with significant changes in electrolyte balance; this is explained by the fact that intestinal secretions contain large volumes of electrolytes, particularly sodium. (Because sodium usually is secreted in greater concentrations than potassium, hyponatremia is seen more commonly than hypokalemia.) Because the main component of secretory diarrhea is intestinal fluid, the secreted electrolytes provide the major osmotic component to the stool. This provides one means of differentiating secretory diarrhea from other types; a stool specimen is obtained, and the electrolyte concentrations and total osmolality are determined. If the electrolyte concentration (determined by the formula $2 \times$

[Na⁺ + K⁺]) is within 40 mOsm/kg of the osmolality value, the diarrhea is considered secretory in nature. Another characteristic of secretory diarrhea is the pH of the stool; bicarbonate that is secreted neutralizes the acids produced by colonic bacteria, so the stool pH is close to neutral.

Osmotic diarrhea is the type seen with most malabsorption syndromes and is the type induced by saline cathartics or unabsorbed glucose loads. In this type of diarrhea, unabsorbable or poorly absorbable substances in the bowel lumen create an osmotic "pull" that interferes with reabsorption of water. The volume of stool typically is less than 1 L per day and is reduced by fasting, since the cause of the diarrhea is unabsorbed substances. Osmotic diarrhea commonly results in hypokalemia and water depletion but does not typically cause hyponatremia; this is because the colon conserves sodium but does not conserve potassium. In osmotic diarrhea the stool osmolality exceeds the electrolyte concentration of the stool by at least 40 mOsm/kg; this is because much of the osmolality is provided by unabsorbed solutes. The pH of the stool usually is acidic, because colonic bacteria act on the unabsorbed nutrients to produce acids.

Mixed-type diarrhea is of unclear origin; the primary etiologic factor is thought to be increased intestinal motility. The rapid transit may cause diarrhea simply by reducing mucosal contact time enough to limit absorption of nutrients and water; however, impaired absorption of nutrients may then trigger a secondary osmotic diarrhea. In addition, bacterial action on incompletely digested nutrients may produce substances that stimulate increased intestinal secretion. The findings in mixed-type diarrhea vary; volumes may be high or low, the pH may be neutral or acidic, and electrolyte concentration may or may not account for most of the stool osmolality. The patient with mixed-type diarrhea may have a variety of fluid-electrolyte derangements; fluid volume deficit, hyponatremia, and hypokalemia may be seen jointly or alone.

Effective management of any diarrheal disorder depends on eliminating or controlling the causative factors; thus the primary focus is on differential diagnosis and control of the underlying disease.

COMPLICATIONS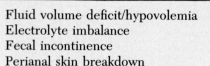

Fluid volume deficit/hypovolemia
Electrolyte imbalance
Fecal incontinence
Perianal skin breakdown

DIAGNOSTIC STUDIES AND FINDINGS

Diagnostic test	Findings
Stool for culture and bacterial toxins	May be positive for infectious agent (e.g., enterotoxigenic *E. coli, V. cholerae, C. difficile, Salmonella* sp., *Shigella* sp., *Campylobacter* sp.)
Stool for leukocytes (Wright's stain)	Positive results indicate infectious process
Stool for ova and parasites	May test positive for parasites (e.g., *Giardia, Amoeba* organisms)
Stool for occult blood	May test positive (e.g., inflammatory bowel disease or acute viral enteritis)
Stool for fat and undigested muscle fibers	May test positive (e.g., fat malabsorption syndromes, exocrine pancreatic insufficiency)
Stool for osmolality and electrolyte concentration	*Secretory diarrhea:* 2 × (Na⁺ + K⁺) approximates osmolality (gap <40 mOsm/kg); *osmotic diarrhea:* 2 × (Na⁺ + K⁺) is less than stool osmolality (gap >40 mOsm/kg) *Note:* Some sources use a gap of 50 or 100 mOsm/kg to identify osmotic diarrhea
Stool pH	Neutral pH indicates secretory diarrhea; acidic pH indicates osmotic diarrhea
Stool for phenolphthalein	May test positive in patient with occult laxative abuse (*Note:* Test is done by adding sodium hydroxide [NaOH] to stool; in presence of phenolphthalein, a common ingredient of laxatives, stool turns red)
Serum electrolytes	May reveal hyponatremia, hypokalemia, or both
Serum levels of vasoactive intestinal peptide (VIP), gastrin, and calcitonin	May be elevated in secretory diarrhea syndromes (e.g., VIP may be elevated in pancreatic cholera, gastrin may be elevated in Zollinger-Ellison syndrome, and calcitonin may be elevated in medullary carcinoma of the thyroid)

DIAGNOSTIC STUDIES AND FINDINGS—cont'd

Diagnostic test	Findings
Hydrogen breath test	Elevated level of hydrogen in lactose intolerance
Upper gastrointestinal series	May show changes consistent with celiac sprue or other malabsorptive disorders (e.g., coarsening of mucosa with edema of mucosal folds, increased volume of secretions); may show changes consistent with Crohn's disease (e.g., rake ulcers, intraluminal narrowing)
Barium enema	May show changes consistent with ulcerative colitis (e.g., mucosal ulcerations and irregularities, colonic shortening) or Crohn's disease (e.g., rake ulcers, strictures, cobblestoning of mucosa)
Endoscopy	May show changes consistent with ulcerative colitis (e.g., mucosal ulcerations, pseudopolyps) or Crohn's disease (e.g., aphthous ulcers, fissures, fistulas) or pseudomembranous colitis (e.g., mucosal edema and ulcerations, yellowish white "membranes")

MEDICAL MANAGEMENT

GENERAL MANAGEMENT

Elimination of causative factors (e.g., removal of fecal impaction; dietary modifications for patient with malabsorption syndrome).

Oral replacement of fluids and electrolytes if tolerated (i.e., no nausea or vomiting and no exacerbation of diarrhea).

IV administration of fluids and electrolytes if patient cannot maintain fluid and electrolyte balance with oral fluid replacement.

Monitoring of intake and output and indicators of fluid and electrolyte status (BP, pulse, urine output, skin turgor).

Scrupulous perianal skin care (gentle cleansing after each bowel movement, application of skin protectants such as moisture barrier ointments).

DRUG THERAPY

Metronidazole: 750 mg PO tid for 5-10 days for intestinal amebiasis; 250 mg PO tid for giardiasis.

Vancomycin: 500 mg-2 g PO daily (in three to four divided doses) for 7-10 days for patient with pseudomembranous enterocolitis.

Sulfasalazine (Azulfidine): Initial therapy, 3-4 g PO daily in divided doses; maintenance therapy, 1.5-2 g PO daily in divided doses, for patient with ulcerative colitis.

Prednisone: 2.5-15 mg PO bid, tid, or qid or prednisolone, 2-30 mg IV q 12 h for patient with inflammatory bowel disease.

Loperamide (Imodium): 4-16 mg PO daily to control diarrhea.*

Diphenoxylate (Lomotil): 2.5-5 mg PO qid to control diarrhea.*

Codeine: 15-60 mg PO bid, tid, or qid to control severe diarrhea.*

*Antiperistaltic agents such as loperamide, diphenoxylate, and codeine should **not** be given to a patient with severe ulcerative colitis because of the risk of toxic megacolon; they also should **not** be given to a patient with pseudomembranous colitis or other infectious diarrheal syndromes because they reduce intestinal motility.)

Kaolin-pectin (Kaopectate): 60-120 ml PO after each loose stool for symptomatic control of diarrhea.

Bulk-forming agent (e.g., Metamucil): 5-10 tsp bid or tid to reduce watery stools.

Antiemetics: As indicated for patient with nausea and vomiting.

1 ASSESS

ASSESSMENT	OBSERVATIONS
Medical history	May report chronic diarrhea; may report other digestive symptoms (e.g., intestinal cramping or increased flatus); may report history of Crohn's disease, ulcerative colitis, pancreatitis, small bowel resection, malabsorption syndromes; may report current or recent treatment with antibiotics; may report frequent use of antacids; may report ingesting large amounts of sugar-free products containing sorbitol
Exposure to amebic dysentery	May report recent travel to southern United States or tropics or exposure to someone who recently has returned from tropics
Gastrointestinal function	May report large-volume stools, watery stools, or frequent stools; may describe stools as watery, bloody, mucoid, or greasy; may report foul-smelling stools; may report cramping, increased flatus, anorexia, nausea, and vomiting
Fluid-electrolyte balance	Output may exceed intake; may exhibit oliguria, postural hypotension, reduced skin turgor, tachycardia, dry mucous membranes; may report dry mouth, thirst, dizziness, and weakness
Perianal skin integrity	May report tenderness, burning, and stinging; perianal area may appear erythematous or denuded

2 DIAGNOSE

NURSING DIAGNOSIS	SUBJECTIVE FINDINGS	OBJECTIVE FINDINGS
Diarrhea related to inflammation, abnormal secretion, or malabsorption	Reports increased volume or frequency of stool (or both); may report malodorous stools; may report cramping, urgency, anorexia, nausea, and vomiting	Stools appear loose and may appear watery, mucoid, bloody, or greasy; volume of stool is >500 ml
High risk for fluid volume deficit related to diarrhea	Reports loose or frequent stools; may report anorexia, nausea, or vomiting; may report feeling thirsty, weak, and dizzy	Output exceeds intake; urine may be concentrated; may have dry skin and mucous membranes, orthostatic hypotension, tachycardia, and reduced muscle tone
High risk for impaired perianal skin integrity related to diarrhea	Reports burning or soreness in perianal area; reports perianal area is sensitive to touch	Erythematous perianal skin that may appear denuded

3 PLAN

Patient goals

1. The patient will regain normal bowel elimination patterns (i.e., soft, formed stools).
2. The patient will maintain balance between fluid intake and fluid losses.
3. The patient will have healthy, intact perianal skin.

4 IMPLEMENT

NURSING DIAGNOSIS	NURSING INTERVENTIONS	RATIONALE
Diarrhea related to inflammation, abnormal secretion, or malabsorption	Monitor stools for frequency, volume, and consistency.	Volume, frequency, and consistency of stools reflect GI tract motility and intestine's ability to digest and absorb nutrients.
	Collaborate with physician, dietitian, and patient to eliminate foods that are malabsorbed or that cause an inflammatory reaction in the intestinal tract.	Eliminating foods that are poorly digested and incompletely absorbed reduces stool volume and consistency.
	Check patient for fecal impaction, and remove if present.	Fecal impaction acts as a partial mechanical obstruction and causes leakage of liquid stool that mimics diarrhea.
	Administer antibiotics as ordered for patient with infectious diarrhea.	Antibiotics eliminate bacteria that cause inflammation of the bowel wall; inflammation causes diarrhea by reducing absorption and increasing motility, and bacterial toxins may increase secretion.
	Administer antiinflammatory agents as ordered to patients with inflammatory bowel disease.	Antiinflammatory agents block the inflammatory process that causes diarrhea.
	Administer antimotility drugs (e.g., loperamide, diphenoxylate, codeine) as ordered. *Note:* Do **not** administer these drugs to patients with infectious diarrhea or patients with severe ulcerative colitis.	Antimotility drugs reduce peristaltic activity and increase transit time, thus improving absorption and reducing stool volume; however, reducing motility may increase damage from bacterial toxins in infectious diarrhea and may precipitate toxic megacolon in severe ulcerative colitis.
	Administer kaolin-pectin medication as ordered and needed.	Kaolin-pectin preparation reduces the water content of stool and acts as an adsorbent and demulcent.
	Administer bulking agents as ordered and needed for patient with watery diarrhea.	Bulking agents absorb water and improve stool consistency.
High risk for fluid volume deficit related to diarrhea	Monitor patient for signs of fluid and electrolyte imbalance (e.g., output exceeding intake, dry mucous membranes, diminished skin turgor, concentrated urine, weakness, dizziness).	Output exceeding intake, dry mucous membranes, diminished skin turgor, and concentrated urine are indicators of fluid volume deficit; weakness and dizziness may indicate electrolyte imbalance.
	Replace fluids and electrolytes with oral fluids as tolerated; encourage fluids that contain a balanced mixture of glucose and electrolytes, and discourage caffeinic fluids.	Fluid and electrolyte replacement is critical to normal tissue perfusion and organ function; balanced electrolyte solutions are more readily absorbed; caffeine increases intracellular levels of cyclic AMP and may increase diarrhea.

→ > >

NURSING DIAGNOSIS	NURSING INTERVENTIONS	RATIONALE
	Administer IV fluids and electrolytes as ordered.	IV fluids and electrolytes restore plasma volume and promote tissue perfusion.
	Administer antiemetics as ordered and needed to control nausea.	Antiemetics reduce nausea and vomiting, thus reducing fluid losses and improving intake.
High risk for impaired perianal skin integrity related to diarrhea	Cleanse skin gently with tap water, mineral oil, or gentle cleanser after each stool.	Diarrheal stool can erode the skin; prevention involves atraumatic cleansing.
	Protect skin with skin sealants or moisture barrier ointment; if skin is denuded, apply pectin-based powder before applying sealant or ointment.	Sealants and moisture barrier ointments provide a protective film over skin; pectin-based powder absorbs moisture and provides a protective "paste" over denuded skin.
	For patient with severe diarrhea and compromised continence: consider applying a perianal fecal incontinence collector.	Use of a perianal pouch contains the stool, protects the skin, and quantifies output.

5 EVALUATE

PATIENT OUTCOME	DATA INDICATING THAT OUTCOME IS REACHED
Patient has regained normal bowel function (i.e., soft, formed stools).	Patient reports resolution of diarrhea; stools are soft to formed; frequency of bowel movements averages one or two daily.
Patient maintains a balance between fluid intake and fluid losses.	Urine output and fluid intake are balanced; patient has no signs or symptoms of fluid-electrolyte imbalance (e.g., dry mucous membranes, diminished skin turgor, concentrated urine, extreme weakness, dizziness, orthostatic hypotension, tachycardia).
Patient's perianal skin is intact and healthy.	Patient states that perianal skin is not sensitive to touch; perianal skin is intact and shows no erythema or denudation.

PATIENT TEACHING

1. Explain the cause of the patient's diarrhea (e.g., intestinal infection, malabsorption of ingested nutrients, production of secretory stimuli that increase production of intestinal secretions).
2. Explain the treatment plan, including dietary modifications (if applicable), medications to correct underlying infection or inflammation (if applicable), medications to control diarrhea, and fluid and electrolyte replacement.
3. Instruct the patient (and caregiver, if applicable) in correct perianal skin care.
4. Explain which oral fluids are most readily absorbed and which are the best source of needed electrolytes.

Constipation

Constipation is the infrequent or difficult passage of hard, dry stool. Constipation has been categorized as colonic constipation or perceived constipation. Colonic constipation can be objectively documented and is characterized by infrequent passage of hard, dry stools as a result of delayed colonic transit. Perceived constipation is subjective in nature; it represents a self-diagnosis based on beliefs about "normal" bowel elimination patterns. Individuals with perceived constipation may routinely use laxatives and enemas to produce the desired "normal" pattern of bowel elimination.

EPIDEMIOLOGY

Constipation is a common problem in the United States, affecting about 4% of the population. Colonic constipation usually is caused by a combination of factors that result in increased colonic transit time and formation of hard, dry stools. The most significant causative factors are reduced colonic motility, reduced dietary bulk, and inadequate fluid intake. Habitual failure to respond to the need to defecate also plays a role in the development of constipation. In some cases incoordination of the pelvic floor muscles is a contributing factor to ineffective elimination and constipation.

Reduced colonic motility contributes to constipation by prolonging fecal contact with the absorptive colonic mucosa, thus causing excessive drying of the stool. Slowed motility may result from loss of innervation or from loss of the normal stimuli for peristaltic activity.

Loss of innervation is the basis for constipation in the patient with Hirschsprung's disease and in the patient with a sacral spinal cord lesion (e.g., spinal cord injury or multiple sclerosis affecting the sacral cord). Peristaltic activity normally is mediated primarily by the intrinsic nervous system of the bowel, which responds to local stimuli such as mechanical stretch or intraluminal irritants. Autonomic innervation serves to modulate the stimuli provided by the intrinsic nervous system; the parasympathetic branches, which stimulate peristaltic activity, exit the cord at the sacral level and synapse on the ganglia of the intrinsic nervous system. Hirschsprung's disease involves total loss of innervation as a result of the absence of ganglion cells in the myenteric plexus (a component of the intrinsic nervous system); loss of innervation causes tonic contraction of the involved segment with dilation of the proximal bowel. Sacral cord lesions cause loss of parasympathetic stimuli; these patients have reduced motility in the distal colon and also have loss of the defecation reflex, which mediates rectal contraction in response to rectal distention.

Reduced motility can also occur without loss of innervation, and in fact most individuals with constipation are neurologically intact. In these patients reduced motility is caused by loss of the normal peristaltic stimuli. Factors known to stimulate peristalsis include eating, physical activity, and dietary bulk; eating and exercise increase the electrical and motor activity of the bowel, and dietary bulk increases the volume of stool and provides mechanical stretch. Thus sedentary individuals and those consuming low-residue diets are at risk for constipation. Individuals taking analgesics (particularly codeine) or central nervous system depressants are also at risk for constipation.

Constipation may also be caused by formation of hard, dry stool. Dry stools are difficult or even painful to eliminate; they do not pass readily through the anal canal, and they typically are small caliber, which means they require increased levels of intraabdominal pressure for evacuation. Hard, dry stools develop when the diet lacks adequate bulk or fluid; dietary bulk, combined with adequate fluid intake, prevents constipation by retaining fluid in the stool. A soft, bulky stool also acts as a peristaltic stimulant, which prevents the excessive drying that occurs with reduced motility.

Habitual failure to heed the "call to stool" is a common contributing factor to loss of normal motility and development of hard, dry stools. Normally rectal distention initiates the defecation reflex, which is mediated by the parasympathetic and intrinsic nervous systems and which causes rectal evacuation unless consciously inhibited. Rectal distention also triggers sensory impulses, which alert a neurologically intact individual to the urge to defecate; the individual can then initiate defecation, if appropriate, or can contract the external sphincter to delay defecation until a socially convenient time. Contraction of the external sphincter maintains continence long enough for the rectum to accommodate the stool; accommodation results in reduced intrarectal pressures and subsidence of the defecation reflex. The reflex is reactivated when additional stool is delivered to the rectum or when the individual "bears down" to voluntarily initiate defecation. When defecation is delayed, the stool becomes hard and dry. If defecation is habitually delayed for long periods, the rectum loses its normal tone and becomes lax; as a result, large volumes of stool are required to initiate the defecation reflex and sensory awareness of rectal filling, and excessive intraabdominal pressure is required to evacuate the rectum. Poor bowel hygiene is common in chronic constipation.

Incoordination of the pelvic floor muscles causes chronic constipation in some individuals. Voluntary defecation is accomplished by a bearing down maneuver, which increases intraabdominal and intrarectal pressure, initiates rectosigmoid contractions, and relaxes the external sphincter. However, some individuals inadvertently *contract* the external sphincter and pelvic floor muscles, thus obstructing rectal evacuation.

Loss of abdominal muscle strength or innervation can also contribute to constipation; abdominal muscle contraction plays a major role in initiation of voluntary defecation and also augments rectal contractions to empty the rectum effectively.

Perceived constipation results when an individual's bowel elimination pattern does not match his expectations of "normal." This is particularly common among individuals who were taught that a daily bowel movement is necessary to health. If the person's bowel pattern does not conform to this expectation, the individual "feels" constipated even if his bowel function is within normal limits. (Some individuals have bowel movements only two or three times a week; this is considered normal so long as the stools are soft and readily eliminated.) Individuals who perceive themselves to be constipated frequently resort to laxatives and enemas to achieve the desired pattern of elimination. Over time this repetitive stimulus can induce bowel dependency and reduced motility, resulting in colonic constipation.

PATHOPHYSIOLOGY

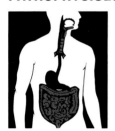

Chronic colonic constipation can result in fecal impaction, abdominal bloating and discomfort, hemorrhoids, perianal fissures, and possibly diverticular disease. Fecal impaction occurs when the fecal mass accumulated in the rectosigmoid becomes too massive to be eliminated spontaneously; the continual rectal distention causes relaxation of the internal sphincter (the rectoanal inhibitory reflex), which permits leakage of liquid stool around the fecal mass. (This liquid stool is sometimes mistaken for diarrhea, with subsequent administration of antidiarrheal medications; fecal impaction should always be ruled out before initiating treatment for diarrhea.)

Abdominal bloating and cramping may occur because retained stool and reduced motility can cause large volumes of stool to accumulate in the proximal bowel. Because the retained stool continues to undergo bacterial action, there is excessive production of flatus, which further contributes to distention and bloating. The patient may complain of excessive "gas."

Chronic straining at stool may contribute to the development of hemorrhoidal disease by causing congestion in the perianal vasculature or by pushing the vascular tissue through the anal canal. Passage of hard, dry stools may also contribute to the development of anal fissures, or tears in the lining of the anal canal.

Diverticular disease is the most serious complication associated with constipation. Constipation is thought to contribute to the development of diverticula because small-caliber stools cause contraction and narrowing of the colonic lumen; the increased intraluminal pressure that is then required to propel the stool through the narrowed lumen is thought to play a role in the development of the diverticular sacs.

COMPLICATIONS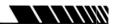

Fecal impaction
Anorectal disease (hemorrhoidal disease, anal fissures)
Diverticular disease

DIAGNOSTIC STUDIES AND FINDINGS

Diagnostic test	Findings
X-ray (flat plate) of abdomen	May reveal large volumes of accumulated stool throughout colon
Colonic transit study	May reveal prolonged transit (i.e., radiopaque markers retained for more than 5 days); may be used to differentiate segmental delays versus generalized colonic motility impairment
Anorectal manometry	May show failure of internal sphincter to relax with rectal distention (denervation syndromes); may show contraction of external sphincter with attempted defecation (incoordination of pelvic floor muscles); may show increased rectal capacity and reduced rectal sensation (rectal laxity); may show inability to effectively empty rectum

MEDICAL MANAGEMENT

GENERAL MANAGEMENT

Removal of fecal impaction (if applicable); cleansing enema.

Addition of dietary bulk as tolerated (titrate to soft, formed stool).

Note: The recommended fiber intake for adults is 28-30 g daily; when adding fiber, the goal is to establish regular evacuation of soft, formed stool (see Table 7-2 on p. 264 for a list of high-fiber foods).

Increased fluid intake (if no contraindications): 2,000-2,400 ml daily.

Increased activity/exercise (within limits of patient's tolerance).

Biofeedback for patient with pelvic floor incoordination or impaired recognition of rectal distention.

Establishment of regular schedule for attempted defecation.

Digital stimulation to initiate rectal evacuation on a routine basis for patient with spinal cord lesion.

Cleansing enema before initiation of program for patient with severe constipation.

Education and counseling regarding normal bowel elimination and effects of repetitive use of laxatives and enemas for patient with perceived constipation.

SURGERY

Resection of aganglionic segment with reanastomosis of proximal and distal bowel for patient with Hirschsprung's disease.

DRUG THERAPY

Bulk laxatives (e.g., Metamucil): 5-10 tsp bid or tid, followed by 8 oz water for patient with hard, dry stools who is unable or unwilling to ingest sufficient dietary bulk.*

Stool softeners (e.g., docusate sodium, docusate calcium, docusate potassium): 240 mg PO daily (docusate calcium or docusate potassium); 50-300 mg PO daily (docusate sodium) for patient with hard, dry stools not corrected by addition of dietary bulk and/or bulk laxatives.*

Softener/stimulant combinations (e.g., docusate with casanthranol, Peri-Colace): 1 capsule (100 mg docusate, 30 mg casanthranol) one to three times daily for patient with constipation related to impaired colonic motility.

Bisacodyl (e.g., Dulcolax): 10-15 mg PO or suppository (1) to cleanse colon or to initiate regularly scheduled defecation (suppository).

Minienema (docusate plus soft soap, ThereVac): To initiate routine rectal evacuation for patient with spinal cord lesion.

Stimulant laxative (e.g., Milk of Magnesia or Fleet's Phospho-Soda): For patient with severe constipation or retained stool.

*Note: Adequate fluid intake is **essential** for preventing obstruction when giving bulk laxatives and is critical for therapeutic effect with both bulk laxatives and stool softeners.

Table 7-2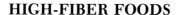

HIGH-FIBER FOODS

Food	Fiber content	Food	Fiber content
Grains		**Vegetables**	
Whole wheat bread (1 slice)	1.3 g	Asparagus (½ cup)	3.5 g
All-Bran cereal (⅓ cup)	8.4 g	Navy beans (½ cup)	8.4 g
Corn Flakes (¾ cup)	2.6 g	Kidney beans (½ cup)	9.7 g
Wheaties (¾ cup)	2.6 g	Lima beans (½ cup)	8.3 g
Shredded Wheat (1 biscuit)	2.8 g	Pinto beans (½ cup)	8.9 g
Rye crackers (3 wafers)	2.3 g	Broccoli (½ cup)	3.5 g
Graham crackers (2 squares)	1.4 g	Brussels sprouts (½ cup)	2.3 g
Brown rice (⅓ cup)	1.6 g	Cabbage (½ cup)	2.1 g
Popcorn (3 cups)	3 g	Carrots, raw (½ cup)	1.8 g
		Cauliflower (½ cup)	1.6 g
Fruits		Corn (½ medium ear)	2.6 g
Apple (½ large)	2 g	Eggplant, raw (½ cup)	2.5 g
Apricots (2)	1.4 g	Kale greens (½ cup)	1.3 g
Banana (½ medium)	1.5 g	Peas, canned (½ cup)	6.7 g
Blackberries (¾ cup)	6.7 g	Potato, white, baked (½ medium)	1.9 g
Orange (1 small)	1.6 g	Potato, sweet (½ medium)	2.1 g
Peach (1 medium)	2.3 g	Radishes (½ cup)	1.3 g
Pear (½ medium)	2 g	Squash, acorn (1 cup)	7 g
Plums (3 small)	1.8 g	Squash, zucchini (½ cup)	2 g
Raspberries (1 cup)	9.2 g	Tomato, raw (1 small)	1.5 g
Strawberries (1 cup)	3.1 g	Turnips (½ cup)	2 g

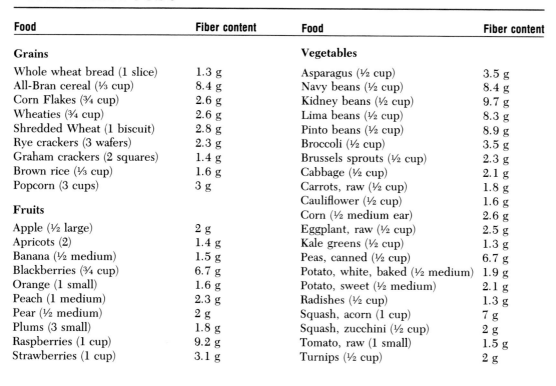

1   ASSESS

ASSESSMENT	OBSERVATIONS
Medical history	May report chronic constipation; may report Hirschsprung's disease or spinal cord lesion (e.g., multiple sclerosis, spina bifida, spinal cord injury)
Medication history	May report chronic use of laxatives; may report use of analgesics or CNS depressants
Diet and fluid intake	May report low-fiber diet and limited fluid intake
Usual physical activity	May report sedentary life-style
Bowel elimination patterns	May report chronic constipation and difficulty eliminating stool; may describe stools as hard and dry; may state that bowel movements occur only with laxative or enema; may complain of excessive flatus
Abdominal assessment	Inspection may reveal distention; palpation may reveal stool throughout colon; palpation may reveal hypotonic abdominal muscles or reduced contractility

ASSESSMENT	OBSERVATIONS
Rectal examination	May reveal large, lax rectal vault; may reveal fecal impaction or large amounts of stool in rectum; may reveal inappropriate contraction of external sphincter (i.e., patient contracts sphincter when instructed to "bear down as if having a bowel movement")
Beliefs about bowel function	May describe rigid expectations of normal bowel function (e.g., daily bowel movement is essential to health and well-being) and may describe measures used to achieve desired pattern (e.g., laxatives or enemas)

2 DIAGNOSE

NURSING DIAGNOSIS	SUBJECTIVE FINDINGS	OBJECTIVE FINDINGS
Colonic constipation related to reduced colonic motility or to formation of hard, dry stool	Reports infrequent bowel movements; describes stools as hard and dry; may describe stools as difficult or painful to eliminate; may complain of bloating or excessive gas	Stools appear hard and dry; abdomen may appear distended; palpation may reveal large volumes of stool in proximal bowel; rectal examination may reveal large amount of stool in rectum
Perceived constipation related to rigid beliefs about normal bowel elimination	Reports being constipated and defines constipation in terms of frequency of bowel movement; describes measures to maintain "normal" bowel movements (e.g., laxatives or enemas)	Nondistended abdomen; no palpable stool in proximal bowel; stools appear soft or loose; rectal examination reveals no retained stool

3 PLAN

Patient goals

1. The patient will regain normal bowel elimination (i.e., regular elimination of soft, bulky stool).

2. The patient will define "normal" bowel elimination patterns as regular elimination of soft stool and will incorporate healthy elimination patterns into life-style.

4 IMPLEMENT

NURSING DIAGNOSIS	NURSING INTERVENTIONS	RATIONALE
Colonic constipation related to reduced colonic motility or to formation of hard, dry stool	Monitor frequency and consistency of stools.	Continual assessment provides information about response to treatment and is the basis for modifying the treatment program.
	Remove any impacted stool, and follow with cleansing enema or oral laxative (e.g., saline cathartic such as Milk of Magnesia).	Impacted stool cannot be eliminated spontaneously and blocks elimination of stool in proximal bowel.

→ › ›

NURSING DIAGNOSIS	NURSING INTERVENTIONS	RATIONALE
	Collaborate with patient and dietitian to provide increased dietary fiber (whole grains, fruits, vegetables) within limits of patient's tolerance.	Fiber retains water and supports formation of soft, bulky stool, which acts as a peristaltic stimulant.
	Collaborate with patient to ensure adequate daily fluid intake (2,000-2,400 ml daily). Work with patient to increase his daily exercise and physical activity (e.g., add a daily walking program).	Adequate fluid intake prevents excessive drying of stool. Exercise and physical activity increase electrical and motor activity in the bowel, increasing peristalsis.
	Administer bran mixture or bulk laxative as ordered for patient who is unable or unwilling to ingest sufficient dietary fiber (collaborate with patient to determine preferred type of bulk agent: powder, wafers, or capsules); begin with 3-6 g of fiber daily, and titrate based on response.	Bran is an effective bulking agent and also helps establish regular bowel movements; bulk laxatives provide fiber, which retains water in stool and promotes formation of soft, bulky stool.
	Note: Adequate fluid intake is **essential** for therapeutic effect and to prevent obstruction.	
	Administer stool softeners as ordered to patient with hard, dry stools (ensure adequate fluid intake to achieve therapeutic effect).	Stool softeners reduce the surface tension of stool and promote water absorption and formation of soft stool.
	Administer softener/stimulant combinations as ordered to patient with reduced colonic motility and hard stools.	These agents help soften stool and stimulate peristaltic activity.
	Establish regular schedule for attempted defecation; scheduled attempt should be made after a meal.	Routine attempts to defecate promote regular bowel movements; attempts should be made after a meal, because eating stimulates peristalsis.
	Teach patient with impaired abdominal muscle contractility to use deep breathing to promote defecation.	Deep breathing causes the diaphragm to descend, which increases intraabdominal and intrarectal pressure.
	Encourage patient to respond promptly to urge to defecate.	Prompt response promotes rectal emptying and prevents drying of stool.
	Collaborate with physician to arrange biofeedback for patient with incoordination of pelvic floor muscles and inappropriate contraction of external sphincter.	Biofeedback has been an effective approach in teaching patients control of pelvic floor muscles.
	Use digital stimulation, suppository, or minienema to stimulate routine rectal evacuation in patient with spinal cord lesion.	Spinal cord lesions cause loss of sensory awareness of rectal filling and reduced motility; sacral lesions cause loss of defecation reflex; routine stimulation of defecation prevents constipation and impaction.

NURSING DIAGNOSIS	NURSING INTERVENTIONS	RATIONALE
Perceived constipation related to rigid beliefs about normal bowel elimination	Explore with patient his concepts and concerns about normal bowel elimination and its importance; provide accurate information about anatomy and physiology of defecation and variations on "normal," and offer "regular elimination of soft stool" as the criterion for "normal" elimination.	Perceived constipation is caused by inaccurate beliefs about what is normal and necessary; correcting inaccurate perceptions is essential to resolve the problem.
	Explain potential adverse effects of routine unnecessary use of peristaltic stimulants; suggest use of natural aids to defecation (e.g., dietary fiber, fluid intake, exercise, and prompt response to defecation urge).	Perceived constipation may progress to colonic constipation if repetitive use of peristaltic stimulants impairs colonic motility and induces bowel dependency.
	Suggest use of a bowel elimination chart to record stools and to determine patient's "normal" pattern.	Address patient's concerns and involve him in developing a healthy, comfortable bowel management program.

5 EVALUATE

PATIENT OUTCOME	DATA INDICATING THAT OUTCOME IS REACHED
Patient has regained a normal bowel elimination pattern	Patient reports regular elimination of soft, formed stool; he states that he no longer has to strain to pass stool; he has no symptoms related to constipation (e.g., bloating, excessive gas); abdomen appears nondistended; there is no palpable stool and no retained stool in rectal vault.
Patient defines "normal" bowel elimination as regular elimination of soft stool and adopts healthy elimination patterns.	Patient verbalizes awareness of individual variations in bowel elimination patterns and states that the criterion for "normal" is regular elimination of soft stool; he states that he no longer takes laxatives or enemas to induce bowel movements, and he describes healthy elimination habits (e.g., increased fiber and fluid intake, increased exercise).

PATIENT TEACHING ■■■■■■■■■■■■■■■■■■■■■■■■■■■■■■■■

1. Explain the normal functioning of the gastrointestinal tract, and teach the patient ways to promote normal bowel elimination (i.e., adequate fiber and fluid intake, routine exercise, prompt response to urge to defecate).
2. Explain the causative factors for the patient's constipation (i.e., loss of normal colonic motility due to denervation or inadequate peristaltic stimuli; formation of hard, dry stools due to inadequate fluid or fiber intake or delayed transit; anorectal obstruction due to incoordination of pelvic floor muscles; inability to eliminate stool effectively due to loss of abdominal muscle strength).
3. Explain the adverse effects of long-term use of peristaltic stimulants such as laxatives and enemas (i.e., potential for reduced colonic motility and creation of dependent bowel).
4. Explain the goal of the bowel management program (regular elimination of soft stool), and explain that normal frequency of bowel movements varies from person to person.
5. Instruct the patient in his individualized bowel management program; include guidelines for fiber and fluid intake, a schedule for attempted defecation, instruction on correct use of any aids to defecation (e.g., digital stimulation or suppository), and information on ways to increase physical activity; stress the importance of prompt response to the urge to defecate.

Fecal Incontinence

Fecal incontinence is the involuntary passage of stool. It is sometimes classified according to severity or duration.

Major incontinence is the involuntary elimination of large volumes of stool, whereas minor or "partial" incontinence involves leakage of small amounts of stool (fecal smearing of underclothes) and inability to control flatus. Transient or "acute" incontinence is characterized by abrupt onset and usually is associated with a sudden change in elimination patterns, such as severe diarrhea, or a sudden change in mentation. Chronic incontinence persists over time and commonly is associated with sphincter dysfunction, neurologic impairment, or chronic changes in mental status.

EPIDEMIOLOGY

Fecal continence is a complex phenomenon affected by many factors: intestinal motility, sensory awareness of rectal distention, anal sphincter function, and rectal capacity and compliance. Because many factors contribute to and "safeguard" continence, a pathologic condition involving only one component does not typically cause incontinence; rather, it usually is a combination of factors that overwhelms the continence mechanisms and results in incontinence. For example, the anal sphincter mechanism is most competent for formed stool; thus the patient with some degree of sphincter dysfunction may remain continent as long as the stool is formed but may experience incontinence during periods of diarrhea.

Normal intestinal motility is essential to the delivery of soft, formed stool to the rectal vault at regular intervals. Increased motility may result in diarrhea, which can exceed rectal capacity and overwhelm the sphincter mechanism. Diarrhea is the most common cause of transient fecal incontinence; it is also a common cause of exacerbation in the patient with chronic fecal incontinence. Any condition that causes diarrhea may also cause fecal incontinence, particularly in a patient who also has reduced sensory awareness, sphincter function, or rectal capacity.

Decreased motility can also compromise fecal continence. Prolonged transit through the bowel increases the time available for water absorption, resulting in hard, dry stools that are difficult to pass and that may form an impaction. The impacted stool causes persistent rectal distention, which results in relaxation of the internal anal sphincter. Bacterial action liquefies the stool above the impaction; this liquid stool can then leak around the impaction and through the relaxed anal sphincter, producing incontinence.

Sensory awareness of rectal distention normally occurs with as little as 15 ml of stool or gas; recognition of rectal filling is the "warning sign" that alerts the individual to find a suitable time and place for defecation. Cognitive awareness of rectal filling is also the stimulus for voluntary contraction of the external sphincter, which maintains continence until defecation is convenient. Any disorder that interferes with sensory recognition of rectal distention may therefore cause incontinence. Conditions that commonly interfere with sensory function include spinal cord lesions and injuries, which disrupt transmission of impulses from the pelvis to the cortex, and mentation disorders, which interfere with cortical interpretation and response. Damage to the pudendal nerve is another common cause of sensory dysfunction; this sensorimotor nerve may be damaged by pelvic trauma, diabetic neuropathy, or difficult childbirth. (Obstetric trauma is thought to cause abnormal "stretching" of the pudendal nerve that can cause a "stretch neuropathy"; this is now thought to be a contributing or causative factor in many cases of fecal incontinence formerly labeled idiopathic.)

Loss of sphincter function is another potential cause of fecal incontinence. Normally the internal anal sphincter is maintained in a state of contraction by the intrinsic nervous system, with modulation by the autonomic nervous system; the internal sphincter relaxes when the rectum is distended (the rectoanal inhibitory reflex). The external sphincter is a skeletal muscle that normally is in a state of tonic contraction; rectal distention and voluntary contraction further increase sphincter tone and anal canal pressure, thus supporting continence. Any lesions or conditions that compromise sphincter function place the individual at significant risk for incontinence. Neurologic lesions such as spinal cord injuries or multiple sclerosis cause loss of voluntary sphincter control, as do cortical lesions that compromise level of consciousness. Sphincter damage and pelvic nerve damage may also contribute to impaired sphincter function and fecal incontinence; causative factors include pelvic trauma and anorectal surgical procedures.

Rectal capacity and compliance affect continence by determining the volume of stool that can be accommodated. Normally the rectum can relax to store stool at low pressures, which supports continence. Loss of normal capacity and compliance, which occurs with fibrotic and inflammatory conditions, causes fecal urgency and an inability to delay defecation once stool has been delivered to the rectal vault; this explains the incontinence commonly experienced by individuals with inflammatory bowel disease. Increased compliance, which can occur in the individual who habitually ignores the "call to stool," can also contribute to incontinence. The individual with an overly compliant and "stretched" rectum may not recognize rectal distention (because it is the rectal "stretch" and increased intrarectal pressure that activate the sensory receptors); in addition, the internal sphincter may fail to relax, since it is rectal distention that triggers internal sphincter relaxation. This individual usually suffers from chronic constipation and may develop an "overflow incontinence" syndrome.

PATHOPHYSIOLOGY

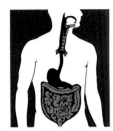 Because many factors contribute to fecal continence, many different patterns of fecal incontinence can occur. The most common patterns are transient incontinence, caused by diarrhea or sudden changes in mentation; neurogenic incontinence, caused by spinal cord injuries or lesions; and "overflow" incontinence, associated with chronic constipation and impaction.

Transient incontinence occurs as a result of a reversible pathologic condition that overwhelms the usual continence mechanisms. The most common causes are diarrhea or changes in mentation. Diarrhea can cause incontinence because the sudden delivery of large volumes of liquid stool can exceed the storage capacity of the rectum and overwhelm the sphincter mechanism. (Maximum contraction of the anal sphincter usually can be maintained for less than a minute; continence beyond this point depends on the rectum's ability to relax and store the stool at relatively low pressures.) Transient incontinence can also be caused by sudden changes in mentation, which may result from metabolic derangements (e.g., renal failure or hepatic encephalopathy) or neurologic lesions (e.g., cerebral edema). The patient may be unaware of rectal distention or may fail to respond to rectal distention appropriately (i.e., with voluntary contraction of the anal sphincter). Patients with clouded sensorium may instead respond to the urge to defecate by relaxing the sphincter and "bearing down" to initiate defecation. Transient incontinence usually is characterized by complete evacuation of rectal contents; if diarrhea is the sole cause, the patient maintains sensory awareness but cannot delay defecation. If altered mental status is a causative or contributing factor, the patient is not consciously aware of rectal filling and does not attempt to delay defecation. Management of transient incontinence is directed toward correcting the underlying disorder.

Neurogenic incontinence results from disorders that interfere with neural regulation of continence mechanisms. Spinal cord lesions (e.g., spina bifida, multiple sclerosis, spinal cord injury) are common causes of neurogenic incontinence. Disruption of the neural pathways causes partial or complete loss of sensory and motor function; the patient is less able or unable to recognize rectal distention and to control the external sphincter. If the lesion is above the sacral cord, the parasympathetic pathways remain intact; this means that parasympathetic stimulation of colonic motility is preserved, as is the defecation reflex. The defecation reflex can initiate rectal evacuation when voluntary control is lost. In this situation, rectal distention causes stimulation of afferent nerves, which synapse on efferent parasympathetic pathways in the sacral cord; parasympathetic stimulation increases rectosigmoid contractility and stimulates rectal emptying. (In a neurologically intact individual, rectal distention is consciously perceived, and voluntary contraction of the external sphincter inhibits the defecation reflex.) Patients with suprasacral lesions experience loss of voluntary control and may also have difficulty with constipation and incomplete rectal evacuation. Constipation is a common problem for patients who are less physically active (e.g., wheelchair-bound patients), because physical activity is a major stimulus for peristalsis. Incomplete rectal evacuation may also be a problem for these patients because effective rectal evacuation usually requires augmentation of the defecation reflex by voluntary contraction of the abdominal muscles (i.e., the Valsalva maneuver). The patient who lacks sensory awareness is less able to coordinate voluntary efforts to defecate with the stimuli resulting from rectal distention; this explains why bowel training programs frequently couple use of a peristaltic stimulant with voluntary efforts to defecate.

Lesions involving the sacral cord (S_2-S_4) cause partial or complete disruption of sensory, motor, and autonomic pathways. These patients have partial or complete loss of sensory awareness and voluntary sphincter control; in addition, colonic motility may be impaired and the defecation reflex may be lost (because the parasympathetic nerve pathways that mediate these functions have been damaged). These patients are particularly prone to constipation and fecal impaction as a result of compromised colorectal contractility; motility and rectal evacuation depend on stimulation of the intrinsic nervous system, which responds to local factors such as mechanical stretch and mucosal irritants. These patients may have "overflow" incontinence and frequent impactions unless an effective bowel training program is established.

"Overflow" incontinence is caused by extreme rectal distention coupled with loss of voluntary defecation; it may or may not be accompanied by fecal impaction. This type of incontinence may occur in a patient with a sacral cord lesion or in a patient who is comatose or semicomatose. The rectum becomes fully distended with stool, because the patient does not recognize rectal distention and does not employ the Valsalva maneuver to initiate defecation; the defecation reflex may or may not be intact but is not able to initiate effective rectal evacuation. Persistent rectal distention causes relaxation of the internal sphincter, which permits passage of stool into the anal canal. The external sphincter may be tonically contracted but cannot be maximally contracted because of the loss of voluntary control; thus there is minimal resistance to stool passage. Because the rectum is not actively contracting, there may be no leakage at rest. However, whenever the intraabdominal and intrarectal pressures rise (e.g., during turning or coughing), the intrarectal pressure overrides the anal canal pressure and some stool leaks out. Because the rectum remains essentially full, this scenario is repeated numerous times throughout the day. If the patient has a fecal impaction, bacterial action liquifies the stool, and liquid stool continuously leaks around the impaction. This is sometimes erroneously interpreted as diarrhea. Appropriate management of "overflow" incontinence involves measures to stimulate routine rectal evacuation.

The three patterns that have been described are the most commonly encountered forms of fecal incontinence, but many types of dysfunction can occur. It is helpful to determine whether the dysfunction involves bowel motility (i.e., What is the consistency and frequency of the stool?), sensory awareness (Does the patient know when a bowel movement is going to occur?), motor sphincter control (Can the patient tighten the sphincter to delay defecation?), or rectal capacity (Does the patient have frequency and urgency for small volumes of stool?). For example, the patient who has sustained damage to the external sphincter muscle might report normal stool frequency and consistency and normal awareness of rectal distention, but an inability to delay defecation effectively; physical examination would reveal a weak, damaged external sphincter muscle. Accurate assessment is essential to management, which is directed toward correcting the underlying problem.

COMPLICATIONS

Breakdown of perianal skin
Fecal impaction
Loss of self-esteem
Social isolation

DIAGNOSTIC STUDIES AND FINDINGS

Diagnostic test	Findings
Stool for ova and parasites	May test positive in patient with diarrhea caused by parasites (e.g., *Giardia* organisms)
Stool for culture	May test positive in patient with bacterial diarrhea (e.g., caused by *C. difficile*)
Stool for occult blood	May test positive in patient with diarrhea and fecal urgency caused by inflammatory bowel disease
Stool for fat	May test positive in patient with diarrhea caused by malabsorption
X-ray (flat plate) of abdomen	May reveal large volumes of accumulated stool throughout colon in patient with constipation
Colonic transit study	May reveal prolonged transit (i.e., radiopaque markers retained for more than 5 days); may be used to differentiate segmental delays versus generalized colonic motility impairment
Anorectal manometry	May reveal reduced sensory awareness of rectal filling; may show failure of internal sphincter to relax with rectal distention; may show inability to voluntarily contract external sphincter
Defecography	May show inability to empty rectum; may show perineal descent
Sphincter electromyography	Reflects external sphincter function; may reveal denervation of external sphincter
Reservoir function study	May reveal increased or decreased rectal capacity and compliance (normal capacity: 250-400 ml)

MEDICAL MANAGEMENT

GENERAL MANAGEMENT

Removal of fecal impaction, followed by cleansing enema (if applicable).

Measures to normalize stool consistency:

Elimination diet for patient with chronic diarrhea not caused by pathogens, parasites, inflammatory disease, or malabsorption.

Increased fiber and fluid intake for patient with constipation: amount of fiber titrated to produce soft, formed stool; 2,000-2,400 ml fluid intake daily if no contraindications.

Establishment of regular schedule for attempted defecation (schedule based on previous patterns and stimuli, attempts scheduled after meals).

Biofeedback for patient with diminished sensory awareness or sphincter control (appropriate only for patient with some intact nerve pathways).

Patient education regarding importance of responding promptly to urge to defecate.

Bowel training programs for patient with neurogenic incontinence (attempted defecation on regular schedule, use of stimulus such as digital stimulation as needed to initiate rectal evacuation).

Application of perianal pouch (fecal incontinence collector) for patient with incontinence secondary to severe diarrhea.

Perianal skin care after each incontinent episode (gentle cleansing followed by application of skin sealant or moisture barrier ointment).

SURGERY

Sphincter repair for patient with structural damage to sphincter.

Gracilis muscle transfer (or gluteus maximus transposition) for patient with severe damage or denervation of external sphincter.

Artificial anal sphincter for patient with neurogenic incontinence.

Electrically stimulated gracilis neoanal sphincter for patient with neurogenic incontinence (transposition of gracilis muscle to create neoanal sphincter with implantation of electrode plate over nerve to muscle and implantation of stimulator that can be switched on and off with hand-held magnet; diverting ostomy). Postoperative stimulation of transposed muscle to effect conversion from type 2 (fatigable) muscle to type 1 (fatigue-resistant) muscle. Stoma closed when satisfactory sphincter function is demonstrated. Sphincter activated and deactivated by use of hand-held magnet over implanted stimulator.

Fecal diversion for intractable incontinence.

DRUG THERAPY

Bulk laxatives (e.g., Metamucil): 5-10 tsp bid or tid, followed by 8 oz water for patient with hard, dry stools who is unable or unwilling to ingest sufficient dietary bulk **or** for patient with chronic watery diarrhea.

Stool softeners (e.g., docusate sodium, docusate calcium, docusate potassium): 240 mg PO daily (docusate calcium or docusate potassium); 50-300 mg PO daily (docusate sodium) for patient with hard, dry stools not corrected by addition of dietary bulk and/or bulk laxatives.

Note: Adequate fluid intake is **essential** for preventing obstruction when giving bulk laxatives and is critical for therapeutic effects with both bulk laxatives and stool softeners.

Softener/stimulant combinations (e.g., docusate with casanthranol, Peri-Colace): 1 capsule (100 mg docusate, 30 mg casanthranol) one to three times daily for patient with constipation related to impaired colonic motility.

Continued.

MEDICAL MANAGEMENT—cont'd

Bisacodyl (e.g., Dulcolax):   10-15 mg PO or suppository (1) to cleanse colon or to initiate regularly scheduled defecation (suppository).

Minienema (docusate plus soft soap):   To initiate routine rectal evacuation for patient with neurogenic incontinence.

Antiinflammatory agents and antibiotics: As needed to treat inflammatory disease or infectious diarrhea.

Antidiarrheal agents (e.g., loperamide, 4-16 mg PO daily; diphenoxylate, 2.5-5 mg PO qid; kaolin-pectin, 60-120 ml PO after each loose stool):   As needed for symptomatic control of diarrhea. *Note:* Antiperistaltic agents such as loperamide and diphenoxylate are **contraindicated** in infectious diarrhea and severe ulcerative colitis, because reduced motility may increase mucosal damage from bacterial toxins or may precipitate toxic megacolon in a patient with ulcerative colitis.

1   ASSESS

ASSESSMENT	OBSERVATIONS
Medical history	May report spinal cord injury, multiple sclerosis, or spina bifida; may report history of ulcerative colitis or Crohn's disease; may report history of pelvic trauma or anorectal surgery
Past and present bowel function	May report: chronic constipation and episodes of fecal impaction; acute or chronic diarrhea; inability to delay defecation; severe fecal urgency and frequency; fecal incontinence that occurs with no sensory warning; incontinence may involve loss of entire stool bolus or may be limited to fecal smearing and difficulty controlling flatus
Rectal examination	May reveal: lax rectum full of stool; fecal impaction; loss of sensory function (i.e., patient does not sense presence of examining finger); diminished resting tone of external sphincter; diminished or absent ability to voluntarily contract external sphincter; diminished or absent ability to relax external sphincter and perform Valsalva maneuver (i.e., patient cannot "push finger out" on command)
Dietary fiber and fluid intake	May report limited intake of fiber-containing foods (i.e., fresh fruits and vegetables, whole grain breads and cereals, bran); may report fluid intake less than 2,000 ml daily
Physical activity level	May report sedentary life-style; may have activity restrictions (e.g., may be wheelchair bound)
Bowel management program (past and present)	May report past or present use of laxatives, suppositories, enemas, or digital stimulation to control defecation; may report unsatisfactory results (persistent accidents, cycles of constipation followed by "purging" and diarrhea, unpredictable results)
Perianal skin status	Inspection may reveal erythematous or denuded skin; may report tenderness and sensitivity
Psychosocial status	May report loss of self-esteem, acute embarrassment, activity restrictions

2 DIAGNOSE

NURSING DIAGNOSIS	SUBJECTIVE FINDINGS	OBJECTIVE FINDINGS
Fecal incontinence related to altered colonic motility, loss of sensory awareness, diminished sphincter function, or altered rectal capacity and compliance	Reports involuntary loss of stool or gas or both; may report sensory awareness with inability to delay defecation due to extreme urgency or diarrhea or both **or** may report loss of stool with no sensory awareness	Incontinent stools; may have large-volume diarrheal stools, normal stools eliminated involuntarily, or frequent leakage of liquid stool due to impaction; rectal examination may reveal loss of sensory awareness or sphincter control
High risk for impaired perianal skin integrity related to diarrhea	Reports burning or soreness in perianal area and that perianal area is sensitive	Perianal skin appears erythematous and may appear denuded
Body image disturbance related to loss of bowel control	Reports feelings of shame, disgust, helplessness; reports concern with odor and cleanliness; reports feeling "like a baby"	Isolates herself from others; appears preoccupied with bowel function; limits activities

3 PLAN

Patient goals

1. The patient will establish an acceptable bowel management program that restores continence.

2. The patient will have healthy, intact perianal skin.
3. The patient will regain a positive body image.

4 IMPLEMENT

NURSING DIAGNOSIS	NURSING INTERVENTIONS	RATIONALE
Fecal incontinence related to altered colonic motility, loss of sensory awareness, diminished sphincter function, or altered rectal capacity and compliance	Establish a monitoring program for bowel function (defecation diary); record volume, consistency, time, and voluntary or involuntary nature of stools.	Continual assessment provides information on patient's response to treatment and guides modification of the treatment program.
	Check patient for fecal impaction, and remove if present; follow with cleansing enema or oral laxative.	Fecal impaction acts as a partial mechanical obstruction and causes leakage of liquid stool around fecal mass.
	For patient with chronic diarrhea of undetermined cause: work with patient and dietitian to record food and fluid intake and fecal volume and consistency. Eliminate foods that cause diarrhea (such as caffeine) and those found "suspect" by diet and defecation diary. Once diarrhea is controlled, reintroduce "suspect" foods one at a time and record results; eliminate foods that cause diarrhea.	Dietary intolerance is a common cause of chronic diarrhea; a diet and defecation record helps identify foods that are poorly tolerated. Eliminating foods thought to cause problems with one-by-one reintroduction of suspect foods permits accurate identification of offending foods.

NURSING DIAGNOSIS	NURSING INTERVENTIONS	RATIONALE
	Administer antidiarrheal medications as ordered to patient with severe or chronic diarrhea (e.g., loperamide, diphenoxylate, kaolin-pectin).	Antidiarrheal medications reduce colonic motility or water content of stool; control of the diarrhea may restore continence.
	Institute measures to normalize stool consistency for patient with diarrhea or constipation.	The anal sphincter is most competent for soft, formed stool.
	Increase dietary bulk *or* administer bulk laxatives (e.g., Metamucil); begin with 3-6 g of fiber daily, and titrate based on response.	Dietary bulk and bulk laxatives retain water and thus help improve stool consistency.
	Ensure adequate fluid intake (2,000-2,400 ml daily) for patient with constipation.	Adequate fluid intake prevents excessive drying of stool.
	Work with patient who is constipated to increase daily activity and exercise.	Exercise and physical activity stimulate peristaltic activity.
	Administer stool softeners as ordered to patient with hard, dry stools (ensure adequate fluid intake to achieve therapeutic effect).	Stool softeners reduce the surface tension of stool and promote water absorption and formation of soft stool.
	Administer softener/stimulant combinations as ordered to patient with reduced colonic motility and hard, dry stools.	These agents help soften stool and also stimulate peristaltic activity.
	Note: Adequate fluid intake is **essential** for therapeutic effect and to prevent obstruction.	
	Collaborate with physician to arrange biofeedback for patient with reduced sensory awareness of rectal distention or reduced contractility of the external sphincter.	Biofeedback helps the individual to recognize rectal distention at an earlier point and to contract the external sphincter more effectively.
	Encourage patient with intact sensation to respond promptly to the urge to defecate.	Prompt response to the urge to defecate promotes rectal emptying and prevents drying of stool.
	Establish bowel training program for patient with neurogenic incontinence.	Bowel training programs compensate for sensory and motor loss by stimulating rectal emptying on schedule, thus preventing involuntary defecation.
	Establish a regular schedule for attempted or stimulated defecation; scheduled attempts should be made after a meal.	Emptying the rectum on schedule prevents reflex defecation and overflow incontinence; eating stimulates peristaltic activity.
	Teach patient to assume upright position for attempted defecation.	Upright position straightens the anorectal angle and increases intraabdominal pressure, which facilitates rectal emptying.
	Teach patient to use Valsalva maneuver (or deep breathing) to initiate defecation.	Valsalva maneuver and deep breathing cause the diaphragm to descend and increase intraabdominal and intrarectal pressures.

NURSING DIAGNOSIS	NURSING INTERVENTIONS	RATIONALE
	Use digital stimulation, suppository, or minienema as needed to stimulate rectal evacuation (digital stimulation may need to be continued for 20 min or even longer when bowel program is first initiated; over time, evacuation occurs with less stimulus).	Digital stimulation, suppositories, and minienemas stimulate rectal evacuation by activating the intrinsic nervous system and the defecation reflex.
	Use suppository or minienema to stimulate routine defecation in a patient with altered level of consciousness and "overflow" incontinence.	Routine stimulation of defecation prevents impaction and "overflow" incontinence.
	Note: The defecation reflex is lost in a patient with a sacral cord lesion; these patients may require more stimulation to effect rectal evacuation.	
High risk for impaired perianal skin integrity related to diarrhea	Cleanse skin gently with tap water, mineral oil, or gentle cleanser after each incontinent stool.	Stool may contain enzymes that damage the skin; prevention includes atraumatic cleansing.
	Protect skin with skin sealants or moisture barrier ointment; if skin is denuded, apply pectin-based powder before applying sealant or ointment.	Sealants and moisture barrier ointments provide a protective film over skin; pectin-based powder absorbs moisture and provides a protective "paste" over denuded skin.
	For patient with severe diarrhea and fecal incontinence: consider applying a fecal incontinence collector (apply to clean, dry skin; if skin is denuded, use pectin-based powder to create a "gummy" surface before application; clip or shave perianal hair before applying collector).	Application of a fecal containment device protects the skin and provides accurate quantification of fecal losses; adhesion requires a dry or tacky surface.
Body image disturbance related to loss of bowel control	Encourage patient and family to share feelings about impact of incontinence on lifestyle and relationships.	Exploring feelings is the first step in dealing with issues and in problem solving; open discussion improves communication and reduces embarrassment.
	Educate and counsel patient and family regarding the principles and options in management of fecal incontinence.	Education involves the patient in problem solving, which improves self-esteem.
	Help patient develop realistic plans for dealing with bowel management program.	Active problem solving improves patient's self-esteem and ability to cope.
	Encourage self-care and grooming activities.	These enhance body image.
	Provide information about support groups (e.g., Help for Incontinent People or spinal cord injury support groups).	Affiliation with others who have similar problems reduces feelings of isolation and enhances self-concept.

_5_ EVALUATE

PATIENT OUTCOME	DATA INDICATING THAT OUTCOME IS REACHED
Patient has established an acceptable bowel management program that prevents incontinence.	Patient states that she has regular bowel movements and no longer has incontinent stools; she describes an appropriate bowel management program (i.e., daily or qod frequency, use of appropriate stimulus as needed to initiate defecation); she describes stool consistency as soft but formed; rectal examination reveals no impacted stool.
Patient has healthy, intact perianal skin.	Patient states that perianal skin is not sensitive to touch; perianal skin is intact without erythema or denudation.
Patient has regained a positive body image.	Patient describes problems with bowel control realistically and describes ways she is coping with these issues; she has resumed her life-style to the extent feasible; she relates positive feelings about her ability to cope and reports improved communication between family members.

PATIENT TEACHING

1. Explain the normal functioning of the gastrointestinal tract, and teach the patient measures to promote normal bowel elimination (e.g., adequate fiber and fluid intake, increased activity, regular schedule for bowel elimination). Explain that the sphincter muscle is most competent for soft, formed stool, and explain that normal functioning depends on intact nerve pathways between the rectum and the brain.

2. Explain the causative factors of the patient's fecal incontinence (i.e., alterations in colonic motility; loss of sensory awareness of rectal distention; loss of ability to tighten voluntary sphincter muscle; loss of normal rectal capacity and compliance). For the patient with neurogenic incontinence, explain that loss of nerve pathways has caused loss of ability to recognize rectal filling and to contract sphincter muscles appropriately.

3. Explain the goal of the bowel management program: regular evacuation of soft, formed stool and prevention of "accidents." For the patient with neurogenic incontinence, explain that effective bowel management depends on keeping the stool soft and formed (so that leakage does not occur and stool can be readily eliminated) and on stimulating rectal evacuation routinely so that reflex defecation and "overflow" incontinence are prevented.

4. Instruct the patient in the rationale and specifics of her individualized bowel management program (i.e., guidelines for fiber and fluid intake; biofeedback program; routine attempts to defecate; measures to stimulate rectal evacuation).

5. Explain the importance of maintaining a defecation record during initial treatment; the record provides the information needed to modify the treatment program appropriately.

Irritable Bowel Syndrome

Irritable bowel syndrome is a symptom complex characterized by abdominal pain, flatulence, and altered fecal elimination patterns (i.e., diarrhea, constipation, or diarrhea alternating with constipation). Other terms used to describe irritable bowel syndrome are *spastic colon, mucous colitis,* and *irritable colon.* Irritable bowel syndrome is the most accurate term, because the symptoms may involve the proximal as well as the distal gastrointestinal tract.

EPIDEMIOLOGY

Surveys indicate that 14% to 22% of the U.S. population has symptoms consistent with irritable bowel syndrome. Some studies indicate that the disorder is more common among women.

The etiology of irritable bowel syndrome is unclear; it is classified as a syndrome because there is no identifiable gastrointestinal pathologic condition to explain the symptoms. Theories about the cause of the disorder include alterations in intestinal motility, increased sensitivity and perception of pain in response to intestinal distention, emotional factors, food intolerance, and intestinal infection.

Considerable evidence supports the theory that changes in intestinal motility are a contributing factor in irritable bowel syndrome. It has been demonstrated that normal individuals respond to pain or stressful events with mucosal engorgement, increased intestinal secretion, and increased motility; it is theorized that people with irritable bowel syndrome show an exaggerated motility response to stress or may respond with increased motility to lesser degrees of stress. Studies have shown that patients with irritable bowel syndrome demonstrate exaggerated motility in response to colonic distention, cholinergic drugs, cholecystokinin, and food. Individuals with irritable bowel syndrome who are symptomatic have been found to have increased colonic activity and altered small bowel motility. (Individuals with diarrhea have increased small bowel motility, whereas those with constipation have reduced small bowel motility.) Patients with irritable bowel syndrome may also demonstrate abnormalities in the proximal gastrointestinal tract; for example, reduced pressure in the lower gastroesophageal sphincter causes gastroesophageal reflux and dyspepsia.

Hypersensitivity to intestinal distention is also hypothesized to play a role in irritable bowel symptomatology. Studies of balloon distention of the colon show that people with irritable bowel syndrome perceive pain at a much lower level of distention than do normal individuals. In addition, the referred pain is more widespread and variable; this indicates that distention of one bowel segment may cause contractions in other bowel segments that are perceived as painful.

Emotional factors have long been thought to play a role in the etiology of irritable bowel syndrome. In the past, studies of patients with irritable bowel syndrome have revealed a significant incidence of depression, insomnia, and anorexia, and patients with irritable bowel syndrome have been classified as neurotic and hypochondriacal. Irritable bowel syndrome has not been proven to be psychogenic in origin; however, stress does seem to play a role in exacerbations, and patients have been found to respond positively to symptom control, empathetic listening, and reassurance that there is no serious underlying disease.

Food intolerance has also been proposed as a causative mechanism. Although some patients experience exacerbations after eating certain foods, there is no definable pathologic response. Thus food intolerances are not thought to be a significant etiologic factor, although individual experiences must be considered when establishing a treatment plan.

Intestinal infections may be an etiologic factor in some cases of irritable bowel syndrome; studies have found that an intestinal infection sometimes is the triggering event for the disorder.

In summary, the etiology of irritable bowel syndrome remains unclear. Currently the symptoms are thought to be caused by a combination of disordered intestinal motility, increased stress response to daily events, and exaggerated sensitivity to intestinal distention.

PATHOPHYSIOLOGY

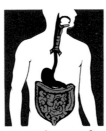

The classic symptoms of irritable bowel syndrome are abdominal pain, increased flatulence, and constipation or diarrhea or both. If the disorder involves the proximal gastrointestinal tract, common symptoms are heartburn, nausea, and belching. The symptom complex varies from individual to individual; common patterns include abdominal pain and constipation, painless diarrhea, diarrhea alternating with constipation, and gastroesophageal symptoms. The onset of symptoms may be abrupt or gradual, and the disorder is characterized by remissions and exacerbations.

Abdominal pain is most commonly seen in patients

with constipation; this symptom complex is sometimes referred to as spastic colon. The constipation is characterized by frequent passage of small, hard stools. The abdominal pain may be described as colicky or as a dull ache; some patients have a chronic dull ache with superimposed episodes of colicky pain. The pain most commonly occurs in the hypogastric area or the left abdomen, but it may also involve the back or the right side or may radiate to the left shoulder. The pain may be relieved temporarily by defecation and may be exacerbated by food intake. Because the pain is sometimes severe, it can mimic acute intraabdominal processes such as appendicitis.

Painless diarrhea is a less common symptom pattern. These patients experience prolonged episodes of diarrhea unassociated with abdominal pain. The diarrhea commonly is low volume (less than 200 g per day) and is characterized by fecal urgency and frequent elimination of semiliquid or ribbonlike stools. This type of diarrhea may be caused by increased colonic motility, which compromises the absorption of water from the stool, and increased anal tone, which produces ribbonlike stools. Bowel movements occur primarily in the morning, particularly after breakfast; this may be due in part to an exaggerated gastrocolic reflex. (Bowel movements do not occur during the night, probably because sleep reduces colonic motility; the absence of nocturnal diarrhea can help differentiate between the functional diarrhea of irritable bowel syndrome and an organic diarrhea.) The diarrhea may be precipitated by eating specific foods, such as fresh fruits or salads, or by excessive intake of coffee or alcoholic beverages. Irritable bowel syndrome can also cause high-volume diarrhea, (more than 200 g per day); this type of diarrhea is thought to be caused by increased motility in the small bowel, which results in the delivery of increased volumes of fluid stool to the colon.

Some patients with irritable bowel syndrome have alternating bouts of constipation and diarrhea. These patients may have abdominal pain during episodes of constipation and may complain of fecal urgency and tenesmus during episodes of diarrhea. The pathologic basis for this symptom pattern is thought to be alterations in colonic motility and increased sensitivity to colonic distention.

It is now recognized that irritable bowel syndrome may involve disturbances in upper tract motility; a common finding is reduced pressure in the gastroesophageal sphincter, which causes esophageal reflux and symptoms of nausea, belching, heartburn, and pain. These symptoms may occur along with lower tract symptoms, or they may predominate, a condition known as functional dyspepsia.

Interestingly, some studies indicate that the motility disturbance may not be confined to the intestinal tract. Patients with irritable bowel syndrome have been found to have an increased incidence of bladder dysfunction, which is reflected by urinary symptoms (e.g., frequency, urgency, and dysuria) and which can be confirmed by urodynamic studies; these patients may also exhibit unusually brisk knee jerks. Systemic symptoms are common in this group of patients; complaints include fatigue, lethargy, inability to concentrate, palpitations, sweating, and backache. Women may complain of dysmenorrhea or dyspareunia or both. Weight loss occurs in about 20% of these patients, and indications of anxiety or depression are common. It is not known whether these symptoms reflect a generalized pathologic condition or unusual sensitivity to distention and contraction phenomena and compromised ability to deal with stressful events.

COMPLICATIONS

Weight loss

DIAGNOSTIC STUDIES AND FINDINGS

Diagnostic test	Findings
Stool studies: guaiac, ova and parasites, culture, fecal fat	Done to rule out inflammatory bowel disease, infectious diarrhea, intestinal parasites, malabsorption syndromes; test results are negative with irritable bowel syndrome
Contrast studies (upper gastrointestinal series, barium enema)	Done to rule out inflammatory bowel disease and other organic conditions; barium enema may be normal or may reveal generalized narrowing of colonic lumen or widespread deep contractions of colonic musculature
Proctosigmoidoscopy	May reveal hyperemic mucosa that does not bleed when rubbed; frequent contractions may be seen, and insufflation of small amounts of air may produce excessive pain (may reproduce patient's usual pain); may reveal spasm of rectosigmoid junction; light touch of rectosigmoid mucosa may cause pain; excessive mucus may be visible

DIAGNOSTIC STUDIES AND FINDINGS—cont'd

Diagnostic test	Findings
Biopsy	Done to rule out other pathologic conditions; test results are normal in irritable bowel syndrome
Hydrogen breath test	Done to rule out lactose intolerance; test results are normal in irritable bowel syndrome
Cholecystography or ultrasound scan of gallbladder	May be done to rule out gallbladder disorder; test results are normal in irritable bowel syndrome
Esophageal manometry	May show reduced pressure in gastroesophageal sphincter
Anorectal manometry and balloon distention studies	May show exaggerated contractile response to balloon distention; patient may complain of pain with balloon distention; may show an increased number of 3 cycles/min contractions and increased frequency of colonic "slow wave" activity

MEDICAL MANAGEMENT

GENERAL MANAGEMENT

Dietary modifications based on symptoms and individual tolerance:

Increased roughage for patient with constipation or alternating constipation and diarrhea (e.g., wheat bran, fruits, and vegetables).

Low-residue diet for patient with diarrhea.

Omission of foods found to cause exacerbations (e.g., coffee, alcoholic beverages).

Patient and family education regarding nature of disorder and rationale for treatment plan.

Emotional support and stress management programs, and psychotherapy when indicated.

DRUG THERAPY

Bulk laxatives (e.g., psyllium products such as Metamucil): 3-12 g daily for patient with constipation or watery diarrhea.

Antidepressants such as amitriptyline (e.g., Elavil), 50-100 mg hs; desipramine (e.g., Norpramin), 75-150 mg daily; or trimipramine (e.g., Surmontil), 50-75 mg daily for patient with anxiety, depression, and abdominal pain. *Note:* Placebo may produce up to 70% reduction in pain.

Anticholinergics such as dicyclomine (e.g., Bentyl): 10-20 mg qid for patients with diarrhea and cramping pain.

Antidiarrheal agents: such as loperamide (e.g., Imodium) 4 mg PO as needed; diphenoxylate (e.g., Lomotil), 5 mg PO as needed; or codeine as needed to control diarrhea and fecal urgency.

1 ASSESS

ASSESSMENT	OBSERVATIONS
Onset of symptoms	May report episodes dating back many years; may report recent onset associated with acute illness; patient with recent onset may report recent travel to areas where intestinal infections or parasites are endemic
Gastrointestinal function	May report constipation (difficult elimination of hard, small-caliber stools), diarrhea (frequent elimination of small-volume, semiliquid or ribbon-like stools *or* high-volume watery diarrhea), or constipation alternating with diarrhea; may report increased elimination of mucus per rectum
Gastrointestinal symptoms	May report abdominal pain, fecal urgency, a sense of incomplete evacuation, increased flatulence, belching, heartburn, and nausea
Other symptoms	May report weight loss, fatigue, inability to concentrate, urinary frequency and urgency, dysuria, dysmenorrhea, dyspareunia, backache, palpitations, or flushing
Emotional status	May report feelings of anxiety or depression; may report concerns about health and fear of serious illness

2 DIAGNOSE

NURSING DIAGNOSIS	SUBJECTIVE FINDINGS	OBJECTIVE FINDINGS
Constipation related to altered colonic motility	Reports difficult elimination of hard, dry stools; may report abdominal pain, back pain, or pain on defecation; may report chronic use of laxatives or enemas	Stools appear small caliber and hard; hard fecal masses may be palpable in left abdominal quadrants
Diarrhea related to increased small bowel motility or increased colonic motility, or both	Reports frequent elimination of small, semi-liquid or ribbonlike stools, or reports large-volume, watery stools; reports urgency and tenesmus; may report attacks after eating particular foods; may report more episodes during morning	Stools appear semiliquid, soft and ribbon-like, or watery; volume varies
Abdominal pain related to increased intestinal motility or hypersensitivity to intestinal distention and contraction, or both	Reports abdominal pain that may be temporarily relieved by defecation; may describe pain as colicky, dull and achy, or dull with superimposed episodes of colicky pain; pain typically is hypogastric but may involve any area of the abdomen as well as the back, sternum, or shoulder	Abdominal palpation reveals abnormal abdominal tenderness over one or more areas of the colon
Anxiety related to abdominal pain and concern about health	Reports feeling worried about health and possibility of serious illness; may report feeling overwhelmed by life events; may recount stressful events that initiate recurrence of symptoms	Patient appears restless; may focus on minor physical complaints and bodily discomfort

_3_ PLAN

Patient goals

1. The patient will regain normal bowel elimination patterns (i.e., regular elimination of soft, formed stool).
2. The patient's diarrhea will resolve or will be effectively controlled.
3. The patient will have no abdominal pain or will be able to control abdominal pain effectively.
4. The patient will be free of anxiety and will be able to cope effectively with daily stressors.

_4_ IMPLEMENT

NURSING DIAGNOSIS	NURSING INTERVENTIONS	RATIONALE
Constipation related to altered colonic motility	Monitor frequency and consistency of stools.	Continual assessment provides information about response to treatment and guides modification of treatment program.
	Collaborate with patient and dietitian to provide increased dietary fiber (whole grains, fruits, vegetables) as tolerated.	Fiber retains water and supports formation of soft, bulky stool, which acts as a peristaltic stimulant.
	Collaborate with patient to ensure adequate daily fluid intake (2,000-2,400 ml).	Adequate fluid intake prevents excessive drying of stool.
	Administer bran or bulk laxative as ordered for patient who is unable or unwilling to ingest sufficient dietary fiber (collaborate with patient to determine preferred type of bulk agent: powder, wafers, or capsules); begin with 3-12 g of fiber daily, and titrate based on response.	Bran is an effective bulking agent and also helps establish regular bowel movements; bulk laxatives provide fiber, which retains water in the stool and promotes formation of soft, bulky stool.
	Note: Adequate fluid intake is **essential** for therapeutic effect and to prevent obstruction	
Diarrhea related to increased small bowel motility or increased colonic motility, or both	Monitor volume and consistency of stools.	Continual assessment provides information about response to treatment and guides modification of treatment plan.
	Collaborate with patient and dietitian to determine any food intolerances (e.g., caffeine and alcoholic beverages) and to eliminate these foods from the diet.	Specific food intolerances may occur in patients with irritable bowel syndrome; ingestion of poorly tolerated foods and fluids may exacerbate symptoms.
	Administer bulk laxatives as ordered to patient with watery diarrhea.	Bulking agents absorb water and improve stool consistency.
	Administer anticholinergic and antidiarrheal agents as ordered and needed (e.g., dicyclomine, loperamide, diphenoxylate, and codeine).	Anticholinergic and antidiarrheal agents reduce peristaltic activity and intestinal motility, thus increasing transit time; increased transit time improves absorption and reduces stool volume.

→ › ›

NURSING DIAGNOSIS	NURSING INTERVENTIONS	RATIONALE
Abdominal pain related to increased intestinal motility or hypersensitivity to intestinal distention and contraction, or both	Monitor pain for severity and for precipitating and relieving factors.	Continual assessment provides information about response to treatment and guides treatment modifications.
	Administer anticholinergic agents (e.g., dicyclomine) as ordered.	Anticholinergic agents reduce intestinal motility and spasticity and thus reduce pain.
	Administer antidepressants (e.g., amitriptyline) as ordered.	Antidepressants have been shown to help reduce pain in individuals with irritable bowel syndrome.
	Teach patient stress management techniques.	Stress is a common precipitating factor for recurrence of irritable bowel symptoms such as pain.
Anxiety related to abdominal pain and concern about health	Provide supportive counseling for patient and family.	Supportive counseling acknowledges the severity of patient's symptoms and establishes a basis for therapeutic intervention.
	Explain nature of irritable bowel syndrome, and explain that there is no evidence of serious illness.	Fear of serious illness contributes to increased anxiety and reduced ability to cope with symptoms.
	Teach patient stress management techniques (i.e., recognition of stressful events and effective management).	Irritable bowel syndrome is thought to be partly caused by the intestine's response to stress; improved stress management may reduce the frequency and severity of episodes by increasing the patient's ability to control autonomic responses.
	Suggest psychotherapy for patient who is anxious or depressed or both.	Psychotherapy has been effective in reducing symptoms of irritable bowel syndrome and in correcting anxiety and depression.
	Administer antidepressants (e.g., amitriptyline) as ordered.	Antidepressants have been effective in reducing anxiety and depression and in relieving pain for patients with irritable bowel syndrome.

5 EVALUATE

PATIENT OUTCOME	DATA INDICATING THAT OUTCOME IS REACHED
Patient has regained normal bowel elimination patterns	Patient reports regular elimination of soft, formed stool; she states that she no longer has to strain to pass stool; no palpable stool is present in descending or sigmoid colon.
Patient's diarrhea has resolved or is effectively controlled.	Patient states that diarrhea has resolved; stools appear soft and formed; *or* patient states that episodes of diarrhea can be controlled by dietary modifications and medications and that diarrhea does not disrupt her life-style.

PATIENT OUTCOME	DATA INDICATING THAT OUTCOME IS REACHED
Patient has no abdominal pain or is able to control pain effectively.	Patient states that pain has resolved *or* states that pain can be effectively controlled by relaxation techniques, dietary modifications, and medications; patient states that pain does not interfere with her daily activities; abdomen is nontender on palpation.
Patient is free of anxiety and is able to cope effectively with daily stressors.	Patient describes improved ability to recognize and manage stressful events; she no longer worries that symptoms of irritable bowel syndrome indicate serious illness; daily conversation does not focus on bodily complaints and functions.

PATIENT TEACHING

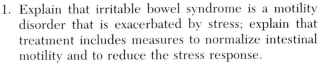

1. Explain that irritable bowel syndrome is a motility disorder that is exacerbated by stress; explain that treatment includes measures to normalize intestinal motility and to reduce the stress response.
2. Teach the patient stress management techniques (routine physical exercise, healthy diet, balance between activity and rest, and relaxation techniques). Encourage her to use relaxation techniques to reduce the severity of abdominal pain.
3. Explain that individuals with irritable bowel syndrome may or may not have food intolerances; encourage the patient to note any relationship between ingested foods and fluids and exacerbation of symptoms. Suggest that she eliminate poorly tolerated foods and fluids from her diet.
4. For the patient with constipation or constipation alternating with diarrhea: Explain the importance of adequate bulk and fluids in the formation of soft, formed stool and the promotion of normal motility.

Explain that laxatives and enemas should be avoided, since they contribute to the motility disorder and may create a dependent bowel. Explain the various types of bulk laxatives available, and explain the importance of an adequate daily intake of dietary fiber or bulk laxatives or both.

5. For the patient with diarrhea: Explain the rationale for dietary modifications (i.e., a low-residue diet), and explain the dosage, schedule, and side effects of any antidiarrheal or anticholinergic medications. Emphasize the daily dosage limitation for medications that are to be taken as needed.
6. For the patient taking an antidepressant for pain control: Explain that the drug is to be taken on schedule rather than as needed. Explain that the effect is cumulative and may not be evident until the drug has been taken for several days or weeks. Emphasize the importance of routine medical follow-up.

CHAPTER 8

Gastrointestinal Intubation and Nutritional Support

Gastrointestinal Intubation and Drainage

Gastrointestinal intubation and drainage may be used to manage gastric distention, small bowel distention, or esophageal or gastric bleeding. The purpose of the therapy directs selection of the tube, intubation procedures, and nursing management.

Gastric distention usually is managed with a double-lumen nasogastric (N/G) tube connected to intermittent suction (e.g., Salem sump). The primary lumen provides for aspiration of gastric contents, and the secondary lumen serves as a "vent" to prevent suction damage to the gastric mucosa. These tubes may be inserted in the operating room (for patients requiring postoperative gastric decompression) or at the bedside by the nurse or physician (see p. 285 for intubation guidelines). Nursing management is directed toward maintaining the placement and functioning of the tube, preventing aspiration and damage to nasal and esophageal tissues, maintaining the fluid and electrolyte balance, and providing comfort measures. Nasogastric suction usually is a short-term therapy; long-term gas-

tric decompression is more commonly accomplished through gastrostomy.

Effective decompression of the small bowel requires insertion of a tube past the pylorus into the appropriate segment of small intestine. The tubes used for small bowel decompression are long and have weighted tips (e.g., Cantor or Miller-Abbott tubes). The tube is passed through the nasopharynx into the stomach; radiologic guidance is then used to advance the tube through the pylorus. Once the tube has been passed through the pylorus, the balloon is filled with air or mercury. The weight of the tube in conjunction with intestinal peristalsis promotes passage through the proximal small bowel to the appropriate segment; follow-up x-rays are used to determine the tube's location, and the tube is taped into place once the desired placement has been achieved. Since peristalsis is the driving force for advancement of the tube, these tubes are not appropriate for managing ileus, and their value in acute mechanical obstruction is controversial. Nursing care includes the measures identified for nasogastric tube

GUIDELINES FOR INSERTION OF NASOGASTRIC TUBE

1. Gather all supplies at the bedside (N/G tube, cup of water, 10- or 20-ml syringe, flashlight, tongue depressor, lubricant, tape, and gloves).
2. Wash hands.
3. Explain the procedure to the patient; stress the importance of the patient's role in facilitating insertion. Assist the patient into a sitting position.
4. Don gloves. Use a flashlight and tongue depressor to examine the patient's nose and oropharynx, looking for obstructions or deformities. Question the patient about previous nasal fractures or nasal surgery.
5. Determine the length of tube to be inserted. Place the insertion end of the tube at the sternoclavicular notch, and measure upward to the tip of the nose; mark the tube at this point (usually about 25 cm).
6. For a tube with a stylet: Irrigate the tube with 5 ml of water to activate the intraluminal lubricant. Insert the stylet, making sure the end does not protrude through the air holes at the (insertion) end of the tube. *Note:* Omit this step if the stylet has already been inserted or if the tube does not require a stylet (review the manufacturer's directions on the cover of the package).
7. Lubricate the insertion end of the tube, or dip the tube in water to activate the lubricant (review the manufacturer's directions).
8. Have the patient tip his head back slightly. Insert the tip of the tube through the chosen nostril, and advance the tube toward the ear and down the nasal passage. Upon reaching the nasopharynx, have the patient bend his head forward (this closes the epiglottis and opens the esophagus). Offer the patient water to sip; advance the tube slowly as the patient swallows.
(*Note:* If the patient begins to cough or has trouble speaking, withdraw the tube until the symptoms disappear and then reinsert.)
When the 25-cm mark is reached, stop and check the tube's position (the tip of the tube should now be in the esophagus); remove the stylet (if applicable), and place the open end of the tube in a cup of water. Observe for bubbling, which indicates an intratracheal position. If bubbling is seen, withdraw the tube completely, reinsert the stylet (if applicable), and begin the insertion procedure again. If no bubbling is seen, continue to advance the tube another 30 to 40 cm into the stomach.
9. Secure the tube to the patient's nose with a commercial attachment device or a piece of tape that has been split to form a Y. (Place the base of the Y on the bridge of the nose, and wrap the two arms of the Y around the tube. The tube should be well secured but should not exert pressure against the nostril.) Confirm placement by obtaining x-ray verification (small-bore tube) or by aspirating gastric fluid (large-bore tube) and testing fluid for pH (gastric fluid has a pH of less than 3).

---

management; in addition, the nurse must monitor the patient for tube advancement and for evidence of balloon rupture or mercury spillage into the bowel (which occurs if a mercury-weighted tip is ruptured).

Gastrointestinal intubation and drainage may also be used to control gastric or esophageal bleeding. Gastric bleeding may be managed with a simple nasogastric tube in conjunction with gastric lavage; this is the approach commonly used for patients with erosive gastritis or bleeding ulcers. Patients with bleeding esophageal or gastric varices usually are managed with balloon tamponade; this involves inserting a tube designed specifically for compression of bleeding varices. Commonly used tubes include the Sengstaken-Blakemore tube and the Linton-Nachlas tube (Figure 8-1). The Sengstaken-Blakemore tube has both an esophageal and a gastric balloon in addition to a gastric aspiration lumen (Figure 8-1, *A*); it permits both esophageal and gastric compression but does not provide for esophageal aspiration. (Since the patient is unable to swallow when the gastric balloon is inflated, patients with a Sengstaken-Blakemore tube require placement of an additional tube for esophageal decompression through the opposite nostril.) The Linton-Nachlas tube has only a gastric balloon but provides ports for both gastric and esophageal aspiration (Figure 8-1, *B*).

Balloon tamponade is initiated by inserting the selected tube through the nasopharynx into the stomach (after anesthetizing the nasopharynx with a topical anesthetic); the stomach is lavaged, and the gastric balloon is inflated with about 50 ml of air. Radiologic confirmation of tube placement should be obtained before inflat-

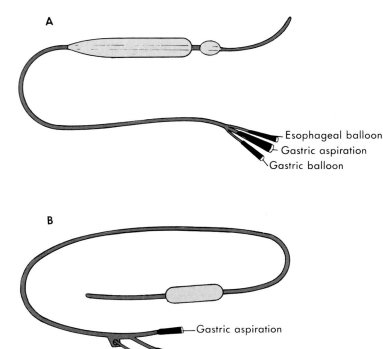

A

B

FIGURE 8-1
A, The triple-lumen, double-balloon Sengstaken-Blakemore tube for tamponade of bleeding esophageal varices. This tube has no port for esophageal aspiration. **B,** The Linton-Nachlas tube, which has not only a gastric balloon but also ports for both gastric and esophageal aspiration.

ing the balloon further; once placement has been verified, the balloon is inflated (usually to about 250 ml of air), pulled snugly against the gastroesophageal junction, and secured in place (e.g., by taping the tube to a football helmet, which the patient must wear). The gastric balloon may be further inflated (to about 450 ml of air) if necessary to control the bleeding. (The Linton-Nachlas tube has a gastric balloon with a 400- to 700-ml capacity.) The Sengstaken-Blakemore tube provides an additional balloon for esophageal compression, which is used as a last resort to control the bleeding; inflation is limited to about 35 mm Hg. These tubes are intended only for short-term therapy; once the bleeding has been controlled for 24 hours, the balloon is deflated and, if

the bleeding does not recur, the tube is removed. Persistent or recurrent bleeding requires alternative therapies. Nursing management of a patient with balloon tamponade involves continual intervention and monitoring to maintain tube placement, prevent aspiration of secretions, and assess the effectiveness of therapy.

INDICATIONS

Gastric Decompression
  Gastric or small bowel surgery
  Paralytic ileus or gastroparesis
  Small bowel obstruction
  Gastric or proximal small bowel fistula
Small Bowel Decompression
  Mechanical obstruction of small bowel
Control of Gastric or Esophageal Bleeding
  Erosive gastritis (N/G tube)
  Bleeding gastric or duodenal ulcer (N/G tube)
  Bleeding esophageal or gastric varices (balloon tamponade)

CONTRAINDICATIONS

No absolute contraindications; use of small bowel tube is not recommended for patient with ileus because advancement of tube depends on peristalsis

COMPLICATIONS

  Gastroesophageal reflux; aspiration
  Esophagitis; esophageal stricture
  Fluid-electrolyte imbalance
  Airway obstruction (balloon tamponade tube, secondary to rupture of gastric balloon with subsequent migration into nasopharynx)
  Aspiration (balloon tamponade tube, secondary to accumulation of secretions in esophagus proximal to gastric and esophageal balloons)
  Esophageal rupture (balloon tamponade tube, secondary to overinflation of esophageal balloon or rupture of gastric balloon with subsequent migration into esophagus)
  Intestinal perforation or mercury toxicity (small bowel tube, secondary to rupture of air-filled or mercury-filled balloon)

PREPROCEDURAL NURSING CARE

NURSING DIAGNOSIS	NURSING INTERVENTIONS	RATIONALE
Knowledge deficit related to GI intubation	Explain rationale for tube placement and intubation procedure; emphasize ways patient can facilitate passage of tube, and arrange communication signals to be used during intubation procedure.	The patient is a critical member of the health care team and must be informed of treatment options and rationale; an informed, cooperative patient contributes to tube placement with minimal discomfort.

POSTPROCEDURAL NURSING CARE

NURSING DIAGNOSIS	NURSING INTERVENTIONS	RATIONALE
High risk for aspiration related to open esophageal sphincters and gastroesophageal reflux or vomiting	Irrigate tube as ordered and needed to maintain patency.	Irrigation maintains tube patency and reduces gastric distention, which reduces the risk of gastroesophageal reflux.
	Monitor patient for evidence of gastric distention (reduced aspirate, increasing abdominal distention, and complaints of nausea or vomiting).	Gastric distention indicates inadequate decompression and must be corrected promptly to prevent reflux, vomiting, and aspiration.
	For patient with compromised level of consciousness: keep head of bed elevated and position patient on side.	Elevating head of bed reduces the risk of gastroesophageal reflux; side-lying position reduces the risk of aspiration should vomiting occur.
	For patient with Sengstaken-Blakemore tube: collaborate with physician to ensure appropriate placement of esophageal catheter; irrigate catheter as needed to maintain patency.	The inflated gastric balloon occludes the gastric inlet and results in pooling of esophageal secretions, which must be removed to prevent aspiration.
High risk for fluid volume deficit related to gastric or intestinal suction	Monitor patient for signs and symptoms of fluid or electrolyte imbalance (output exceeding intake, concentrated urine, decreased skin turgor, postural hypotension, dry mucous membranes, diminished muscle tone, dizziness, weakness, muscle cramps).	Early detection of abnormalities permits prompt intervention and helps prevent complications.
	Irrigate tube with normal saline; do not use tap water.	Isotonic saline prevents the electrolyte shifts that could occur with hypotonic solutions such as water.
	Limit oral intake to occasional ice chips or "electrolyte" (e.g., Gatorade) chips.	Oral intake stimulates gastric secretion and increases the fluids and electrolytes lost through suction.
	Administer IV fluids and electrolytes as ordered.	Fluid balance must be maintained to maintain blood volume and tissue perfusion.

NURSING DIAGNOSIS	NURSING INTERVENTIONS	RATIONALE
Alteration in oral mucous membranes related to mouth breathing and drying of mucous membranes and friction caused by N/G tube	Provide oral care q 4 h and as needed for complaints of dry mouth or sore throat.	Frequent rinsing maintains hydration of mucous membranes.
	Provide hard candy or anesthetic lozenges for patient to suck on.	Sucking on hard candy stimulates production of saliva; anesthetic lozenges also provide topical analgesia.
	Lubricate lips with petroleum jelly or similar product.	Lubrication prevents drying and cracking.
High risk for suffocation related to airway obstruction by balloon tamponade tube	Maintain accurate positioning of tube: secure tube in correct position (e.g., by taping tube securely to football helmet that patient wears); monitor patient for tube position and indicators of airway obstruction.	Upward migration of inflated or partially inflated gastric (or esophageal) balloon can cause airway obstruction.
High risk for alteration in tissue integrity related to taping of tube against nares	Secure N/G or small bowel tube to nares in a manner that prevents nares compression (e.g., with a commercial tube holder, or a Y-shaped piece of tape).	Friction and pressure are common causes of tissue damage when the tube is taped up against the nostril.

PATIENT TEACHING

1. Explain the purpose of the tube (to decompress the stomach and prevent vomiting, to permit gastric lavage for control of bleeding, to compress bleeding varices, or to decompress the small bowel).
2. Describe the procedure for intubation (if the tube is to be placed at the bedside), and identify measures used to prevent gagging, vomiting, and discomfort (positioning and swallowing sips of water; use of topical anesthetic before insertion of the balloon tamponade tube).
3. Explain the reason for limiting oral intake of ice, water, and other fluids (promotes gastric secretion, which may cause chemical imbalance); explain the use of oral care measures, hard candy, lozenges, and lip lubricants to prevent dry mouth and sore throat.

Enteral Nutritional Support

Enteral nutritional support involves administration of nutrients directly into the stomach or small bowel; enteral feedings are used to maintain nutritional status or to correct nutritional deficits in a patient with functional small bowel who is unable or unwilling to ingest sufficient nutrients orally.

Enteral feedings can be used as total nutritional support or as a supplement for other forms of nutrient intake and can be provided on a temporary or a long-term basis. Enteral feedings may be delivered to the stomach or to the proximal small bowel by way of nasally placed or abdominally placed tubes. Formulas used for enteral feedings vary; the selection of a formula and the volume and rate of feeding are determined primarily by the patient's nutrient needs and nutritional status and by the route of administration.

Enteral feedings are used to provide total nutritional support for patients with intact small bowel function who cannot ingest nutrients orally (e.g., patients with esophageal strictures, swallowing disorders, or altered level of consciousness preventing oral intake). These patients are administered pureed foods or commercial formulas in sufficient volumes to meet all their nutrient needs. Enteral feedings can also be used as one component of a broad nutritional support program. For example, enteral feedings may be used to supplement oral intake until oral intake is adequate to meet nutrient needs. Patients receiving total parenteral nutrition (TPN) may also benefit from low-volume enteral feedings; simultaneous administration of an enteral formula prevents atrophy of the villi and maintains integrity of the gut wall, which is thought to play a role in immune system functioning.

Enteral feedings may be delivered to the stomach or directly into the proximal small bowel. A major advantage associated with gastric feedings is the ability to administer bolus feedings, since the reservoir function of the stomach and the pyloric sphincter are maintained. The major disadvantage to gastric feedings is the increased risk of gastroesophageal reflux and aspiration in the patient who is prone to gastric distention. In contrast, small bowel feedings bypass the stomach and thus reduce the risk of reflux and aspiration; however, they require continuous-drip administration because the gastric reservoir has been bypassed.

Enteral feedings may be administered through nasally inserted tubes or abdominal tubes. Nasally inserted tubes include nasogastric tubes and nasoduodenal tubes. Historically most nasally placed tubes were nasogastric, and standard decompression tubes (e.g., Levine or Salem sump) were commonly used. In current practice, the small-bore silicone elastomer tube is the tube of choice in most situations. The advantages associated with these tubes include reduced incidence of mucosal trauma and minimal compromise of the gastroesophageal sphincter, which reduces the risk of gastric reflux and aspiration. In addition, passage of these tubes through the pylorus into the duodenum permits nasoduodenal feedings, which further reduces the risk of aspiration. Disadvantages associated with the small-bore tubes are the increased risk of tube obstruction from feedings or medications and the inability to aspirate consistently to check for placement and gastric residual.

Long-term enteral feedings usually are administered through a gastrostomy or jejunostomy tube; these abdominally placed tubes eliminate some of the risks associated with nasal tubes (e.g., mucosal trauma and

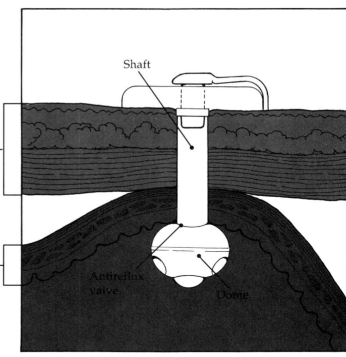

FIGURE 8-2

Gastrostomy button demonstrating how stability is achieved by use of correct shaft length so that dome is positioned against anterior stomach wall. (From Bryant.[8])

gastroesophageal reflux). In the past, creation of a gastrostomy or jejunostomy required an open surgical procedure; however, the trend is toward percutaneous placement of feeding tubes under endoscopic or radiologic guidance (unless the procedure is carried out in conjunction with an open surgical procedure). Table 8-1, p. 292, provides a brief description of the various approaches to gastrostomy and jejunostomy. Tubes used for gastrostomy and jejunostomy include large-bore latex tubes (e.g., Foley catheters), polyurethane tubes (e.g., Ross Sacks-Vine, Sheridan-Moss, or Silk), and silicone tubes (e.g., MIC tubes from Medical Innovations Corporation). The polyurethane and silicone tubes are more expensive but are associated with longer use and less soft tissue reaction. A gastrostomy "button" is also available; this is a short silicone tube with a skin-level flip-top opening and a one-way antireflux valve that prevents leakage of stomach contents when the tube is closed (Figure 8-2). The button device is inserted into a previously constructed and well-established gastrostomy tract; the tube remains closed except for feedings, when an adapter is passed through the one-way valve to provide access to the stomach.

PROCEDURE FOR POUCHING AROUND A LEAKING GASTROSTOMY TUBE

1. Obtain a two-piece fecal pouch (e.g., ConvaTec SurFit system or Hollister two-piece system). Size the barrier wafer to fit around the gastrostomy tube, allowing at least ⅛-inch clearance between the insertion site and the barrier.
2. Attach a catheter support device to the anterior surface of the pouch.
   Place one strip of paper tape over the site where the tube is to be brought through the pouch (this prevents tearing of the pouch material when it is cut to accommodate the tube support device and the tube).
   Cut an **X** in the anterior wall of the pouch where the tape has been placed.
   Attach the tube support device (e.g., feed a baby nipple through the **X** from the inside of the pouch to the outside of the pouch, and secure on both the inside and outside with tape; **or** attach NuHope catheter holder (NuHope, Los Angeles, California) over the **X**; **or** omit the tape and use a Hollister Universal Catheter Access Device (Hollister, Libertyville, Illinois) to establish the exit site and support system for the tube (follow the manufacturer's instructions). Cut an appropriate-size opening in the top of the support device (baby nipple or commercial device).
   Note: As an alternative to using a support device, attach a piece of tape to the tube exit site, cut an **X** opening, and feed the catheter through. Use pectin-based paste (e.g., Stomahesive) and waterproof tape to secure the tube to the anterior surface of the pouch and prevent leakage.
3. Clean and dry the skin. Treat any skin damage by applying a light coat of pectin-based powder (e.g., Stomahesive) and then blotting lightly over the powder with a wet gloved finger or skin sealant (e.g., Skin Prep).
4. Peel the paper backing off the wafer; plug the tube and fit the wafer into place around the tube. Press firmly to obtain a secure seal. Apply a thin layer of skin barrier paste (e.g., Stomahesive) to any exposed skin; allow to dry until nonsticky.
5. Remove the plug from the tube. Pass lubricated hemostats through the support device on the anterior wall of the pouch, and grasp the drainage lumen of the tube; slowly and steadily pull the tube through the anterior wall of the pouch and the support device, being careful not to exert excessive pressure and dislodge the tube.*
6. Once the tube has been brought through the anterior wall of the pouch, reinsert the plug to prevent further leakage.
7. Snap the pouch onto the flange of a two-piece system.
8. Secure the tube to the support device with tape.

*Note: The hemostats should be inserted from outside the pouch to inside the pouch to grasp the tube; the tube is then passed from the inside surface of the pouch to the outside surface of the pouch.

PROCEDURE FOR STABILIZING TUBE WITH BARRIER WAFER AND BABY NIPPLE

1. Cut out the barrier wafer (e.g., Stomahesive) to fit around the abdominal tube (be sure to allow at least ⅛-inch clearance between the wafer and the insertion site). Slit the wafer along the top side to facilitate placement around the tube.
2. Clean and dry the skin. Treat any damaged skin by applying a light coat of pectin-based powder (e.g., Stomahesive) and then blotting lightly over the powder with a wet gloved finger or skin sealant (e.g., Skin Prep).
3. Peel the paper backing off the wafer, and apply the wafer to the skin around the tube. Press firmly into place to ensure a good seal.
4. Slit a baby nipple up one side, and cut an opening in the top of the nipple to accommodate the tube. Fit the baby nipple into place around the tube, and secure the nipple to the barrier wafer with four strips of tape. Tape the junction between the tube and the baby nipple securely.
5. The nipple may be untaped and removed daily for site care and inspection. The barrier wafer is changed q 5-7 days as needed.

A major problem associated with all feeding tubes is maintaining the tube's position. Nasal tubes are secured proximally with tape or a commercial device to the nose, but this does not completely prevent proximal migration in the alimentary canal; the nurse or caregiver must continually monitor the patient for evidence of tube displacement or aspiration. Abdominal tubes are stabilized either with inflatable intraluminal balloons or with internal and external "bumpers," domes, or discs (Figure 8-3). Jejunal "balloon" tubes should be left deflated to prevent obstruction of the relatively narrow jejunal lumen.

Enteral nutritional support can be provided by using pureed foods or commercial formulas. Pureed diets are most appropriate for patients with normal small bowel function and a large-bore feeding tube. Commercial formulas are a better approach for patients with compromised small bowel function, specific nutrient or metabolic needs, or small-bore feeding tubes. Most commercial formulas are lactose free, since many malnourished patients are lactose intolerant. They may be categorized as protein intact, chemically defined, or specialty formulas. Protein-intact formulas (e.g., Osmolite, Isocal) are nutritionally complete "liquid diets"; the nutrients in these formulas require enzymatic digestion before they can be absorbed. These diets are more appropriate for patients with normal small bowel function. Chemically defined diets (e.g., Citrotein) contain nutrients that are partially broken down, or "predigested"; for example, the protein may be supplied as peptides or amino acids. Because these formulas are essentially "ready to absorb," they may be used for patients with compromised small bowel function. Specialty formulas (e.g., Pulmocare or Stresstein) are designed for patients with specific diseases or metabolic demands.

Selection of a specific formula and determinations regarding volume to be administered depend on assessment of the patient's nutrient needs, current nutrient intake by the oral or parenteral route, and factors affecting tolerance of specific nutrients or formulas (e.g., liver function and renal function). These decisions are best made by a qualified dietitian or nutritional support team. Continual assessment of the patient's progress and tolerance is essential, and the nutritional support plan is altered as needed.

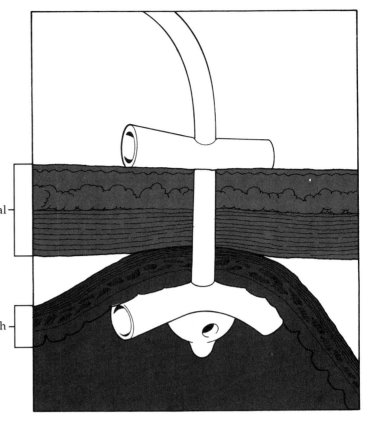

Abdominal wall

Stomach wall

FIGURE 8-3
Percutaneous endoscopic gastrostomy (PEG). Notice internal bumper against anterior stomach wall and external bumper at skin level. (From Bryant.[8])

Table 8-1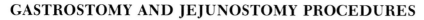

GASTROSTOMY AND JEJUNOSTOMY PROCEDURES

Name of procedure	Description	Advantages
Stamm gastrostomy	Subcostal incision is made through abdominal wall; anterior wall of stomach is sutured to abdominal wall for stabilization; balloon-tipped catheter is inserted through abdominal wall into stomach and sutured into place; balloon is inflated and rests snugly against abdominal wall to stabilize tube	Can be performed under local anesthesia; can use large-bore catheter, which is less likely to obstruct
Percutaneous endoscopic gastrostomy (PEG)	Gastroscope is inserted through oral cavity into stomach; stomach is insufflated with air and transilluminated at desired puncture site; 16 Fr. needle is passed through abdominal wall into stomach; long suture is passed through needle into stomach; one end of suture is grasped by endoscopic snare and pulled up through mouth (endoscope is removed) while other end of suture is held securely at abdominal wall; oral end of suture is tied securely to distal end of feeding tube; suture and feeding tube are pulled down through esophagus and stomach and out onto abdominal wall and anchored with internal and external bumpers	Requires no anesthesia; cost-effective; lower complication rate than surgical gastrostomy
Percutaneous gastrostomy under radiologic guidance	Stomach is distended with air; needle is inserted percutaneously into stomach; J-wire is threaded into stomach under radiologic guidance and needle is removed; small incision is made at exit site of wire; when entry into stomach is confirmed, tract is gradually dilated, and permanent catheter is inserted; catheter usually is stabilized in stomach by inflatable balloon and stabilized at skin level by suture or tube stabilization device	Can be performed under local anesthesia
Janeway gastrostomy	Rectangular flap is lifted from midanterior stomach wall; stomach defect is closed; rectangular flap is used to create mucosa-lined tube that is brought to abdominal wall as stoma	Creates permanent stoma that can be intubated as needed for feedings; eliminates risk of tube displacement
Spivak gastrostomy	Modification of Janeway gastrostomy; fundoplication at base of mucosa-lined gastric "tube" provides improved continence	Same as Janeway plus improved continence
Button gastrostomy	Requires established gastrostomy tract with at least an 18 to 20 Fr. diameter; special measuring device provided by manufacturer is inserted into tract to determine appropriate shaft length (internal "dome" must fit snugly against stomach wall, and external flip-top opening must fit securely against abdominal surface to prevent reflux around the tube); obturator is inserted into button to straighten the internal "dome"; button is lubricated and inserted; obturator is removed, and flip-top opening is closed	Creates a skin-level tube that can be closed between feedings
Witzel jejunostomy	Catheter is inserted into jejunum; exterior serosal layer of bowel is folded over catheter and sutured in place (forms subserosal tunnel); catheter is brought through stab wound in abdominal wall and sutured in place; jejunum is secured to abdominal wall (parietal peritoneum)	Can be performed in conjunction with open abdominal procedure or under local anesthesia; larger-bore catheter can be used
Needle catheter jejunostomy	Percutaneous insertion of large-bore needle through abdominal wall into jejunum; small catheter is threaded through needle, and needle is removed; catheter is sutured in place (small-bore catheter)	Done in conjunction with open abdominal procedure with minimal additional operating time
Percutaneous endoscopic jejunostomy	Percutaneous endoscopic gastrostomy is performed; small-bore feeding tube is passed through PEG into duodenum under endoscopic guidance; tube is advanced by peristalsis into jejunum and stabilized with internal and external "bridges"	Simple procedure that can be performed without anesthesia; reduced incidence of reflux (compared to PEG)

INDICATIONS

Dysphagia

Esophageal stricture

Loss of continuity between mouth and stomach (e.g., surgery for head and neck cancer necessitating esophageal resection)

Esophagogastric obstruction (e.g., patient with obstructing gastric tumor)

Altered level of consciousness precluding oral intake (e.g., patient who is comatose or semicomatose)

Anorexia

Short bowel syndrome (*Note:* Must be given in conjunction with TPN until small bowel adaptation permits adequate absorption of enteral nutrients)

To maintain bowel wall integrity in patient receiving TPN

CONTRAINDICATIONS

Severe hypoproteinemia and hypoalbuminemia (resulting bowel wall edema precludes effective nutrient absorption and causes severe diarrhea; enteral feedings should be delayed until protein deficit has been partially corrected, or albumin should be administered intravenously in conjunction with enteral feedings)

Ileus or mechanical small bowel obstruction

Small bowel fistulae (*Note:* Chemically defined low-residue formulas may be used for patient with proximal small bowel fistula if feeding can be delivered distal to the fistula *or* for patient with very distal small bowel fistula)

Small bowel dysfunction (malabsorption, inflammatory diseases, short bowel syndrome)

Severe gastroesophageal reflux, gastric atony, or pyloric obstruction (gastric feedings)

COMPLICATIONS

Gastroesophageal reflux and aspiration (gastric feedings)

Tube blockage

Diarrhea

Constipation

Hyperglycemia

Tube-feeding syndrome

Tract erosion and peritubular skin breakdown (abdominal tubes)

PREPROCEDURAL NURSING CARE

NURSING DIAGNOSIS	NURSING INTERVENTIONS	RATIONALE
Knowledge deficit related to enteral feedings and tube placement	Explain rationale for enteral feedings and procedure for tube placement; for N/G or nasoduodenal tube, emphasize ways the patient can facilitate tube passage, and arrange communication signals to be used during intubation procedure.	The patient and family are critical members of the health care team and must be informed of treatment options and rationale; an informed, cooperative patient contributes to tube placement with minimal discomfort.
High risk for alteration in skin integrity related to peritubular leakage (percutaneous tubes)	Mark site for placement of percutaneous tubes (if feasible); site chosen should be away from costal margins and on a flat surface.	Locating the tube site on a flat surface away from the costal margins facilitates tube stabilization, which reduces the risk of tract erosion and peritubular leakage.
High risk for infection related to percutaneous tube insertion	Prepare the site for percutaneous tube placement with an antiseptic solution (e.g., Betadine or Hibiclens). Maintain sterile technique during percutaneous tube insertion.	Skin antiseptics reduce bacterial counts and thus reduce the risk of infection. Sterile technique prevents introduction of pathogens.
	Administer antibiotics as ordered before and after percutaneous tube placement.	Antibiotics interfere with bacterial replication and help prevent infection.

➤ ➤ ➤

POSTPROCEDURAL NURSING CARE

NURSING DIAGNOSIS	NURSING INTERVENTIONS	RATIONALE
High risk for aspiration related to incorrect tube position or gastric distention and reflux or vomiting	Ensure accurate position of nasally placed tube before administration of feeding. For firm large-bore tubes: aspirate gastric fluid (most accurate test), or auscultate epigastric area while rapidly injecting 10 ml of air into stomach, or place proximal end of tube into water and observe for bubbling that coincides with respirations. Repeat confirmation of tube position before each feeding. For soft small-bore tubes: obtain radiologic confirmation of tube position after initial placement and "as needed" for evidence of tube migration or any concerns regarding tube position. Attempt aspiration before each feeding; if unable to aspirate, observe closely for any respiratory distress during feedings.	Nasally placed tubes can be inadvertently inserted into the respiratory system or can migrate out of the stomach into the esophagus or respiratory system. Accurate placement can be verified by aspiration of gastric fluid or by radiologic confirmation of tube placement. Rapid insufflation of air into stomach can usually be auscultated over epigastric area but is not consistently reliable. Bubbling with respirations may indicate migration into the respiratory system. Aspiration may cause collapse of small-bore tubes, so verification of tube position before each feeding may not be feasible; careful monitoring of patient tolerance is essential.
	Attempt aspiration before each feeding (or q 4 h for patient receiving continuous-drip feedings); delay feedings when residual exceeds 150 ml (or the volume established for this patient) *or* when there is evidence of intolerance (e.g., absent bowel sounds, distention, or complaints of nausea).	Gastric distention is a major risk factor for gastroesophageal reflux, vomiting, and aspiration; monitoring of patient tolerance and adjustment of feeding rates to prevent gastric distention reduce the risk of aspiration.
	Elevate head of bed during bolus feedings and for 1 hour after feeding; keep head elevated 30 degrees for patient on continuous feedings.	Elevating the head of the bed reduces the risk of gastroesophageal reflux.
	Gradually advance volume of bolus feedings or rate of continuous feedings based on patient tolerance.	Gradual advancement of feeding volume and rate permits assessment of patient tolerance and reduces the risk of gastric distention and aspiration.
Diarrhea related to bacterial contamination, edema of bowel wall (resulting in compromised absorption), administration of osmotic laxatives (e.g., sorbitol), or impaction	Monitor patient's stools for volume, frequency, and consistency.	Patients given enteral feedings normally have mushy stools once or twice a day; continual monitoring permits prompt recognition of excessive stool volume and allows early intervention.
	Observe strict aseptic technique in setting up and administering enteral feedings.	Strict aseptic technique minimizes the risk of bacterial contamination.
	Keep unused formula refrigerated until the next feeding; for patients receiving continuous-drip feedings, limit amount of formula "hung" at one time to the amount that can be infused in 4-6 h.	Refrigeration prevents bacterial proliferation; limiting "hang time" of formula reduces exposure of formula to room temperature, thus limiting bacterial proliferation.
	Change administration sets q 24 h.	Daily change of administration sets reduces the chance for bacterial growth.

NURSING DIAGNOSIS	NURSING INTERVENTIONS	RATIONALE
	For patients with hypoproteinemia (e.g., serum albumin < 2.8) and for patients who have been NPO for prolonged periods or who have short bowel syndrome: initiate feedings at a slow rate (e.g., 20-50 ml/h) and advance according to patient tolerance.	Hypoproteinemia causes bowel wall edema; prolonged NPO status results in atrophy of the villi, and short bowel syndrome results in reduced absorptive surface; rapid feeding in these patients will cause diarrhea due to reduced absorption; gradual advancement of the feeding rate permits adaptation by the bowel and reduces diarrhea.
	Dilute hypertonic formulas (osmolarity >400 mOsm/kg) to half strength and advance strength gradually (*Note:* Isosmotic formulas do *not* require dilution).	Hypertonic formulas may act as a cathartic by retaining fluid in the bowel lumen.
	For patient who develops diarrhea: evaluate for causative factors (fecal impaction, medications containing sorbitol, superinfection with *Clostridium difficile,* hypoproteinemia). (*Note:* Stool culture is recommended for patient who has been taking antibiotics and has unexplained diarrhea.)	Diarrhea in tube-fed patients is not usually a result of the tube feedings; common etiologies are impaction, sorbitol (unabsorbable solute that acts as an osmotic laxative), *C. difficile* infection, and hypoalbuminemia.
	Treat causative factors: Eliminate fecal impaction. Modify medications to eliminate sorbitol; Administer antibiotics as ordered to patient with *C. difficile* infection. Administer albumin or protein solution as ordered to patient with hypoproteinemia. Administer Lactinex as ordered to patient with diarrhea resulting from antibiotic therapy and overgrowth of yeast organisms.	Treatment of any pathologic condition must always address causative factors.
	Collaborate with physician and dietitian to use formula with fiber or to add nongelling fiber to formula.	High-fiber formulas and fiber supplements retain water and thus reduce diarrhea.
	Administer antidiarrheal medications as ordered and needed (e.g., kaolin-pectin products, loperamide, diphenoxylate). *Note:* Kaolin-pectin products may be used for patients with suspected or proven bacterial infections (e.g., *C. difficile*), but antimotility agents should not be used for infectious states.	Antidiarrheal agents reduce intestinal motility or increase absorption and thus reduce diarrhea. Kaolin-pectin products absorb toxins and are appropriate for infectious diarrheas; antimotility agents increase mucosal contact with bacteria and bacterial toxins.
	For patient with severe diarrhea: collaborate with physician and nutritional support team regarding use of TPN.	Severe diarrhea may further compromise nutritional status and may cause fluid and electrolyte imbalance.
Constipation related to inadequate fiber and fluid intake	Monitor stools for frequency, volume, and consistency.	Prompt detection of constipation permits early intervention.
	Ensure adequate daily fluid intake (30 ml/kg body weight minimum intake).	Adequate fluid intake is essential for maintaining soft, bulky stools.

→ ⟩ ⟩ ⟩

NURSING DIAGNOSIS	NURSING INTERVENTIONS	RATIONALE
	Collaborate with physician and dietitian to provide adequate fiber (e.g., with use of fiber-based formula or addition of nongelling fiber supplement).	Fiber retains water and supports formation of bulky stool; bulky stool promotes peristaltic activity.
	Administer mild laxative or suppository as ordered to patient who is constipated.	Mild laxatives and suppositories promote peristalsis and colonic evacuation.
Altered nutrition: less than body requirements related to obstructed feeding tube and reduced nutrient intake	Use feeding pump to administer continuous-drip feedings through small-bore tubes.	Feeding pumps provide positive pressure to ensure constant flow of solution and prevent tube occlusion.
	Flush feeding tubes with at least 50 ml of water after each bolus feeding (or each time formula is added to a continuous-drip system).	Thorough flushing removes residual formula from the tube, which helps maintain tube patency.
	Collaborate with pharmacist to determine the most appropriate form of prescribed medications; thoroughly flush tube before and after administration of any medications.	Administration of pulverized medications is a common cause of tube occlusion; when possible, elixir or parenteral medications should be substituted for tablets that require crushing, and tablets should *never* be crushed without a pharmacist's approval.
	Use warm water to flush obstructed tubes.	Warm water has proved as effective as carbonated drinks in restoring tube patency.
	Notify physician if tube becomes occluded.	Occluded tubes must be removed and replaced.
Alteration in skin integrity related to tract erosion and subsequent peritubular leakage	Stabilize abdominal tubes to prevent lateral and "in-out" tube migration (*Note:* Tubes can be stabilized at skin level with commercial devices or with a baby nipple and barrier wafer, as shown on p. 290).	Lateral or "in-out" tube movements may result in tract erosion, a common cause of peritubular leakage.
	Protect peritubular skin with a pectin-based barrier cut to fit around the tube; if skin is denuded, treat raw area with light coat of pectin-based powder (e.g., Stomahesive) and blot over powder with skin sealant (e.g., Skin Prep) or water before applying barrier wafer.	A pectin-based barrier wafer is resistant to intestinal drainage; pectin-based powder absorbs drainage and forms a protective coating over the denuded area.
	Apply pouching system for persistent or severe leakage, as shown on p. 290.	A pouching system contains the drainage and protects the peritubular skin.
Fluid volume deficit related to hyperglycemia and resulting serum hyperosmolarity or to tube-feeding syndrome	Monitor patient for hyperglycemia (i.e., via serum studies or urine checks) during initiation of feedings.	Hyperglycemia may occur during initiation of enteral feedings containing significant carbohydrate loads.

NURSING DIAGNOSIS	NURSING INTERVENTIONS	RATIONALE
	Reduce the carbohydrate concentration of the feeding and gradually advance (for patient with hyperglycemia).	Reducing the carbohydrate concentration usually corrects the hyperglycemia; gradual advancement of the carbohydrate concentration permits the pancreas to adapt to the increased demand for insulin.
	Administer insulin as ordered for patient with persistent hyperglycemia.	Insulin promotes glucose utilization and prevents hyperglycemia.
	Monitor hyperglycemic patient for signs and symptoms of fluid volume deficit (output exceeding intake, dry mucous membranes, oliguria, postural hypotension, weakness, tachycardia, reduced skin turgor).	Hyperglycemia increases serum osmolarity, which causes fluid to shift from the intracellular compartment into the plasma, where it is subsequently lost in the urine in the process of glucose elimination; the end result is fluid volume deficit.
	Administer enteral or IV fluids and electrolytes as ordered.	Replacement of fluids and electrolytes is essential to maintain plasma volume and tissue perfusion.
	Ensure an adequate fluid intake for patients receiving high-protein hyperosmolar formulas (i.e., at least 30 ml/kg body weight per day); if the patient is unable to ingest sufficient fluids orally, fluids should be administered enterally.	High-protein, hyperosmolar formulas require adequate fluid intake to prevent fluid volume deficit, hypernatremia, hyperchloremia, and azotemia (tube-feeding syndrome).

PATIENT TEACHING

1. Explain the purpose of enteral feedings and the importance of positive nutritional status.
2. Describe the options for delivery of enteral feedings (i.e., nasally placed tubes or abdominally placed tubes), and explain the option that is being recommended and why. (For example, explain that nasally placed tubes usually are preferred for short-term support because they are simpler to insert, *or* explain that abdominal tubes usually are better for long-term use because there is less risk of aspiration and damage to the esophagus.)
3. Explain the intubation or insertion procedure, including any preprocedural and postprocedural care. Explain that feedings will be initiated once placement has been confirmed and gastrointestinal activity has returned to normal.
4. For a patient with a small-bore or enteral tube: Explain the rationale for using a pump device (if applicable).
5. Explain measures used to prevent complications (e.g., verifying the position of the tube before feedings are administered, elevating the head of the bed during feedings, and delaying feeding if significant residual or signs of poor tolerance, such as nausea, distention, or absent bowel sounds, develop).
6. For patients with abdominal tubes: Explain the importance of stabilizing the tube, and describe ways this is achieved.
7. For a patient who is discharged home with enteral feedings: Teach the caregiver how to check tube placement and gastric residual, how to administer feedings (including pump function if applicable) and medications, how and when to flush the tube, how to recognize and manage tube occlusion, and how to care for the equipment used for feedings. Stress the importance of aseptic technique in handling the formula and equipment. Have the caregiver return all demonstrations, and be sure he or she understands the potential complications and preventive measures. Collaborate with the physician to ensure home health care follow-up for a patient who is discharged with enteral feedings.

Parenteral Nutritional Support

Parenteral nutritional support involves intravenous administration of nutrient solutions; parenteral support is indicated for patients whose nutrient needs cannot be met by oral or enteral feedings. There are two approaches to parenteral nutritional support: use of peripheral veins (peripheral parenteral support) and use of large "central" veins such as the subclavian vein (total parenteral nutrition, or TPN). Each approach has advantages and disadvantages.

Peripheral parenteral nutrition involves the use of large peripheral veins for administering nutrients. This approach has several advantages: peripheral veins are more easily accessed, and peripheral parenteral support is associated with a much lower rate of infection and catheter-related complications. However, administration of hyperosmolar solutions via peripheral veins results in a significant incidence of phlebitis and thrombosis, due to the lower flow rates in these veins. In addition, peripheral veins do not provide secure venous access; they are prone to infiltration. Therefore, peripheral parenteral support usually is used as a supplement for patients who are consuming some nutrients orally; amino acid solutions can be given to supplement protein intake, and lipid emulsions can be used to provide calories. Peripheral parenteral nutrition can also be used to provide total nutritional support on a very short-term basis; in this case, protein needs are met through amino acid solutions, and caloric needs are met through lipid emulsions and 10% dextrose solutions.

Long-term administration of total parenteral nutrition requires a large central vein, such as the subclavian. TPN solutions commonly contain 25% to 35% dextrose in addition to amino acids, vitamins, minerals, trace elements, and electrolytes. The high flow rates in central veins provide immediate dilution of these hypertonic solutions, which prevents the phlebitis and thrombosis associated with administration of these formulas through peripheral veins. Central veins also provide secure venous access, which is essential for long-term support. However, total parenteral nutrition via central venous line is a complex therapy associated with a number of serious complications. If the patient does not already have a central line in place, a surgical procedure is required to establish central venous access; complications of the insertion procedure include pneumothorax and hemothorax. There is also a significant risk of catheter-related sepsis; the amino acid–dextrose solution is a potential growth medium for yeast organisms, and bacteria thrive in lipid solutions. Therefore

scrupulous technique is essential in providing catheter care and in administering the prescribed solutions. Additional complications include central vein thrombosis, catheter occlusion, air embolism, and metabolic complications (e.g., hyperglycemia and hypoglycemia). Hepatic dysfunction, characterized by elevated liver function tests and varying degrees of fat infiltration, has been a serious complication in children; it occurs in adults also but is more likely to be benign and reversible. The mechanism whereby total parenteral nutrition causes hepatic dysfunction is thought to be the delivery of excess glucose, which is converted to intrahepatic fat. Measures that can be used to reduce hepatic dysfunction include avoiding excess glucose, providing nonglucose calories (e.g., lipids), ensuring a calorie-to-protein ratio no higher than 200:1, and incorporating a glucose-free infusion into the daily infusion cycle.

Parenteral nutritional support must be closely monitored by the nutritional support team; modifications in prescribed formulas and administration rates are based on the patient's response to therapy. Meticulous management is critical in preventing complications.

INDICATIONS

Small bowel disease precluding use of the enteral route for feeding or necessitating bowel rest (e.g., multiple small bowel fistulae or fistula located in mid-small bowel; severe inflammatory conditions; short bowel syndrome; severe malabsorption syndromes; prolonged ileus)

Severe pancreatitis

Hypermetabolic states in which nutrient intake via the oral or enteral route is insufficient to meet nutrient needs (e.g., burns, multiple trauma, or sepsis)

Severe hypoproteinemia resulting in severe bowel wall edema and inability to absorb enteral nutrients

High-dose chemotherapy and radiation therapy (e.g., before bone marrow transplantation) resulting in inability to ingest or absorb enteral nutrients

CONTRAINDICATIONS

Terminal illnesses (when death is imminent or patient and family do not desire nutritional support)

Inability to establish or maintain venous access

Short-term loss of nutrient intake in well-nourished patient (e.g., patient who will be able to resume oral intake in 5 to 7 days)

Patient with a functional small bowel who can be maintained on enteral feedings

COMPLICATIONS

Insertion procedure
  Pneumothorax
  Hemothorax
Catheter related
  Sepsis
  Air embolism
  Catheter occlusion
  Catheter breakage
  Central venous thrombosis

Metabolic
  Hyperglycemia
  Hypoglycemia
  Hepatic dysfunction
  Azotemia

PREPROCEDURAL NURSING CARE

NURSING DIAGNOSIS	NURSING INTERVENTIONS	RATIONALE
Knowledge deficit related to parenteral nutritional support and establishment of venous access	Explain rationale for parenteral nutritional support and procedure for establishing venous access (i.e., peripheral venipuncture or insertion of central venous catheter); for patient undergoing central venous catheter insertion, stress the importance of following positioning and breathing instructions to prevent lung injury.	The patient and family are critical members of the health care team and must be informed of treatment options and rationale; an informed, cooperative patient is less likely to sustain pleural injury from sudden movements or erratic breathing.
High risk for infection related to venipuncture or insertion of central venous line	Prepare site for venipuncture or central venous line insertion with antiseptic solution (e.g., Betadine or Hibiclens).	Skin antiseptics reduce bacterial counts and thus reduce the risk of infection.
	Maintain strict sterile technique (gowns, masks, gloves) during insertion of central venous catheter.	Strict adherence to sterile technique prevents introduction of pathogens.

POSTPROCEDURAL NURSING CARE

NURSING DIAGNOSIS	NURSING INTERVENTIONS	RATIONALE
High risk for infection related to central venous catheter and administration of TPN	Maintain strict aseptic technique when handling or hanging solutions or manipulating tubing.	Strict aseptic technique prevents introduction of pathogens.
	Maintain dry occlusive dressing (i.e., dry gauze and occlusive tape or transparent adhesive dressing with high moisture vapor transmission rate); change dressing immediately for known or suspected contamination.	Dry occlusive dressing reduces the risk of bacterial invasion.

→ > >

NURSING DIAGNOSIS	NURSING INTERVENTIONS	RATIONALE
	Change dressing over central venous catheter according to institutional protocol using strict sterile technique (usually three times weekly). *Note:* Protocol should include application of a skin antiseptic (e.g., Betadine or alcohol).	Routine changes permit cleansing and inspection of insertion site and promote maintenance of a bacterial barrier; strict sterile technique prevents introduction of pathogens. Antiseptics inhibit bacterial proliferation.
	Limit "hang time" for solutions to no more than 24 h.	Limiting hang time reduces the potential for bacterial proliferation (dextrose–amino acids support growth of yeast organisms; lipids support bacterial growth).
	Avoid using central line for other therapies if at all possible (e.g., administration of blood, IV fluids, and medications; attachment of monitoring devices; drawing blood); if a multilumen central venous catheter is used, use scrupulous technique whenever manipulating or accessing the catheter.	Multiple-use lines are more vulnerable to bacterial contamination.
	Monitor patient for local or systemic signs of infection (erythema, tenderness, and drainage at insertion site; edema of neck, shoulder, and arm on side corresponding to catheter placement; fever and chills).	Prompt recognition of infection permits early intervention.
	For suspected infection or thrombosis: remove catheter and administer antibiotics and anticoagulants as ordered.	Removing the catheter eliminates the source of infection or inflammation; antibiotics reduce bacterial proliferation and help eliminate infection; anticoagulants reduce clot formation and sludging in the damaged vessel.
Ineffective breathing pattern related to pneumothorax or air embolism	Observe patient for evidence of pneumothorax after insertion of central venous catheter (chest pain, dyspnea, hypotension, anxiety).	Pneumothorax may result from pleural injury during insertion of central venous line; prompt recognition permits early intervention.
	Notify physician of suspected pneumothorax; monitor patient's vital signs; assist with needle aspiration of air or insertion of chest tube.	Significant pneumothorax usually requires insertion of a chest tube to reexpand the lung.
	Secure all tubing connections in air-tight manner.	Secure connections prevent entry of air and reduce the risk of air embolism.
	Consider use of a 0.22-micrometer filter to administer dextrose–amino acid solutions.	A 0.22-micrometer filter traps any in-line air.
	Instruct patient in performance of Valsalva maneuver during tubing changes, *or* change tubing at end of expiration for patient on a ventilator.	The Valsalva maneuver increases intrathoracic pressure and prevents entry of air during tubing changes (expiration also increases intrathoracic pressure).

NURSING DIAGNOSIS	NURSING INTERVENTIONS	RATIONALE
	Maintain occlusive dressing over insertion site for at least 24 h after removal of catheter.	An occlusive dressing prevents air from entering.
	Monitor patient for signs of air embolism (dyspnea, cyanosis, tachycardia, hypotension, apnea).	Prompt recognition permits early intervention.
	For suspected air embolism: immediately place patient in left lateral Trendelenburg position; notify physician; administer oxygen and CPR as indicated.	This position traps air in the apex of the right ventricle and away from the outflow tract; emergency aspiration may be required to remove air from the heart.
Fluid volume deficit related to hyperglycemia and resulting serum hyperosmolarity	Gradually advance drip rate of concentrated dextrose solutions *or* administer lesser dextrose concentrations (10% dextrose) before beginning administration of concentrated dextrose solutions.	Gradual advancement of carbohydrate load permits pancreas to adapt to increased demand for insulin and reduces the risk of hyperglycemia.
	Monitor serum glucose levels at least daily when initiating concentrated dextrose solutions and until glucose levels normalize, then two to three times per week.	Prompt recognition of hyperglycemia permits early intervention; hyperglycemia is most likely to occur during initiation of therapy.
	Use an infusion pump to ensure consistent delivery of solution at prescribed rate.	Infusion pumps or monitors prevent erratic delivery of solution (sudden administration of large volumes of concentrated dextrose can cause hyperglycemia).
	Administer insulin (or add insulin to solution) as ordered for patient with persistent hyperglycemia.	Insulin promotes cellular uptake of glucose, which prevents hyperglycemia.
	Monitor hyperglycemic patient for signs and symptoms of fluid volume deficit (output exceeding intake, dry mucous membranes, oliguria, postural hypotension, reduced skin turgor, weakness, tachycardia).	Hyperglycemia increases serum osmolarity, which causes fluid to shift from the intracellular compartment into the plasma, where it is subsequently lost in the urine in the process of glucose elimination; the end result is fluid volume deficit.
	Administer additional fluids and electrolytes as ordered.	Replacement of fluids and electrolytes is essential for maintaining plasma volume and tissue perfusion.
Altered protection related to hypoglycemia and resulting alteration in mental acuity	Use an infusion pump or monitor to ensure continuous administration of solution at prescribed rate.	Infusion pumps and monitors prevent erratic delivery of solution; a sudden reduction in flow rate could cause hypoglycemia.
	Wean patient from concentrated dextrose solutions by gradually slowing the rate *or* by administering a lesser concentration of dextrose (e.g., 10%) before discontinuing.	Sudden discontinuation of concentrated dextrose solutions causes an imbalance between pancreatic insulin production and available glucose.

→ ❭ ❭

NURSING DIAGNOSIS	NURSING INTERVENTIONS	RATIONALE
	Monitor patient for signs and symptoms of hypoglycemia (diaphoresis, tachycardia, confusion, tremors, anxiety, altered LOC).	Prompt recognition of hypoglycemia permits early intervention.
	Administer oral or IV glucose to patient with suspected or proven hypoglycemia.	Prompt administration of glucose corrects hypoglycemia.
Altered nutrition: less than body requirements related to catheter occlusion	Use an infusion pump or monitor to ensure constant delivery of solutions at ordered rate.	Infusion pumps and monitors provide continuous infusion and thus prevent occlusion of catheter.
	Flush catheter with heparinized solution whenever infusion is temporarily discontinued or interrupted.	Thorough flushing with heparinized solution prevents clot formation in catheter lumen.
	Attempt to aspirate line if catheter becomes occluded; do not irrigate.	Aspiration may permit safe removal of clotted blood; irrigation is contraindicated because it could force a clot into the bloodstream and cause an embolism.
	Notify physician of occluded catheter, and instill streptokinase or urokinase into catheter as ordered (or assist with instillation).	Streptokinase and urokinase are thrombolytic agents that may restore patency.

1. Explain the purpose of parenteral nutritional support and the importance of positive nutritional status.
2. Explain the procedure for establishing venous access (if applicable); for the patient undergoing central venous catheter placement, stress the importance of cooperating with positioning and breathing instructions to prevent inadvertent injury to the lungs.
3. For the patient receiving concentrated dextrose–amino acid solutions as a component of a total parenteral nutrition program: Explain the purpose of gradually advancing the rate of administration, and explain the importance of monitoring serum glucose levels. If hyperglycemia occurs, explain the physiologic basis and the rationale for administering insulin. (For the patient who was previously normoglycemic, explain that the development of hyperglycemia during initiation of therapy does not mean that the patient has developed diabetes mellitus.)
4. Teach the patient how to hold her breath and "bear down" (Valsalva maneuver) during tubing changes, and explain the rationale for this maneuver. Explain that the tubing connections are tight, that the in-line filter will remove any small air bubbles, that air embolism is not common, and that the entry of air during tubing changes can be prevented by the Valsalva maneuver.
5. Explain the purpose of the infusion monitor or pump, and describe the various safety alarms; explain that the alarm alerts the nurse to provide needed care and does not indicate an emergency.
6. Explain the importance of strict technique in hanging solutions, changing or manipulating tubing, and providing catheter care. Instruct the patient to notify the nurse of any discomfort at the insertion site or any contamination of the catheter dressing.
7. For a patient who is discharged home with total parenteral nutrition: Teach the caregiver how to hang solutions, how to operate the infusion pump or monitor, how to change the catheter dressing and provide site care, how to flush and cap the infusion catheter (if the patient is receiving cyclic therapy), and how to handle potential complications (e.g., catheter obstruction or breakage). Instruct the patient and caregiver in the signs and symptoms that should be reported to a physician or nurse. Stress the importance of strict sterile technique in catheter site care and strict aseptic technique in hanging solutions. Have the caregiver return all demonstrations, and ensure that he or she understands potential complications and preventive measures. Work with the physician, discharge planner, and home infusion company to ensure home health care follow-up and access to supplies after discharge.

CHAPTER 9

Surgical Procedures

Abdominal Surgery

The routine care required by any patient undergoing abdominal surgery is outlined in the general care plan for abdominal surgery. Specific care requirements are addressed in the care plans for the particular procedures.

COMPLICATIONS

Atelectasis and pneumonia	Wound infection
Adynamic ileus	Bleeding and hemorrhage
Small bowel obstruction	Urinary retention
Thrombophlebitis and deep vein thrombosis	

PREPROCEDURAL NURSING CARE

NURSING DIAGNOSIS	NURSING INTERVENTIONS	RATIONALE
Anxiety related to surgery and anesthesia	Encourage patient to express concerns and feelings about anesthesia and surgery.	Ventilation provides emotional relief and is the first step in dealing with feelings and concerns.
	Provide information as patient and family demonstrate readiness for learning (e.g., postoperative pain management).	Understanding what is to be done and the care routines reduces fear of the unknown.
	Administer preoperative sedation.	Preoperative sedation helps reduce anxiety and promotes rest.
High risk for infection related to abdominal incision	Complete skin preparation as ordered (e.g., antiseptic showers or scrubs).	Showering or scrubbing with skin antiseptics reduces bacteria on the skin.

Patient teaching regarding planned procedure is essential for informed consent. See Patient Teaching section for Abdominal Surgery, p. 307.

POSTPROCEDURAL NURSING CARE

NURSING DIAGNOSIS	NURSING INTERVENTIONS	RATIONALE
High risk for ineffective airway clearance related to anesthesia, inactivity, and incisional pain limiting inspiratory effort	Monitor patient for signs and symptoms of atelectasis (tachycardia, tachypnea, fever, rales, or diminished breath sounds).	Prompt detection of pulmonary compromise permits early intervention.
	Administer pain medication as ordered and indicated (or instruct patient in use of patient-controlled analgesia).	Analgesics reduce incisional pain, which reduces splinting and improves inspiratory depth and volume.
	Help patient with deep-breathing exercises at least q 2 h.	Deep-breathing exercises increase lung expansion and help prevent atelectasis.
	Help patient to cough as needed; splint incision when coughing.	Coughing clears the airways of mucus and supports deep breathing; incisional splinting reduces pain and improves cough effort.
	Reposition patient at least q 2 h until patient can reposition self.	Frequent position changes maintain ventilatory function in all lung fields.
	Collaborate with physician and respiratory therapist to provide additional respiratory support for patients with signs and symptoms of atelectasis (or patients who are at high risk for pneumonia, such as those who smoke).	Aggressive pulmonary toilet (e.g., intermittent positive-pressure breathing treatments) promotes lung expansion and helps prevent pneumonia.
Pain related to abdominal incision and sore throat (secondary to endotracheal intubation or oxygen administration or both)	Monitor patient for location and severity of pain and effectiveness of analgesics.	Continual assessment of pain and response to analgesics guides appropriate intervention.
	Administer analgesics as ordered and needed (or instruct patient in patient-controlled analgesia).	Analgesics reduce incisional pain and increase patient's comfort.
	Use nursing measures to reduce discomfort (e.g., positioning and oral care).	General comfort measures reduce pain and the need for analgesics.
High risk for infection related to abdominal incision or intraabdominal contamination	Monitor patient for signs and symptoms of incisional or intraabdominal infection (fever, incisional erythema and tenderness, purulent drainage from incision, increasing abdominal tenderness and pain).	Prompt detection of infection permits early intervention.
	Use strict aseptic technique for incisional care.	Aseptic technique prevents introduction of pathogens.
	Administer antibiotics as ordered.	Antibiotics kill bacteria and help control infection.
	Notify physician of signs and symptoms of infection; prepare patient for possible incisional drainage or placement of abdominal drain under radiologic or CT guidance.	Effective treatment of infection requires adequate drainage of purulent material or abscess cavities.

NURSING DIAGNOSIS	NURSING INTERVENTIONS	RATIONALE
High risk for urinary retention related to intraoperative bladder distention or sympathetic stimulation	Monitor patient for evidence of urinary retention: inability to void, frequent voiding of small amounts (measure all voids until bladder function and fluid balance are normal), bladder distention, sensation of incomplete emptying.	Urinary retention may occur as a result of (1) overdistention of the bladder during surgery, which causes temporary loss of tone in the bladder; (2) sympathetic stimulation, which increases tone in the bladder neck and inhibits voiding; or (3) the effects of regional anesthesia.
	Catheterize patient as indicated and ordered; explain that difficulty voiding is a temporary problem that usually resolves spontaneously and that catheterization prevents further complications.	Catheterization prevents further bladder distention and loss of tone and also eliminates urinary stasis, which reduces the risk of urinary tract infection; retention usually resolves in less than 48 hours.
Potential alteration in tissue perfusion (renal, cerebral, cardiopulmonary, gastrointestinal, peripheral) related to postoperative hemorrhage or to pulmonary embolus resulting from thrombophlebitis or deep vein thrombosis	Monitor patient for signs and symptoms of hypovolemia (tachycardia, tachypnea, hypotension, oliguria, diaphoresis, anxiety) and for indications of intraabdominal or incisional bleeding (increasing abdominal girth, large volume of bloody output from surgical drains, incisional bleeding).	Prompt detection of complications permits early intervention.
	Administer IV fluids and blood replacement as ordered; observe for transfusion reactions if blood is given.	IV fluids are administered to maintain plasma volume; blood may be required for replacement of RBCs and platelets during episodes of massive bleeding.
	If patient fails to respond to above measures, prepare for emergency surgery.	Surgery may be needed to control bleeding.
	Institute measures to prevent thrombophlebitis and deep vein thrombosis: leg exercises (extension and flexion) at least q 2 h and assisted ambulation at least two to three times daily until patient can ambulate independently.	Routine flexion and extension of the feet and legs promotes venous return and reduces venous stasis.
	Implement compression therapy as ordered (elastic bandages or elastic antiembolism stockings for the legs or sequential compression therapy device); if stockings or elastic wraps are used, remove daily and inspect legs and feet.	Compression of the superficial veins increases blood flow into the deep veins and back to the heart; increased blood flow reduces venous stasis, which reduces platelet aggregation and clot formation.
	Administer anticoagulant medications (e.g., heparin) as ordered; monitor patient for evidence of bleeding (e.g., hematuria, epistaxis).	Anticoagulant medications reduce platelet aggregation and help prevent clot formation; bleeding indicates excessive anticoagulation and the need to reduce the dosage.
	Monitor patient for signs and symptoms of deep vein thrombosis or thrombophlebitis (prominent distended veins; calf or thigh tenderness and pain on dorsiflexion; edema in affected leg; increased warmth in affected leg).	Prompt detection of complications permits early intervention, which is essential for preventing pulmonary embolus.

→ ❯ ❯ ❯

NURSING DIAGNOSIS	NURSING INTERVENTIONS	RATIONALE
	For patient with clinical indicators of deep vein thrombosis or thrombophlebitis: place patient on bed rest with legs elevated, and discontinue compression therapy and leg exercises.	Ambulation and compression therapy are contraindicated, because increasing the volume of blood flow through the veins may disrupt the thrombus and cause emboli.
	Monitor patient for signs and symptoms of pulmonary emboli (sudden onset of chest pain and dyspnea, tachypnea, tachycardia, hypotension, bloody sputum).	Prompt detection of serious complications permits early intervention.
	For patient with clinical indicators of pulmonary embolus: initiate emergency measures as ordered to include oxygen.	Pulmonary emboli alter $\dot{V}/\dot{Q}$, producing hypoxemia.
High risk for constipation related to postoperative ileus	Monitor patient for evidence of peristaltic activity (audible bowel sounds, passage of flatus, bowel movements).	Ileus is a common complication of abdominal surgery, resulting from the inhibiting effects of bowel manipulation and narcotic analgesics on bowel motility.
	Implement measures to increase activity (repositioning, in-bed exercises, assisted ambulation) until patient can ambulate independently.	Physical activity increases the electrical and motor activity in the bowel, increasing peristalsis.
	Keep patient NPO or limit oral intake to sips of clear liquids (as ordered) until peristalsis resumes.	Oral intake stimulates intestinal secretions; in the absence of peristalsis, the increased volume of intraluminal fluids may cause distention, nausea, and vomiting.
	If applicable (patient with N/G tube placed intraoperatively): monitor function of N/G tube and irrigate tube q 2 h and prn to maintain patency.	N/G tube patency must be maintained to prevent accumulation of intestinal fluids, distention, nausea, and vomiting.
	For patient with severe distention or persistent nausea: place N/G tube as ordered (or assist with placement); irrigate tube q 2 h and prn to maintain patency.	Decompression of the stomach and proximal small bowel may be required to control distention, nausea, and vomiting.
Potential fluid volume deficit related to vomiting, nasogastric suction, or reduced fluid intake	Monitor patient's intake and output (including emesis and N/G aspirate).	Output exceeding intake may indicate fluid volume deficit.
	Monitor patient for signs of hypovolemia or electrolyte imbalance (dry mucous membranes, oliguria, hypotension, reduced skin turgor, extreme weakness, confusion).	Prompt recognition of fluid-electrolyte imbalance permits early intervention.
	Provide IV fluid and electrolyte replacement as ordered.	Maintaining fluid volume and electrolyte balance is essential for normal tissue perfusion and neuromuscular function.

PATIENT TEACHING

1. Explain the surgical procedure, its purpose, and any impact it may have on digestive tract functioning.
2. Advise the patient to avoid strenuous activity and lifting until the abdominal muscles have healed (usually about 2 to 3 months after surgery); he may then begin exercises to strengthen abdominal muscles.
3. Teach the patient how to care for his incision (if applicable): keep incision clean and dry until sutures or staples are removed; report signs of infection (i.e., redness, swelling, or pain around incision; purulent drainage from incision) to physician.
4. Explain the purpose, dosage, schedule, and side effects of any prescribed medications.
5. Teach the patient the signs and symptoms to report to the physician (increasing abdominal pain and swelling, persistent nausea and vomiting, fever, and signs of incisional infection).

Gastrectomy (Partial or Total)

Gastrectomy may be required to control inflammatory processes such as peptic ulcer disease or to remove or palliate gastric malignancies.

Gastrectomy may be partial or total; inflammatory processes usually can be managed by partial gastrectomy, whereas malignancies may require total gastrectomy. The Billroth I and Billroth II procedures are the two most common approaches to reanastomosis between the gastric remnant and the small bowel following partial gastrectomy. Partial gastrectomy frequently is performed in conjunction with a vagotomy, which may in turn require pyloroplasty to prevent obstruction of the gastric outlet.

Partial gastrectomy is most appropriately performed for lesions or processes confined to the distal or proximal regions of the stomach. Peptic ulcer disease is the most common indication for partial gastrectomy; in these patients, removal of the distal stomach reduces the parietal cell mass, which reduces the stimulus for secretion of hydrochloric acid (HCl) and thus helps prevent recurrent ulceration. It may also be possible to resect the ulcer itself; resection is advantageous, because ulcers tend to recur in the same location. Gastric ulcers are more amenable to resection than duodenal ulcers, because duodenal ulcers are adjacent to many vital structures, which may be damaged in the resection. Partial gastrectomy is also appropriate for patients with gastric tumors in the distal or proximal stomach. Tumors in the midstomach require total gastrectomy for adequate surgical clearance.

Partial gastrectomy usually involves removal of the distal 50% to 60% of the stomach, leaving about a 40% gastric remnant. Anastomosis of the gastric remnant to the distal small bowel may be accomplished by either a Billroth I or a Billroth II procedure; factors determining the anastomotic approach include the extent of the gastric resection, the viability of the gastric remnant (stump), and the amount of tension produced by an end-to-end anastomosis.

The Billroth I procedure is the procedure of choice for gastric ulcers proven to be benign; it may also be used to manage duodenal ulcers (in combination with vagotomy), erosive gastritis, trauma, or benign tumors involving the distal stomach. In a Billroth I procedure, the distal stomach is removed and the gastric remnant is anastomosed directly to the duodenum. To accomplish this, the surgeon creates three lines of resection: a vertical incision across the body of the stomach, a shorter, "angled" incision from the greater curvature to the vertical incision, and a duodenal incision. The vertical incision is closed to form the new "lesser curvature," and the angled incision forms the gastric outlet, which is anastomosed to the duodenal stump (see figure on p. 308). (The specific placement of the gastric lines of resection is determined in part by the location of the ulcer to be excised.)

A Billroth II procedure may be required for duodenal or combined gastric and duodenal ulcers, for early gastric cancer or distal gastric cancers with negative lymph nodes, for trauma to the distal stomach and duodenum, or for bleeding erosive gastritis. A Billroth II procedure is also preferred when a Billroth I anastomosis cannot be constructed without tension on the suture line or when the viability of the gastric remnant and duodenal stump is questionable. In a Billroth

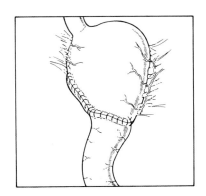

Billroth I operation; completed anastomosis.

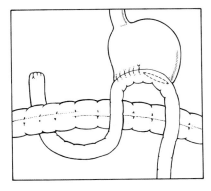

Billroth II operation.

controlled emptying, many patients can resume fairly normal eating habits within a few months.

Vagotomy involves surgical interruption of the gastric vagal nerve fibers, which are the parasympathetic nerves that stimulate gastric secretion and also mediate gastric motility. Vagotomy may be performed alone or in conjunction with partial gastrectomy to promote healing and prevent recurrence of duodenal ulcers, which are caused primarily by gastric hyperacidity. Vagotomy may be "truncal," "selective," or "highly selective." Truncal vagotomy involves removal of sections from the anterior and posterior vagal trunks, resulting in complete denervation of the stomach; innervation to the gallbladder is also lost, and an increased incidence of cholelithiasis is now a recognized complication. Selective vagotomy spares the vagal fibers innervating the gallbladder but results in complete denervation of the stomach. Since the vagus nerve mediates gastric motility as well as secretion, both truncal vagotomy and selective vagotomy must be accompanied by a pyloroplasty to enlarge the gastric outlet and maintain gastric emptying. Highly selective vagotomy is the surgical interruption of vagal fibers to the gastric antrum with preservation of the fibers innervating the pyloric region; acid production is effectively reduced, and gastric motility is maintained, which obviates the need for pyloroplasty. This is now the procedure of choice when vagotomy is indicated.

INDICATIONS

Gastric ulcer (usually partial gastrectomy with Billroth I anastomosis)

Duodenal ulcer or combined gastric and duodenal ulcers (highly selective vagotomy and vagotomy in conjunction with Billroth I anastomosis are the most common procedures)

Gastric cancer (usually total gastrectomy)

Benign gastric tumors (partial gastrectomy, usually Billroth I anastomosis)

Bleeding erosive gastritis (vagotomy with partial gastrectomy; may be Billroth I or Billroth II anastomosis, depending on extent of resection)

Gastric trauma (usually partial gastrectomy)

CONTRAINDICATIONS

Billroth I procedure is contraindicated with proximal or distal gastric cancer

COMPLICATIONS (EARLY)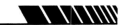

Anastomotic breakdown, resulting in intraabdominal abscess and possibly sepsis

Necrosis of gastric remnant

Obstruction of gastroduodenal or gastrojejunal suture line (secondary to edema, intraabdominal

II procedure, the distal stomach and possibly the proximal duodenum are resected; the open duodenal stump is sutured closed, and the gastric remnant is anastomosed to the jejunum with an end-to-side or side-to-side anastomosis. Billroth II procedures have been associated with significant long-term complications related to loss of controlled gastric emptying and loss of duodenal absorption of minerals; these complications include "dumping," vomiting, diarrhea, iron-deficiency anemia, and osteoporosis. Therefore this procedure usually is carried out only as a last resort.

Total gastrectomy is most commonly performed for cancer of the stomach. A radical dissection usually is required, involving removal of the entire stomach, distal esophagus, and a proximal duodenal "cuff"; depending on the location of the tumor, it may also involve removal of the spleen, the body and tail of the pancreas, the greater and lesser omenta, and the gastric lymph nodes. Reconstruction of the gastrointestinal tract most commonly involves a "Roux-en-Y" esophagojejunostomy. In this approach, the duodenal stump is closed and the bowel is divided at the level of the proximal jejunum. The distal jejunal stump is closed, and the esophagus is anastomosed to this segment of jejunum by means of an end-to-side anastomosis. The end of the proximal jejunal loop is then connected to the side of the distal jejunal segment. Ideally the jejunojejunal anastomosis is constructed about 40 cm distal to the esophagojejunal anastomosis, because this length of intervening bowel prevents biliary reflux into the esophagus. This surgical procedure yields satisfactory results in most cases; despite loss of the gastric reservoir with

inflammation, or adhesions)

Pancreatitis (secondary to intraoperative trauma)

Injury to common bile duct (secondary to intraoperative trauma)

Obstruction of afferent jejunal limb (Billroth II procedure or total gastrectomy)

Jejunal loop herniation (Billroth II procedure)

COMPLICATIONS *(LATE)*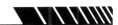

Alkaline reflux gastritis with/without esophagitis

Dumping syndrome (immediate postprandial response and late hypoglycemic response)

Postvagotomy diarrhea (most common with truncal vagotomy)

Malabsorption

Bezoar formation

Delayed gastric emptying (truncal vagotomy or selective vagotomy without pyloroplasty)

Carcinoma of gastric remnant

Recurrent ulceration

Chronic afferent loop obstruction (Billroth II procedure or total gastrectomy)

Chronic efferent loop obstruction (Billroth II procedure)

Internal hernia (herniation of afferent or efferent loop through defects in mesentery, causing obstruction and possible ischemia)

PREPROCEDURAL NURSING CARE

See Preprocedural Nursing Care under Abdominal Surgery, p. 303.

POSTPROCEDURAL NURSING CARE

NURSING DIAGNOSIS	NURSING INTERVENTIONS	RATIONALE
Altered renal, cerebral, cardiopulmonary, gastrointestinal, and peripheral tissue perfusion related to intraabdominal infection and septic shock	Monitor patient for signs and symptoms of anastomotic breakdown, gastric remnant necrosis, jejunal loop herniation, pancreatitis, intraabdominal abscess, and sepsis (increasing abdominal tenderness and distention, tachycardia, tachypnea, fever, hypotension, drainage of gastric fluid through sump or Penrose drain).	Prompt detection of complications permits early intervention.
	Monitor patient for increasing abdominal distention; insert N/G tube as ordered (or assist with placement); irrigate tube prn to maintain patency.	Gastric decompression prevents tension on the suture lines and helps prevent anastomotic breakdown.
	Administer antibiotics as ordered.	Antibiotics reduce bacterial proliferation and help control infection.
	Administer IV fluids as ordered.	Fluid balance must be maintained to provide adequate tissue perfusion.
	Monitor patient's hemodynamic status (Swan-Ganz or CVP readings, urine output, BP, and pulse).	Continual monitoring provides data that guide modification of the treatment plan.
	If patient fails to respond to above measures, prepare her for surgery.	Immediate surgical intervention may be needed for anastomotic repair, resection of gangrenous bowel, or drainage of intraabdominal abscess.

NURSING DIAGNOSIS	NURSING INTERVENTIONS	RATIONALE
Altered nutrition: less than body requirements, related to dumping syndrome (early postprandial symptoms or late reactive hypoglycemia)	Initiate oral feedings (when ordered and tolerated) with small, frequent feedings.	Small feedings at frequent intervals produce less distention of the gastric remnant and are better tolerated.
	For patient with signs of postprandial dumping syndrome (sweating, weakness, nausea, vomiting, diarrhea): provide frequent, small feedings low in carbohydrates and high in fats and proteins.	Loss of the pylorus results in rapid gastric emptying; liquids and carbohydrates are associated with more rapid gastric emptying, whereas proteins and fats retard gastric emptying.
	For patient with postprandial dumping: administer medications as ordered (e.g., Sandostatin and anticholinergic drugs).	Sandostatin relieves dumping symptoms by altering intestinal motility and reducing the hormonal response to gastric distention; anticholinergics reduce intestinal motility.
	For patient with reactive hypoglycemia: provide high-protein, low-carbohydrate meals, and administer foods containing glucose between meals.	Reactive hypoglycemia occurs because "dumping" causes hyperglycemia, which stimulates increased production of insulin; low-carbohydrate meals reduce dumping and hyperglycemia. Glucose between meals helps prevent hypoglycemia.
	For patient with reactive hypoglycemia: administer insulin as ordered before meals.	Giving insulin before meals helps prevent hyperglycemia, which prevents overproduction of insulin.
	Monitor patient's nutrient intake, nutrient tolerance, and nutritional status (weight, general appearance, and laboratory data).	Continual assessment of nutritional intake and nutritional status provides the data needed to guide the treatment plan.
	Collaborate with dietitian, physician, and patient to develop an acceptable plan for nutritional support.	Nutritional status must be maintained to promote healing, prevent infection, and maintain health.
	For patient with total gastrectomy: instruct patient in essential nature of routine parenteral administration of vitamin B_{12}.	Total gastrectomy eliminates the sites for production of intrinsic factor, which is essential for absorption of vitamin B_{12}; a deficiency of this vitamin produces pernicious anemia.
Diarrhea related to gastric hypoacidity with resultant bacterial overgrowth and malabsorption and to rapid gastric emptying	Monitor frequency, volume, and consistency of stools.	Diarrhea is a major symptom of malabsorption and intestinal dysfunction; stool volume and consistency are indicators of intestinal function and nutrient absorption.
	Instruct patient to avoid liquids during meals.	Fluid intake enhances gastric emptying, which contributes to diarrhea.
	Administer antibiotics as ordered (e.g., neomycin or tetracycline).	Antibiotics inhibit bacterial proliferation, thus reducing malabsorption and diarrhea.
	Administer antidiarrheal medications as ordered (e.g., codeine, loperamide or diphenoxylate, cholestyramine).	Antidiarrheal medications reduce intestinal motility and thus help control diarrhea; cholestyramine binds with bile acids and reduces the diarrhea caused by bile acids in the colon.

NURSING DIAGNOSIS	NURSING INTERVENTIONS	RATIONALE
	Administer pectin- or psyllium-based preparations as ordered.	Bulking agents absorb water in the intestine and help prevent diarrhea.
	For patient with severe diarrhea unresponsive to above measures: discuss surgical options as indicated.	Severe diarrhea in patients with postvagotomy diarrhea usually can be treated effectively by surgically reversing a 10-12 cm segment of jejunum at a level 90-100 cm below the Treitz' ligament.

PATIENT TEACHING ■

1. For the patient with a partial or total gastrectomy: Explain the "anti-dumping" diet: small, frequent meals of low-carbohydrate, high-fat, and high-protein foods; liquids omitted during meals. Explain that dietary tolerance differs from one individual to another, and instruct the patient in gradual dietary advancement based on her ability to tolerate various foods.
2. For the patient with reactive hypoglycemia: Explain the rationale for a low-carbohydrate, high-protein diet; frequent small feedings; eating glucose-containing foods between meals. Teach patient the signs and symptoms of hypoglycemia and the appropriate response (ingestion of a rapidly absorbed carbohydrate followed by a complex carbohydrate or protein).
3. For the patient with a total gastrectomy: Explain the need for lifelong injections of vitamin B_{12}, the impact of vitamin B_{12} deficiency (i.e., pernicious anemia with potentially irreversible peripheral neuropathy), and early signs of vitamin B_{12} deficiency (fatigue, activity intolerance, and tingling and numbness in the hands and feet).
4. Instruct the patient to notify the physician of any complications (e.g., increasing abdominal pain or tenderness, fever, nausea and vomiting, persistent or worsening diarrhea, inability to tolerate foods and fluids, weight loss).

Colostomy

Colostomy is the surgical creation of an opening between the colon and the abdominal wall to provide fecal diversion. A colostomy can be constructed in any segment of the large intestine, but the transverse colon and the descending or sigmoid colon are the most common sites. Cecostomy occasionally is required for obstructing lesions in the ascending colon.

The location of the colostomy determines the consistency and volume of the output, which significantly affect management options. For example, the output from a cecostomy or ascending colostomy occurs throughout the day, usually is semifluid to mushy, and contains residual enzymes that are potentially damaging to the skin; these patients must wear a correctly sized pouch at all times and must pay particular attention to peristomal skin care. A transverse colostomy drains mushy stool at irregular intervals (usually after meals), but the stool usually does not contain enzymes; these patients must also wear a correctly sized pouch at all times, but they are less likely to develop peristomal skin breakdown. Output from a descending or sigmoid colostomy usually is soft to formed and has a frequency similar to the patient's preoperative bowel elimination patterns; these patients may be able to regulate their bowel elimination through routine colostomy irrigations. Patients who are not candidates for irrigation or do not wish to irrigate manage their stomas with a correctly sized pouch worn at all times. (The volume and consistency of the stool from *any* colostomy are affected by the length and function of the proximal bowel, by medications, and by dietary intake; these factors must

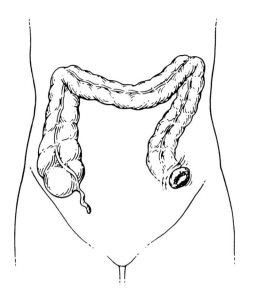

FIGURE 9-1
Abdominal view of sigmoid colostomy with rectum and anus removed, as with abdominal perineal resection. (From Hampton, Bryant.[27])

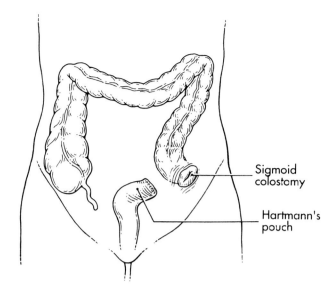

FIGURE 9-2
Sigmoid colostomy. Distal bowel is oversewn and left in place to create Hartmann's pouch. (From Hampton, Bryant.[27])

always be assessed before establishing a management plan for an individual patient.)

Colostomy may be performed on either a temporary or a permanent basis. A colostomy is considered temporary if reanastomosis is possible (i.e., if the distal rectum and anus remain intact). Temporary colostomy may be performed to promote healing of a traumatic injury, surgical incision, or inflammatory process in the distal bowel, or to provide bowel decompression in the presence of an obstructing lesion such as a tumor. (Definitive management of the underlying obstructive process is delayed until the bowel can be decompressed and a "bowel prep" can be completed; resection and reanastomosis in an unprepared colon carries an unacceptable risk of fecal contamination and peritonitis.) Temporary colostomy may also be performed after segmental colon resection when reanastomosis is thought to carry an unacceptable risk of anastomotic breakdown (e.g., with ischemic conditions or in the presence of massive intraabdominal inflammation). A permanent colostomy is required when the distal bowel, rectum, and anus are removed (Figure 9-1); most commonly this is due to a malignancy involving the rectum.

A colostomy may be constructed as a single end stoma, a double-barrel stoma, or a loop stoma. A single end stoma is constructed by dividing the bowel and bringing the proximal end of the bowel through an opening in the abdominal wall; the bowel is everted and sutured to the dermis or subcutaneous tissue. The distal bowel segment may be removed (as in abdomino-

perineal resection of the rectum) or may be sutured closed and left in place (Hartmann's pouch) (Figure 9-2). If the distal segment is removed, the patient will have a perineal incision or wound, and the colostomy is permanent. If a Hartmann's pouch is constructed, the potential for reanastomosis exists; these patients will continue to produce mucus in the retained segment and may periodically feel the urge to evacuate the rectum. If they are unable to eliminate the mucus, they may require a low-volume enema to cleanse the rectal segment.

A double-barrel colostomy usually is constructed after segmental resection when reanastomosis is deemed inadvisable because of ischemia or infection (e.g., following a gunshot wound to the abdomen with colonic perforation and intraabdominal contamination). In this case, both ends of the bowel are brought to the abdominal surface as two separate end stomas; the stomas may be constructed side by side or at widely separated points on the abdominal wall. The proximal stoma drains stool and requires a pouch, whereas the distal stoma (also known as a "mucous fistula") drains only mucus and can be managed by using a gauze pad or other absorptive cover (Figure 9-3); if the stomas are constructed side by side, both will have to be incorporated into the pouching system. Because the distal bowel remains intact, the patient may continue to have bowel movements until all residual stool has been eliminated from the distal segment. A double-barrel colostomy is intended to be temporary; once the ischemia or infection has resolved, the stomas can be "taken down"

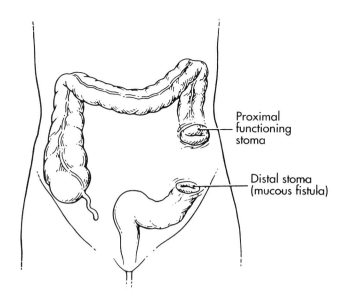

FIGURE 9-3
Abdominal view of descending colostomy with distal bowel in place and exiting to skin as mucous fistula. (From Hampton, Bryant.[27])

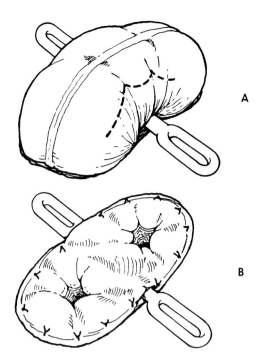

FIGURE 9-4
Loop colostomy construction is much the same as construction of loop ileostomy. **A,** Stoma is created with longitudinal incision through sacculations in colon. **B,** Loop colostomy matured. (From Hampton, Bryant.[27])

and the proximal and distal segments can be anastomosed to reestablish intestinal continuity.

A loop colostomy usually is constructed when immediate fecal diversion is required and a minimal operative procedure is desired (e.g., to provide decompression above an obstructing tumor or to divert the fecal stream away from an area of intense inflammation when no definitive procedure can be safely performed). A loop colostomy is constructed by making an incision through the abdominal wall to access the abdominal cavity; a loop of bowel is brought through the incision and stabilized on the abdominal wall. Stabilization is necessary to prevent retraction of the exteriorized loop until granulation to the abdominal wall has taken place (usually in about 1 week). Stabilization is most commonly accomplished by securing a plastic or latex rod, bridge, or catheter to the abdominal wall underneath the loop of bowel. Alternative approaches include the construction of a skin and fascial bridge that provides support for the bowel, or placement of a whistle-tip catheter through a subcutaneous "tunnel" underneath the exteriorized loop of bowel, with the ends of the catheter brought to the surface and sutured in place some distance from the stoma. (These alternative approaches have been devised to simplify pouch application, which can be difficult with bulky external stabilization devices. However, external devices are now available that are relatively flat and compatible with most pouching systems.) The anterior wall of a loop colostomy may be opened at surgery or later at the bed-

side (the posterior wall remains intact). One advantage to opening the bowel at surgery is the opportunity to surgically "mature" the stoma; surgical maturation involves eversion of the bowel (so that the mucosal layer is exposed) and suturing of the stoma to the underlying dermis or subcutaneous tissue. If the bowel is opened at the bedside, it is done with electrocautery; the patient must be properly grounded and must be assured that this is a painless procedure. Stomas opened at the bedside usually are allowed to "self-mature"; this means that the stoma gradually self-everts to expose the mucosal layer. Self-eversion occurs because the exposed serosa becomes inflamed and begins to slough; the inflamed serosal surfaces adhere to each other and cause the bowel to roll back on itself. Loop colostomies provide access to both the proximal and distal bowel (Figure 9-4); however, they usually provide almost complete fecal diversion, because the normal haustrations of the bowel wall tend to prevent spillage of stool into the distal bowel. Because the distal bowel remains intact, the patient may continue to have bowel movements through the rectum until all residual stool has been eliminated from the distal bowel. Loop colostomies are intended to be temporary diversions.

INDICATIONS

Cancer of the rectum (permanent end sigmoid colostomy for lesions in the distal rectum)

Low anterior resection (temporary colostomy may be done to protect the suture line)

Crohn's disease of the colon and perianal tissues (may require rectal resection with permanent colostomy; may require temporary colostomy to allow fissures and fistulas to heal)

Diverticulitis with perforation and abscess formation or peritonitis (temporary diverting colostomy)

Gunshot wound or stab wound to abdomen causing colonic perforations (temporary diverting colostomy)

Blunt trauma to abdomen causing colonic perforations (temporary diverting colostomy)

Ischemic or gangrenous processes affecting colon; e.g., volvulus or infarction of mesenteric artery (temporary diverting colostomy)

Obstructing lesions such as tumors (temporary diverting colostomy or palliative diverting colostomy)

Trauma to anorectum with loss of sphincter function (temporary or permanent colostomy)

Fistulas involving colon or rectum; e.g., rectovaginal fistula (temporary diverting colostomy)

CONTRAINDICATIONS

Chronic ulcerative colitis (requires total colectomy)

COMPLICATIONS

Mucocutaneous separation	Stomal prolapse
Stomal ischemia or necrosis	Stomal stenosis
Peristomal hernia	

PREPROCEDURAL NURSING CARE

NURSING DIAGNOSIS	NURSING INTERVENTIONS	RATIONALE
Anxiety related to construction of colostomy	Acknowledge negative feelings as normal, and emphasize the importance of honestly confronting one's feelings.	Recognizing that negative feelings are normal reduces feelings of guilt and improves the ability to cope.
	Explain the availability of ostomy visitors (trained volunteers from United Ostomy Association), and arrange a visitor if desired.	Sharing concerns with others who have had similar experiences reduces patient's sense of isolation and provides additional support.
High risk for impaired skin integrity (postoperative) related to suboptimal stoma placement with resultant difficulty in maintaining pouch seal	Collaborate with ostomy care nurse and physician to select and mark optimum site for stoma (within rectus muscle, within patient's visual field, and on flat pouching surface); evaluate patient in lying, sitting, and standing positions.	An appropriately sited stoma facilitates self-care by improving pouch seal security and preventing frequent and unplanned pouch changes.
High risk for infection related to opening of large bowel	Complete bowel preparation as ordered (e.g., laxatives, enemas, oral antibiotics); monitor results and notify physician if preparation does not produce clear returns.	Cleansing the colon of stool and bacteria reduces the risk of intraabdominal contamination and sepsis.

POSTPROCEDURAL NURSING CARE

NURSING DIAGNOSIS	NURSING INTERVENTIONS	RATIONALE
High risk for impaired skin integrity related to frequent fecal contamination of skin or frequent disruption of pouch seal	Select appropriate pouching system based on patient's abdominal contours and type of colostomy (ascending, transverse, or descending): Patient with flat or gently rounded abdominal contours may use a flexible or a rigid pouching system; Patient with deep peristomal creasing usually requires an all-flexible pouching system; Patient with a retracted stoma usually requires a convex pouching system and may need a belt or binder for support; Patient with an ascending or a transverse colostomy usually gets better wear time with pouch that has pectin- or gelatin-based barrier and may also benefit from use of skin barrier paste to caulk around stoma and keep stool from undermining pouch seal; Patient with descending or sigmoid colostomy may use pectin-, gelatin-, or karaya-based barriers; Patient who irrigates colostomy and has only mucoid drainage may use closed-end pouch without barrier ring.	Effective protection of peristomal skin depends on a securely adhered pouch that prevents fecal contamination of skin and does not require frequent changes. Adherence of pouch is promoted by a close match between the pouch and the abdomen. Pectin and gelatin barriers are very resistant to fecal drainage. The paste form of skin barriers effectively caulks the junction between the pouch and the skin and improves the pouch seal. Barriers protect the skin from fecal contamination; barriers are not required for a colostomy that is regulated by irrigation.
	Size pouch opening so that barrier ring fits closely around stoma (may "clip" barrier ring if stoma is edematous) *or* size pouch opening so that barrier "clears" stoma by ⅛ inch, and protect exposed skin with skin barrier paste.	Pouch opening must be sized so that it prevents stomal constriction and fecal contamination of peristomal skin.
	Change pouch approximately q 5 days and prn for leakage or complaints of peristomal skin pain.	Routine pouch changes help prevent accidental disruption of pouch seal; pouch must be changed immediately for leakage or skin pain to prevent prolonged fecal contact with skin.
	Incorporate skin protective measures into pouch change procedure: gently remove pouch by pushing down on skin while lifting up on pouch; cleanse skin with water and pat dry.	Peristomal skin is subjected to repetitive trauma. Routine care should be designed to minimize mechanical trauma, shear force, and chemical irritants.
	Remove peristomal hair by shaving in direction of hair growth and away from stoma: may use electric shaver or safety razor with wet or dry lubricant (shaving cream or powder).	Folliculitis is caused by trauma to hair follicles and can be prevented by routine gentle removal of hair.

→ 〉 〉

NURSING DIAGNOSIS	NURSING INTERVENTIONS	RATIONALE
	If needed, apply skin barrier paste around stoma and to any skin defects to create a smooth pouching surface.	Skin barrier paste is an effective caulking agent and can be used to fill irregularities in the skin's surface.
	Treat minor peristomal skin breakdown by dusting on skin barrier powder; seal powder if needed by blotting with water or skin sealant.	Skin barrier powders absorb drainage and provide a protective coating; it may be necessary to seal the powder to create a nonpowdery surface.
	Empty pouch when it is one third to one half full: remove clip and cuff bottom of pouch; drain stool from pouch; clean spout with toilet paper or disposable wipes (may rinse pouch if desired); uncuff pouch and reattach clip.	Pouch should be emptied before it gets full enough to disrupt the seal. The pouch spout must be kept clean to prevent odor. Rinsing is an option but is not necessary since the pouch is odor-proof.
Altered gastrointestinal tissue perfusion related to stomal necrosis	Monitor stoma for color and turgor q 8 h until moist and pink for 72 hours.	Stomal ischemia may occur during early postoperative period as a result of edema, tension on the mesentery, or excessive stripping of the mesentery during surgery.
	Size pouch to prevent stomal constriction.	Stomal constriction increases edema.
	Monitor patient for increasing abdominal distention; insert N/G tube as ordered (or assist with insertion); irrigate tube with saline as needed to maintain patency.	Abdominal distention causes tension on the mesentery, which reduces blood flow to the stoma.
	Use lubricated test tube and flashlight to inspect mucosa of proximal bowel for viability; notify physician promptly of necrosis extending past fascia level.	Stomal necrosis extending past fascia level is a surgical emergency because of the risk of perforation.
Impaired tissue integrity related to mucocutaneous separation	Assess integrity of mucocutaneous suture line at each pouch change.	Mucocutaneous separation may occur as a result of nutritional compromise or steroid therapy.
	Promote healing of separated areas: flush area with saline; fill area with absorptive powder or granules; cover powder or granules with SteriStrips or paper tape to create pouching surface; apply paste and pouch (pouch should fit around stoma and cover area of separation).	Optimum wound healing requires absorption of excess exudate, maintenance of a moist wound surface, and prevention of fecal contamination.
Knowledge deficit related to management options and irrigation procedure (*Note:* Applicable only to patient with descending or sigmoid colostomy)	Assess patient's candidacy for management by irrigation (descending or sigmoid colostomy, ability to learn and perform procedure, desire to regulate bowel elimination, absence of stomal complications such as prolapse or hernia, patient not receiving radiation). Other considerations are length and function of proximal bowel and usual bowel elimination patterns (patients with history of regular bowel movements or tendency toward constipation are more likely to respond positively).	Irrigation is a management option only for patients who have descending or sigmoid colostomies; the nurse must determine the patient's candidacy for irrigation and counsel him regarding management options.

NURSING DIAGNOSIS	NURSING INTERVENTIONS	RATIONALE
Body image disturbance related to colostomy	Encourage patient to express his feelings and concerns about colostomy and its anticipated impact on his health status and life-style.	Exploring feelings provides emotional relief and is the first step in dealing with concerns and issues.
	Teach patient measures for controlling gas: identify gas-producing foods, discuss lag time between ingestion of gas-forming foods and actual flatulence (4-6 h) and implications (omission of these foods versus selective ingestion at "safe" times), and explain measures for muffling the sound of flatus (e.g., hand or arm pressure against stoma).	The ability to control gas improves the patient's confidence in his ability to manage the colostomy and promotes adaptation.
	Teach patient measures for controlling odor: using odor-proof pouch, prompt pouch change in the event of leakage, keeping pouch spout clean, using room deodorants when pouch is emptied and oral deodorants as desired.	The ability to control odor is essential for comfort in social and business situations; this in turn promotes comfort with one's self and adaptation.
Sexual dysfunction related to change in body appearance and function (colostomy)	Encourage patient and partner to be open about their feelings about colostomy; help them separate their feelings about the stoma from their feelings about the patient.	Open communication reduces misunderstanding and fosters intimacy.
	Discuss with patient (and partner, if appropriate) measures to enhance patient's self-esteem and to reduce focus on pouch and stoma: general self-care activities and grooming; measures to secure and conceal the pouch (e.g., special underwear, tube tops); measures to enhance intimacy (e.g., shared activities).	Measures to improve comfort with self and to reduce focus on the pouch and stoma enhance feelings of sexual attractiveness and allow the patient and partner to refocus on shared pleasure and intimacy.
	If patient has long-standing sexual issues, refer him to a sex therapist.	Sex therapists can help the patient and partner deal with their issues and establish a satisfactory relationship.

Note: A patient who has undergone wide rectal resection for rectal cancer may have organic dysfunction (see care plans under Abdominoperineal Resection of the Rectum, pp. 319-320).

See also Preprocedural Nursing Care and Postprocedural Nursing Care under Abdominal Surgery, pp. 303-306.

PATIENT TEACHING

1. Describe normal colostomy function and normal stomal characteristics (involuntary elimination of stool and gas at intervals, with consistency of stool dependent on type of colostomy; stoma normally pink to red, moist, and insensate with tendency to bleed slightly when cleaned).

2. Teach the patient how to empty the pouch and clean the spout, and how to change the pouch and provide peristomal skin care. Have the patient return the demonstrations before discharge.

3. Provide dietary guidelines: no absolute restrictions; importance of adequate fiber and fluid intake to pre-

→ > >

vent constipation; measures to control gas (identification of gas-forming foods, explanation of lag time between ingestion of gas-forming foods and actual flatulence, measures to muffle gas).

4. Teach the patient how to manage constipation and diarrhea (this may be done on an outpatient basis). Constipation: increase fiber and fluids and take an over-the-counter laxative unless contraindicated. Diarrhea: adhere to bland, "constipating" diet, omit irrigation (if applicable), increase fluid intake (sports drinks and fruit juices are good fluids, since they replace electrolytes as well as water), take over-the-counter antidiarrheal medicines unless contraindicated.

5. Teach the patient how to obtain needed supplies.
6. Teach the patient the signs and symptoms that should be reported to the ostomy nurse specialist. Arrange follow-up with ostomy nurse specialist.
7. Discuss ways to manage the colostomy in business, recreational, social, and sexual situations.

Abdominoperineal Resection of the Rectum

Abdominoperineal resection (APR) involves removal of the rectum through a combined abdominal and perineal approach. This procedure is most commonly performed for cancer of the distal rectum, but it may also be done for Crohn's disease affecting the rectum and perianal tissues. Inflammatory disease affecting the entire colon and rectum necessitates total colectomy as well as abdominoperineal resection of the rectum, a procedure called proctocolectomy.

Abdominoperineal resection involves an abdominal incision and a perineal incision. The proximal rectal dissection is carried out through the abdominal incision, and the distal dissection is completed through the perineal incision. If the resection is being done for benign disease, a "narrow" rectal resection is performed, meaning that the perirectal tissues are disturbed as little as possible. If the resection is being done for rectal cancer, however, a wide dissection is carried out to excise the regional lymph nodes. This wider dissection is associated with a reduced rate of local recurrence, but also with an increased incidence of sexual dysfunction, because the pathways for the autonomic nerve fibers controlling erection and ejaculation in men pass through the perirectal tissues in the plane of dissection.

In the past the perineal defect created by removal of the rectum usually was left to close by secondary intention, and perineal wounds that did not heal were a common complication of abdominoperineal resections. The current standard of practice is to perform primary closure of the perineal wound, with placement of closed suction drains to prevent fluid accumulation and abscess formation. However, in some situations primary closure is not feasible (e.g., hemorrhage); in these cases the wound is packed open and allowed to close by secondary intention. Meticulous wound management is required to promote healing and prevent complications in these patients.

Abdominoperineal resection always necessitates creation of a permanent fecal diversion. If the resection is limited to the rectum, an end sigmoid colostomy is constructed. If the resection is performed in conjunction with a colectomy, an ileostomy must be created. The surgical techniques and considerations involved in construction of a fecal diversion are discussed under the Colostomy and Ileostomy sections.

INDICATIONS

Cancer of distal rectum (lesions within distal 4 to 5 cm of rectum)
Crohn's disease affecting rectum and perianal tissues (when disease is refractory to medical management or proximal fecal diversion or both)
Crohn's disease affecting entire colon and rectum, necessitating proctocolectomy
Familial polyposis or ulcerative colitis requiring proctocolectomy when sphincter-saving procedure is not feasible or not desired

CONTRAINDICATIONS

Chronic ulcerative colitis (unless performed in conjunction with proctocolectomy)
Familial polyposis (unless performed in conjunction with proctocolectomy)

COMPLICATIONS

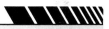

Sexual dysfunction (in men, loss of erectile or ejaculatory function or both; in women, possible loss of vaginal lubrication, and possible dyspareunia related to change in angle of vaginal vault or to vaginal distortion caused by formation of excessive perineal scar tissue)

Voiding dysfunction (retention related to damage to parasympathetic nerve fibers that cause bladder contraction and to change in urethrovesical angle)
Delayed wound healing (open perineal wound)

PREPROCEDURAL NURSING CARE

NURSING DIAGNOSIS	NURSING INTERVENTIONS	RATIONALE
Anxiety related to surgery, anesthesia, and creation of ostomy	Encourage patient to express concerns and feelings about surgery, anesthesia, and construction of ostomy.	Ventilation provides emotional relief and is the first step in dealing with feelings and concerns.
	Provide information as patient and family demonstrate readiness for learning (e.g., postoperative pain management and ostomy management).	Understanding what is to be done and the care routines reduces fear of the unknown.
	Administer preoperative sedation.	Preoperative sedation helps reduce anxiety and promotes rest.
High risk for infection related to abdominal incision and opening into colon and rectum	Complete skin preparation (e.g., antiseptic showers or scrubs).	Showering or scrubbing with skin antiseptics reduces bacteria on the skin.
	Complete bowel preparation (e.g., laxatives, enemas, oral antibiotics); monitor results and notify physician if preparation does not produce clear results.	Cleansing the colon and rectum of stool and bacteria reduces the risk of intraabdominal contamination and sepsis.

POSTPROCEDURAL NURSING CARE

NURSING DIAGNOSIS	NURSING INTERVENTIONS	RATIONALE
High risk for sexual dysfunction related to autonomic nerve damage (if applicable: male undergoing wide rectal resection for rectal cancer)	Explain to patient that the nerves controlling erection and ejaculation pass through the perirectal tissue and may be damaged by the wide rectal excision required for attempted curative resection; explain that dysfunction may be temporary or long term. Explain that sensation and the potential for orgasm are controlled by different nerve fibers that are not damaged.	Informed consent includes information about potential complications. Erection and ejaculation are mediated by autonomic pathways that pass through the perirectal tissue. Sensation and orgasm are mediated by sensorimotor nerves that innervate the perineum and that remain intact.

→ > >

NURSING DIAGNOSIS	NURSING INTERVENTIONS	RATIONALE
	Counsel patient and partner about ways to maintain intimacy: nonsexual sharing, touching and kissing, alternatives to intercourse (e.g., manual stimulation, oral stimulation, use of vibrators).	This helps the patient and partner maintain a satisfactory sexual relationship.
	Collaborate with physician to provide information on options for regaining erectile function and the potential for intercourse (vacuum pump devices, surgically implanted penile prostheses, and penile papaverine injections).	Restoring erectile function restores the ability to have intercourse.
Potential impaired tissue integrity related to delayed healing of perineal wound	Monitor perineal wound for approximation of incision, volume and character of drainage, and evidence of infection (redness, induration, heat in surrounding tissues).	Prompt detection of complications permits early intervention.
	Maintain patency of wound suction catheters or drains (if applicable).	Accumulation of fluid in the wound bed promotes bacterial proliferation and abscess formation.
	Administer antibiotics as ordered.	Antibiotics reduce bacterial proliferation and help prevent infection.
	Use aseptic technique in wound care.	This prevents the introduction of pathogens.
	Keep wound edges shaved to prevent hair from growing into wound.	Hair acts as a foreign body, prolonging inflammation and delaying healing.
High risk for altered patterns of urinary elimination related to damage to autonomic nerves controlling bladder and sphincter function	Monitor patient for urinary output, voiding patterns, and evidence of retention (bladder distention, frequent voiding of small amounts, feeling of incomplete emptying).	Prompt detection of complications permits early intervention.
	Check postvoid residual volume of urine if patient has signs and symptoms of urinary retention.	High postvoid residual urine volume indicates incomplete bladder emptying and retention.
	Collaborate with physician to obtain diagnostic workup for any patient with persistent postoperative voiding dysfunction.	This provides the data needed to determine an appropriate management plan.
	Instruct patient in measures to promote bladder function (based on diagnostic workup and established management plan): e.g., scheduled voiding and double voiding (voiding and then voiding again within 5 min), or clean intermittent catheterization.	Management of bladder dysfunction focuses on restoration of function; scheduled voiding, clean intermittent catheterization, and double voiding are used for the patient who has difficulty with retention.

See also Preprocedural Nursing Care and Postprocedural Nursing Care for Colostomy, pp. 314-317, or Ileostomy, pp. 326-330, and for Abdominal Surgery, pp. 303-306.

PATIENT TEACHING ▪▪

1. Explain that the surgical procedure involves both an abdominal and a perineal (rectal) incision and that a permanent fecal diversion will be required.
2. Men: Explain the pathways for nerves controlling erection, ejaculation, and sensation and orgasm. Explain that rectal dissection may cause temporary or long-term damage to these nerves; explain that long-term damage is very unlikely with a narrow rectal resection (as is done for familial polyposis or inflammatory disease) but is more likely with a wide rectal resection (as is required for removal of cancer). Explain that if damage does occur, it may involve loss of erectile function or loss of ejaculatory function or both; explain that sensation and the potential for orgasm are retained. Discuss options for management based on the patient's level of concern; make him aware that several options do exist should this complication occur.
3. For the patient discharged with an open perineal wound: Instruct the patient or family member in prescribed procedures for wound care. Stress the importance of aseptic technique. Teach the patient and family the signs and symptoms of wound infection, and instruct them to report such symptoms to the physician promptly.
4. For the patient with bladder dysfunction: Instruct the patient in the treatment plan, including specific procedures, their rationale, the expected outcomes, and the time frame for improvement. Establish a plan for follow-up care.

Bowel Resection

Bowel resection involves the removal of an intestinal segment; common indications are malignant lesions, inflammatory processes, obstructive conditions, ischemia, or traumatic injury.

Resection for benign disease involves removal of the involved segment with anastomosis of the proximal and distal ends of the remaining bowel. If the anastomosis is between small bowel and colon (ileocolic), an end-to-side anastomosis is performed; an anastomosis between two small bowel or two colonic segments is fashioned in an end-to-end manner. (If anastomosis is deemed inadvisable because of ischemia of the remaining segments or extensive peritoneal contamination, the proximal and distal ends of the remaining bowel may be brought to the abdominal wall as an ileostomy or colostomy and a mucous fistula.)

Resection for malignant disease involves a much more radical approach. The principles determining the lines of resection include removal of the lesion itself with adequate margins of resection, and removal of the lymphatics draining the involved segment of bowel. For a small bowel malignancy, this usually can be accomplished by resecting the area of the tumor and at least 6 cm of bowel both proximal and distal to the tumor, along with the mesentery supplying that segment of bowel; if the mesenteric dissection results in devascularization of a wider segment of bowel, a more radical resection is performed. Since the lymphatics draining colonic segments are located adjacent to major arteries and veins, a curative resection for colon cancer involves removal of all lymphatics and vessels draining the involved segment of bowel. The bowel supplied by the resected vessels must also be removed, since collateral blood flow is inadequate to maintain viability of the devascularized bowel. For tumors in the distal sigmoid colon, adequate resection requires at least 15 cm of bowel proximal to the tumor and at least 5 cm of bowel distal to the tumor. For tumors elsewhere in the colon, much more radical resections are required to remove all the involved lymphatics.

A low anterior resection involves a subtotal resection of the rectum through an abdominal incision, with a colorectal or coloanal anastomosis. This procedure is indicated for most tumors in the midrectum or proximal rectum (i.e., at least 5 cm from the anal verge). (Curative resection of midrectal tumors that are bulky, invasive, or virulent may still require abdominoperineal resection.) Anastomosis between the rectal stump (or anal canal) and the proximal colon usually is accomplished by means of a stapling device; this provides a secure anastomosis in an area where a secure hand-sewn anastomosis is difficult to achieve. A proximal colostomy may be constructed for temporary diversion of the fecal

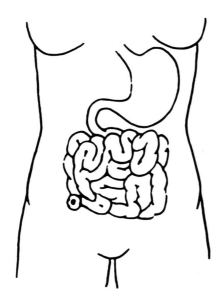

● **FIGURE 9-5**
Abdominal view of ileostomy with colon, rectum, and anus removed, as with total proctocolectomy. However, ileostomy can be constructed and rectum, colon, and anus left intact. (From Hampton, Bryant.[27])

stream if the security of the anastomosis is in doubt; in most cases no diversion is required.

Total colectomy may be required for management of premalignant or inflammatory conditions involving the entire colon. If the pathologic process is confined to the colon, the colon can be resected and the small bowel can be anastomosed to the rectum (ileorectal anastomosis). If the disease process involves the rectum as well as the colon, curative resection involves either a proctocolectomy (total colectomy with abdominoperineal resection of the rectum) (Figure 9-5) and end ileostomy, or a total colectomy, subtotal proctectomy (partial rectal resection) with or without mucosal stripping, creation of a proximal small bowel reservoir, and anastomosis of the reservoir to the anal canal (ileal reservoir–anal anastomosis).

Segmental bowel resection usually has minimal impact on gastrointestinal function, because the bowel has tremendous reserve capacity. However, repetitive or massive small bowel resections may produce short bowel syndrome; this is most likely to occur when more than 75% of the small bowel has been resected and the remaining bowel is less than 100 cm long. If most of the terminal ileum is resected, the patient is at risk for loss of vitamin B_{12} absorption and may require lifelong parenteral replacement. Total colectomy with ileorectal anastomosis or ileal reservoir with anal anastomosis alters the consistency and frequency of bowel movements.

INDICATIONS

Diverticulitis
Crohn's disease
Ischemic or necrotic processes affecting the bowel (e.g., strangulated hernia, infarction of mesenteric artery, volvulus)
Traumatic injury (gunshot wound, stab wound, or blunt trauma to abdomen) causing bowel ischemia or perforation
Fistulas
Small bowel or colon cancer
Chronic ulcerative colitis (total proctocolectomy, or colectomy with partial proctectomy and creation of small bowel reservoir with anastomosis to anal canal)
Rectal cancer in midrectum or proximal rectum (localized and noninvasive lesions)
Familial polyposis (total proctocolectomy, or colectomy with partial proctectomy and creation of small bowel reservoir with anastomosis to anal canal)

CONTRAINDICATIONS

None

COMPLICATIONS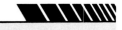

Anastomotic breakdown, resulting in intraabdominal infection and peritonitis
Short bowel syndrome (massive or repetitive small bowel resections)
Vitamin B_{12} deficiency (resection of terminal ileum)

PREPROCEDURAL NURSING CARE

NURSING DIAGNOSIS	NURSING INTERVENTIONS	RATIONALE
High risk for infection related to opening of small or large bowel	Complete bowel preparation as ordered (e.g., liquid diet, laxatives, enemas, oral antibiotics); monitor results and notify physician if preparation does not produce clear results (patient scheduled for colon resection).	Cleansing the bowel of stool and bacteria reduces the risk of intraabdominal contamination and sepsis; small bowel has lower bacterial counts and therefore requires less vigorous preparation.

POSTPROCEDURAL NURSING CARE

NURSING DIAGNOSIS	NURSING INTERVENTIONS	RATIONALE
Altered renal, cerebral, cardiopulmonary, gastrointestinal, and peripheral tissue perfusion related to intraabdominal infection and septic shock	Monitor patient for signs and symptoms of anastomotic breakdown, intraabdominal infection, and sepsis (increasing abdominal tenderness and distention, tachycardia, tachypnea, fever, hypotension, and prolonged ileus).	Prompt detection of complications permits early intervention.
	If patient has an N/G tube, monitor function of tube and irrigate with saline as needed to maintain patency.	Decompression of the stomach and proximal small bowel prevents tension on the suture lines and helps prevent anastomotic breakdown.
	If patient does not have an N/G tube: monitor for increasing abdominal distention; insert N/G tube as ordered (or assist with placement).	Accumulation of gastric and small bowel secretions causes distention and can cause tension on the suture lines, which contributes to anastomotic breakdown.
	Administer antibiotics as ordered.	Antibiotics reduce bacterial proliferation and help control infection.
	Administer IV fluids and electrolytes as ordered.	Fluid and electrolyte balance must be maintained to ensure tissue perfusion and neuromuscular function (including peristalsis).
	Monitor patient's hemodynamic status (Swan-Ganz or CVP readings, urine output, BP, and pulse).	Continual monitoring provides data to guide modification of treatment plan.
	If patient's clinical condition worsens, prepare him for surgery.	Immediate surgical intervention may be needed for anastomotic repair or drainage of intraabdominal abscess.
High risk for altered nutrition: less than body requirements, related to significant small bowel resection or resection of terminal ileum	When oral feedings are initiated, monitor patient for nutrient intake and evidence of compromised nutrient absorption (diarrhea, flatulence, cramping, nausea, anorexia).	Prompt detection of complications permits early intervention.

→ > >

NURSING DIAGNOSIS	NURSING INTERVENTIONS	RATIONALE
	For patient with evidence of malabsorption: collaborate with physician, nutritional support team, and patient to develop and implement a nutritional support plan (parenteral, enteral, or modified oral formulas).*	Positive nutritional status is essential for life, health, and immune system function; parenteral support may be required until adequate nutrients can be absorbed through the gut.

*(*Note:* See care plan under Short Bowel Syndrome pp. 233-237.)

See also Preprocedural Nursing Care and Postprocedural Nursing Care under Abdominal Surgery, pp. 303-306.

PATIENT TEACHING

1. Explain the surgical procedure and rationale (need to remove damaged or diseased segment of bowel). If colostomy or ileostomy is performed, explain the reason; if the ostomy is temporary, discuss plans for closure and the factors that determine readiness for closure.
2. Explain that the bowel has tremendous reserve capacity and that most bowel resections are well tolerated, with no real change in the ability to eat and absorb nutrients.
3. If the patient has had massive or repetitive small bowel resections, explain the effect on nutrient digestion and absorption, and explain the nutritional support plan and rationale. (*Note:* See care plan under Short Bowel Syndrome, pp. 233-237.)
4. If the patient has had large segments of colon removed, explain that it is normal to have more frequent bowel movements of more liquid consistency. Explain that the remaining bowel gradually will adapt and begin to absorb more water from the stool and that bowel elimination will become more normal.
5. If the patient has had most or all of the terminal ileum resected, explain that the terminal ileum contains the only sites for absorption of vitamin B_{12} and that vitamin B_{12} is essential for preventing anemia and peripheral neuropathy. Explain that because the liver stores vitamin B_{12}, deficiencies do not appear immediately. Explain the need to monitor vitamin B_{12} levels and to begin lifelong parenteral administration when these levels begin to drop. Teach the patient the signs and symptoms of vitamin B_{12} deficiency, and emphasize the importance of *promptly* reporting these signs and symptoms to the physician.
6. If the patient has had coloanal anastomosis following low anterior resection, explain that urgency and some fecal leakage are normal during the early postoperative period and that sphincter function gradually will become more normal. Instruct the patient in sphincter exercises. (Tell the patient to squeeze as if trying to prevent a bowel movement and to hold the contraction for a count of 10; repeat this at least 10 to 15 times several times a day.)

Ileostomy

Ileostomy is the surgical creation of an opening between the ileum and the abdominal wall for the purpose of fecal diversion. An ileostomy may be temporary or permanent and may be constructed as an end stoma, a loop stoma, or a double-barrel stoma.

An ileostomy is permanent when the distal bowel, rectum, and anus are removed; permanent ileostomy is most commonly performed for inflammatory bowel disease involving the entire colon and rectum (e.g., Crohn's disease). An ileostomy is considered temporary when reanastomosis is possible (i.e., when the distal

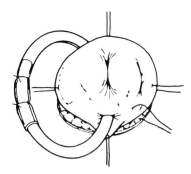

FIGURE 9-6
Loop ileostomy matured with protruding functional limb. (From Hampton, Bryant.[27])

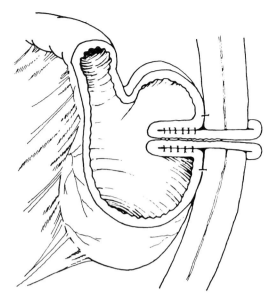

FIGURE 9-7
Distal limb is intussuscepted into reservoir to create one-way valve and accomplish continence. Sutures or staples, or both, are placed to stabilize and maintain intussuscepted nipple. Anterior surface of reservoir is anchored to anterior peritoneal wall. (From Hampton, Bryant.[27])

rectum and anus remain intact). A temporary ileostomy is most commonly constructed for protection of a distal anastomosis (e.g., a newly constructed ileal reservoir with anal anastomosis). A temporary ileostomy may also be created after segmental ileal resection (when ischemia makes reanastomosis inadvisable), to provide bowel rest for an inflamed distal segment, or to relieve obstruction.

An end ileostomy is constructed by dividing the bowel and bringing the end of the proximal bowel through an opening in the abdominal wall; the bowel is everted and sutured to the dermis or subcutaneous tissue. The distal segment may be removed (total proctocolectomy) or may be sutured closed and left in place (Hartmann's pouch). If the distal segment is removed, the patient will have a perineal incision or wound, and the ileostomy is permanent. If the distal segment is closed and left in place, reanastomosis is possible; these patients continue to produce mucus in the retained segment and may periodically feel the urge to evacuate the rectum. If they are unable to eliminate the mucus, they may require a low-volume enema to cleanse the rectal segment.

A loop ileostomy usually is constructed when temporary diversion is required, as in the case of a newly constructed ileal reservoir with anal anastomosis. A loop ileostomy is constructed by bringing a loop of ileum to the abdominal surface, where it is stabilized with a support device (commonly a plastic rod or bridge or a soft rubber catheter) until granulation has taken place. The loop of bowel usually is opened and matured at the time of surgery (i.e., the bowel is everted and sutured to the dermis or subcutaneous tissue in a manner that creates a well-budded proximal [functioning] end and a less prominent distal [mucous fistula] end) (Figure 9-6). The external support device is removed when the stoma has granulated to the abdominal wall, usually about 1 week after surgery.

A double-barrel ileostomy is uncommon; indications include segmental resection when reanastomosis is deemed inadvisable (e.g., ischemic process) and situations in which complete fecal diversion is required. A double-barrel ileostomy is constructed by bringing both ends of the bowel to the abdominal surface as two separate end stomas; the stomas may be constructed side by side or at widely separated points on the abdominal wall. The proximal stoma drains stool and requires a pouch; the distal stoma (also known as a mucous fistula) drains only mucus and can be managed by a gauze pad or other absorptive cover. If the stomas are constructed side by side, both will have to be incorporated into the pouching system. Because the distal bowel remains intact, the patient may continue to have bowel movements until all residual stool has been eliminated from the distal segment. A double-barrel ileostomy is intended to be temporary.

The drainage from an ileostomy is mushy, occurs at frequent intervals, and contains proteolytic enzymes; thus peristomal skin protection is a major concern.

A continent ileal reservoir (Kock pouch) is an alternative to standard ileostomy for selected patients. This procedure involves construction of an internal ileal pouch that is connected to the abdominal wall by a stoma; continence is provided by intussuscepting a portion of the ileum between the abdominal stoma and the internal reservoir (Figure 9-7). For the first few weeks after surgery, the reservoir is drained continuously by an indwelling reservoir catheter; this allows the long suture lines and the continence mechanism to heal. Once healing has occurred, the indwelling catheter is removed and the patient is taught to intubate the reservoir at gradually lengthened intervals. Long-term management involves intubation at 4- to 6-hour intervals and daily irrigation of the reservoir with tap water or saline to prevent bacterial overgrowth and inflammation of the reservoir (pouchitis). An external pouch is not required; instead, the patient wears a light dressing over the stoma to absorb mucus. This procedure usually is contraindicated for patients with Crohn's disease, because recurrence involving the reservoir is common and results in loss of a significant segment of bowel. The most common complication after this procedure is nipple valve dysfunction, which requires reoperation in as many as 25% of patients. Since the advent of the ileal reservoir–anal anastomosis procedure, the continent ileal reservoir has been used less frequently. In many centers the continent ileal reservoir is reserved for patients who have had a proctocolectomy and standard ileostomy but now desire conversion to a continent procedure. Management of the patient with a continent ileal reservoir is not discussed in this text.

INDICATIONS

Crohn's disease affecting the entire colon and rectum (proctocolectomy with end ileostomy)

Chronic ulcerative colitis (proctocolectomy with end ileostomy when continent diversion is not feasible or desired; temporary loop ileostomy for protection of newly constructed ileal reservoir with anal anastomosis)

Obstructing lesion in the ascending colon (loop ileostomy)

Ischemic process involving the ileum (double-barrel ileostomy)

CONTRAINDICATIONS   None

COMPLICATIONS

Peristomal skin breakdown	Stomal prolapse
Mucocutaneous separation	Peristomal hernia
Stomal ischemia or necrosis	Food blockage
Stomal stenosis	

PREPROCEDURAL NURSING CARE

NURSING DIAGNOSIS	NURSING INTERVENTIONS	RATIONALE
Anxiety related to creation of ileostomy	Acknowledge negative feelings as normal, and emphasize the importance of honestly confronting one's feelings.	Recognizing that negative feelings are normal reduces guilt and improves ability to cope.
	Explain the availability of ostomy visitors (trained volunteers from the United Ostomy Association), and arrange for a visitor if desired.	Sharing concerns with others who have had similar experiences reduces the patient's sense of isolation and provides additional support.
High risk for impaired skin integrity (postoperative) related to suboptimal stoma placement with resultant difficulty in maintaining pouch seal	Collaborate with ostomy care nurse and physician to select and mark optimum site for stoma placement (within rectus muscle, within patient's visual field, on flat pouching surface); evaluate patient in lying, sitting, and standing positions.	An appropriately sited stoma facilitates self-care by improving pouch seal security and preventing frequent and unplanned pouch changes.

NURSING DIAGNOSIS	NURSING INTERVENTIONS	RATIONALE
High risk for infection related to opening of large bowel	Complete bowel preparation as ordered (e.g., laxatives, enemas, oral antibiotics); monitor results and notify physician if preparation does not produce clear returns.	Cleansing the bowel of stool and bacteria reduces the risk of intraabdominal contamination and sepsis.

See also Preprocedural Nursing Care under Abdominal Surgery, p. 303.

POSTPROCEDURAL NURSING CARE

NURSING DIAGNOSIS	NURSING INTERVENTIONS	RATIONALE
High risk for impaired skin integrity related to frequent disruption of pouch seal and exposure of peristomal skin to proteolytic drainage or trauma resulting from frequent pouch changes	Select appropriate pouching system based on patient's abdominal contours: Patient with flat or gently rounded abdominal contours may use either a flexible or a rigid pouching system; Patient with deep peristomal creasing usually requires an all-flexible pouching system; Patient with a retracted stoma usually requires a convex pouching system and may need a belt or binder for additional support; Patient with an ileostomy usually gets better wear time with a pouch that has a pectin- or gelatin-based barrier and also usually benefits from use of a skin barrier paste to caulk around the stoma and keep stool from undermining the pouch seal; these patients must always use a pouch with a barrier.	Ileostomy drainage contains proteolytic enzymes that can cause severe skin damage. Effective skin protection requires a secure pouch seal that prevents leakage and does not require frequent pouch changes. Adherence of the pouch is promoted by a close match between the pouch and the abdomen. Pectin and gelatin barriers are very resistant to small bowel drainage (much more resistant than karaya). The paste form of skin barriers effectively caulks the junction between the pouch and skin and improves the pouch seal. Barriers are essential for protection from enzymatic output.
	Size pouch opening so that barrier ring fits closely around stoma (may clip barrier ring if stoma is edematous) *or* size pouch opening so that barrier clears stoma by ⅛ inch and protect exposed skin with skin barrier paste.	Pouch opening must be sized so that it prevents stomal constriction and fecal contamination of peristomal skin.
	Change pouch approximately q 5 days and prn for leakage or complaints of peristomal skin pain.	Routine pouch changes help prevent accidental disruption of pouch seal; the pouch must be changed immediately for any sign of leakage (e.g., skin pain) to prevent prolonged contact between stool and skin.
	Incorporate skin protection measures into pouch change procedure: Gently remove pouch by pushing down on skin while lifting up on pouch; Cleanse skin with water and pat dry.	Peristomal skin is subjected to repetitive trauma. Routine care should be designed to minimize mechanical trauma, shear force, and chemical irritants.

NURSING DIAGNOSIS	NURSING INTERVENTIONS	RATIONALE
	Remove peristomal hair by shaving in direction of hair growth and away from stoma (may use electric shaver or safety razor with wet or dry lubricant such as shaving cream or powder).	Folliculitis is caused by trauma to hair follicles and can be prevented by routine gentle hair removal.
	If patient has fragile skin, apply skin sealant (e.g., Skin Prep) under tape.	Skin sealants add a copolymer film that helps prevent mechanical damage from tape removal.
	If indicated, apply skin barrier paste around stoma and to any skin defects to create a smooth pouching surface.	Skin barrier paste is an effective caulking agent and can be used to fill irregularities in the skin's surface.
	Treat minor peristomal skin breakdown by dusting on skin barrier powder; seal powder if needed by blotting with water or skin sealant.	Skin barrier powders absorb drainage and provide a protective coating; it may be necessary to seal the powder to create a nonpowdery surface.
	Empty pouch when it is one third to one half full. Remove clip and cuff bottom of pouch; drain stool from pouch; clean spout with toilet paper or disposable wipes (may rinse pouch if desired); uncuff pouch and reattach clip.	Pouch should be emptied before it gets full enough to disrupt the seal. Pouch's spout must be kept clean to prevent odor. Rinsing is an option but is not required, because the pouch is odor proof.
Altered gastrointestinal tissue perfusion related to stomal necrosis	Monitor stoma for color and turgor q 8 h until moist and pink for 72 hours.	Stomal ischemia may occur during early postoperative period as a result of edema, tension on the mesentery, or excessive stripping of the mesentery during surgery.
	Size pouch to prevent stomal constriction.	Stomal constriction increases edema and reduces blood flow.
	Monitor patient for increasing abdominal distention; insert N/G tube as ordered (or assist with insertion). If patient has an N/G tube, irrigate tube with saline as needed to maintain patency.	Abdominal distention causes tension on the mesentery, which reduces blood flow to the stoma.
	Use lubricated test tube and flashlight to inspect mucosa of proximal bowel for viability; notify physician promptly of necrosis extending to fascia level.	Stomal necrosis extending past fascia level is a surgical emergency because of the risk of perforation.
Impaired tissue integrity related to mucocutaneous separation	Assess integrity of mucocutaneous suture line at each pouch change.	Mucocutaneous separation may occur as a result of nutritional compromise or steroid therapy.
	Promote healing of separated areas. Flush area with saline; fill area with absorptive powder or granules; cover powder or granules with SteriStrips or paper tape to create pouching surface; apply paste and pouch (pouch should be sized to fit around stoma and cover separation).	Optimum wound healing requires absorption of excess exudate, maintenance of a moist wound surface, and prevention of fecal contamination.

NURSING DIAGNOSIS	NURSING INTERVENTIONS	RATIONALE
Knowledge deficit related to preventing food blockage*	Explain how food blockage can occur (i.e., undigested high-fiber food can clump just proximal to the stoma, causing partial or complete obstruction; also, the thick fluid consistency of small bowel drainage permits fibrous components of stool to separate from fluid components, creating a "mass" effect).	Patient must be knowledgeable about potential complications to effectively manage self-care.
	Teach patient preventive measures: (1) avoid high-fiber foods until stomal edema subsides (usually 6 weeks after surgery); (2) add high-fiber foods one at a time in small amounts; (3) *chew all food thoroughly;* (4) maintain adequate fluid intake; (5) monitor tolerance to newly added foods (cramping and diarrhea indicate poor tolerance to a particular food, so that food should be eaten in very limited amounts or omitted until tolerance improves).	Food blockage can be prevented by limiting intake of high-fiber food based on individual tolerance.
Potential fluid volume deficit related to loss of colonic absorption of fluids and electrolytes	Monitor patient for intake and output (including ileostomy output) and signs of fluid and electrolyte imbalance (output exceeding intake, oliguria, dry mucous membranes, diminished skin turgor, orthostatic hypotension, dizziness when standing, extreme weakness, tachycardia).	Patients with ileostomies are at increased risk for fluid volume deficit because they no longer have the absorptive surface of the colon.
	Provide fluid replacement (IV and oral) as ordered and tolerated.	Fluid and electrolyte balance must be maintained to ensure tissue perfusion and neuromuscular function.
	Instruct patient to increase daily fluid intake to at least 10 8-oz. glasses (2,400 ml).	Average daily ileostomy output is 500 to 750 ml; this represents an increased daily loss of about 400 to 500 ml.
	Instruct patient to increase fluid intake during periods of increased loss (e.g., diarrhea, sweating). Replace volume (e.g., drink an extra glass of fluid each time pouch is emptied). Replace components (e.g., replace water, sodium, and potassium by drinking fruit juices, vegetable juices, broth, and sports drinks as well as water).	Increased fluid losses must be balanced by increased intake to prevent fluid volume depletion. In replacing fluid, it is essential to replace both volume and components to prevent fluid deficits and electrolyte imbalance; small bowel drainage contains large amounts of sodium and potassium.
	Teach patient to recognize and promptly report to physician signs and symptoms of fluid and electrolyte imbalance (thirst, dry mouth and skin, reduced urine output and increased urine concentration, extreme weakness and fatigue, dizziness) *or* increased fluid losses and inability to replace fluid (e.g., diarrhea and vomiting).	Fluid and electrolyte imbalance must be corrected promptly to maintain adequate tissue perfusion and normal neuromuscular function.

*Note: See page 331 for ileostomy lavage procedure.

NURSING DIAGNOSIS	NURSING INTERVENTIONS	RATIONALE
Body image disturbance related to ileostomy	Encourage patient to express feelings and concerns about ileostomy and anticipated impact on health status and life-style.	Exploring feelings provides emotional relief and is the first step in dealing with concerns and issues.
	Teach patient ways to control gas: measures to reduce swallowed air (e.g., not using straws), identifying gas-producing foods, recognizing lag time between ingestion of gas-forming foods and actual flatulence (2-4 hours) and the implications of this (omitting foods or eating them at "safe" times), and measures for muffling the sound of flatus (e.g., hand or arm pressure against the stoma).	The ability to control gas improves the patient's confidence in her ability to manage the ileostomy and promotes adaptation.
	Teach patient measures for controlling odor: using odor-proof pouch, changing pouch promptly if leak occurs, keeping pouch spout clean, using room deodorants when emptying pouch, using oral deodorants as desired.	The ability to control odor is essential for comfort in social and business situations, which in turn promotes adaptation.
	Provide information about additional resources for support for adaptation, such as support groups (United Ostomy Association) and professional counselors.	Support groups reduce the patient's sense of isolation and expand her support system; professional counselors can help her deal with feelings and issues.
Sexual dysfunction related to change in body appearance and function (ileostomy)*	Encourage the patient and partner to be open about their feelings about ileostomy; help each of them deal with their feelings and acknowledge their partner's feelings. Help the partner separate feelings about the stoma from feelings about the patient.	Open communication reduces misunderstandings and fosters intimacy.
	Discuss with patient and partner ways to enhance patient's self-esteem and to reduce focus on the pouch and stoma: general self-care activities and grooming; measures to secure and conceal the pouch (e.g., special underwear, tube tops); measures to enhance intimacy (e.g., shared activities, emotional openness).	Measures to improve comfort with self and to reduce focus on the pouch and stoma enhance feelings of sexual attractiveness and allow patient and partner to refocus on shared pleasure and intimacy.
	Refer patient with long-standing sexual issues to sex therapist.	Sex therapists can help patient and partner deal with their issues and establish a satisfactory relationship.

*Note: Patient who has undergone rectal resection (proctocolectomy) may have organic dysfunction, which usually is temporary. Long-term dysfunction is rare. (See care plans under Abdominoperineal Resection of the Rectum, pp. 319-320.)

PATIENT TEACHING

1. Describe normal ileostomy function and stomal characteristics (involuntary elimination of mushy stool and gas at intervals: a stoma that normally is pink or red, moist, and insensate, with a tendency to bleed slightly when cleaned).
2. Teach the patient how to empty the pouch and clean the spout. Have the patient return the demonstration before discharge.
3. Teach the patient how to size the stoma, change the pouch, and provide peristomal skin care. Emphasize the importance of protecting all peristomal skin from proteolytic output. Have the patient return the demonstration before discharge.
4. Provide dietary guidelines for preventing food blockage: identifying high-fiber foods; omitting high-fiber foods until stomal edema has subsided; adding high-fiber foods to the diet one at a time in small amounts; chewing foods thoroughly and drinking adequate fluids; and recognizing indicators of intolerance (e.g., cramping or diarrhea).
5. Teach the patient ways to control gas: reducing swallowed air (e.g., forgoing straws, smoking, chewing gum); identifying gas-forming foods and lag time between ingestion of gas-forming foods and actual flatulence; and measures to muffle gas.
6. Teach the patient ways to manage diarrhea and prevent fluid-electrolyte imbalance: a daily fluid intake of at least 10 8-oz. glasses; a bland diet, constipating foods, over-the-counter antidiarrheal medications and increased fluid intake during episodes of diarrhea; the importance of replacing both water and electrolytes during periods of increased loss (diarrhea or sweating); food and fluid sources of electrolytes; the signs and symptoms of fluid-electrolyte imbalance; and the importance of notifying the physician of signs of fluid-electrolyte imbalance or increased fluid losses with inability to replace (i.e., diarrhea with vomiting).
7. Teach the patient the signs of food blockage and the appropriate response. Partial blockage: symptoms (foul-smelling liquid output, cramping, distention, stomal swelling); management (liquid diet, peristomal massage, warm bath, pouch change). Complete blockage: symptoms (no output, severe cramping, nausea and vomiting, distention); management (nothing by mouth, peristomal massage, warm bath, pouch change). Instruct patient to promptly report signs of complete blockage not responding to above measures (ileostomy lavage is indicated).
8. Explain to the patient that certain medications are contraindicated—time-released medications, enteric-coated tablets, and large tablets, because they may be incompletely and unpredictably absorbed; laxatives also should be avoided because they may cause severe fluid and electrolyte imbalance. Teach the patient to consult the pharmacist routinely about the best form of medication to take and to notify all prescribing physicians and dentists of the ileostomy and removal of the colon. Tell the patient *never* to crush pills without the pharmacist's approval.
9. Teach the patient how to obtain needed supplies.
10. Teach the patient the signs and symptoms to report to the ostomy nurse specialist. Arrange follow-up with the ostomy nurse specialist.
11. Discuss ways to manage the ileostomy in business, recreational, social, and sexual situations.

ILEOSTOMY LAVAGE

1. Remove the pouch and attach an irrigation sleeve around the stoma.
2. Lubricate a no. 14 or no. 16 French catheter and insert it into the stoma until the blockage is reached (usually about 2 to 4 inches, just past the fascia level).*
3. Instill 30 ml of saline.
4. Remove the catheter and wait for returns.
5. Repeat steps 2 through 4 until the blockage has been removed.
6. Advance the catheter and check for proximal blockage.

*If the catheter can be advanced 4 to 6 inches without encountering the blockage, the obstruction probably is caused by something other than a food bolus (e.g., adhesions).

Ileal Reservoir–Anal Anastomosis

An ileal reservoir with anal anastomosis is an alternative to a permanent ileostomy for a patient who has a premalignant or inflammatory condition involving the colon and rectum. In the past these patients were treated with total proctocolectomy, which removed the diseased tissue but also left the patient unable to store and voluntarily eliminate stool. With the ileal reservoir procedure, a pelvic reservoir is created from loops of the terminal ileum and is anastomosed to the anal canal, which is preserved; thus the patient can still store and voluntarily eliminate stool.

Candidates for this procedure include patients with chronic ulcerative colitis and those with familial adenomatous polyposis. Crohn's disease generally is considered a contraindication, because it can affect the small bowel as well as the colon; recurrence involving the reservoir is a significant risk and could result in loss of a large segment of small bowel (which contributes to the development of short bowel syndrome). Obesity is a relative contraindication to this procedure; the mesentery is less mobile in obese individuals, so it is difficult to mobilize the ileum enough to achieve a tension-free anastomosis deep in the pelvis. (Obese patients who wish to have this procedure done may delay the operation until they can lose weight, or they may undergo a staged procedure.) Any degree of anal sphincter incompetence is another contraindication, because continence depends on the anal sphincter's ability to retain liquid stool. In some settings anorectal manometry studies are performed routinely before surgery to verify the competence of the anal sphincter.

The procedure may be performed in one, two, or three stages. The most common approach is the two-stage procedure. Stage 1 of this approach is a lengthy and complex surgical procedure that involves removal of the diseased tissue, construction of an ileal reservoir with anastomosis to the anal canal, and a temporary diverting ileostomy. Removal of the diseased tissue involves a colectomy, subtotal proctectomy, and distal rectal mucosectomy. The colon and proximal rectum are removed through an abdominal incision. The distal portion of the rectum and the anorectal junction are left intact to preserve the anorectal sphincter musculature. (However, the mucosal layer of the distal rectum usually is "stripped out" through a transanal approach; this eliminates the tissue layer involved in polyp formation and ulcerative colitis, preventing recurrence of the disease.) The ileal reservoir is then constructed by anastomosing adjacent loops of terminal ileum to form a pouch; the pouch is brought down to the pelvis and anastomosed to the anal canal. Finally, a proximal ileo-

stomy is constructed to divert the fecal stream; this protects the newly constructed reservoir and the ileal-anal anastomosis. The ileostomy is most commonly constructed as a loop; it may also be done as an end stoma, with the distal ileum sutured or stapled closed and secured within the abdominal cavity. Stage 2 involves "takedown" of the ileostomy; this is done when the reservoir and anastomosis have healed, usually about 3 months after the first procedure. (A "pouch-o-gram" usually is done before the ileostomy takedown to confirm anastomotic healing, and in some centers anorectal manometry is also done to verify sphincter function.)

A three-stage procedure may be indicated for a patient who is acutely ill at the time of initial surgery or for an obese patient who is unable to lose weight before the initial surgical procedure (either because of high-dose steroids or because the emergent nature of the colectomy does not permit planned weight loss). The first stage of a three-stage procedure involves colectomy with closure of the rectal stump (Hartmann's pouch) and an end ileostomy. This eliminates most of the diseased tissue; for the patient with ulcerative colitis, it also permits weaning from steroids. Stage 2 can be delayed until the patient's physical status improves or until weight loss can be accomplished. Stage 2 involves removal of the proximal rectum (unless this was done with the initial surgery), distal rectal mucosectomy, takedown of the ileostomy, construction of the ileal reservoir, anastomosis of the reservoir to the anal canal, and creation of a proximal diverting ileostomy. (Although the ileostomy usually is located in the same site as the original ileostomy, it frequently is more difficult to manage, because it commonly is constructed as a loop and because it is a more proximal stoma with higher volume, more enzymatic output.) Stage 3 involves takedown of the ileostomy.

In some settings and for some patients, the procedure may be performed in one stage: colectomy and subtotal proctectomy, distal rectal mucosectomy, construction of an ileal reservoir, and anastomosis of the reservoir to the anal canal. A diverting ileostomy is not created, and therefore no additional surgical procedures are required. Because this approach may carry increased risk of anastomotic breakdown, it is commonly reserved for low-risk patients (i.e., slender, well-nourished patients who are not taking steroids).

Some variations in surgical technique affect postoperative patient care and therefore should be considered. One variation is the type of ileal reservoir constructed. The two most common reservoirs are the J-reservoir and the S-reservoir. The J-reservoir, also

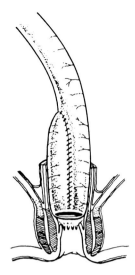

FIGURE 9-8
J-shaped configuration for IAR. Distal ileum is aligned in J shape; antimesenteric surface of J shape is opened, and adjacent bowel walls anastomosed. Side-to-end anastomosis of bowel to dentate line is evident. (From Hampton, Bryant.[27])

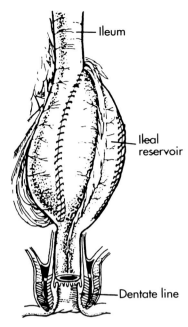

FIGURE 9-9
S-shaped configuration for IAR. Three 10-cm limbs of ileum are used, antimesenteric surface of each limb opened, and adjacent bowel walls anastomosed. (From Hampton, Bryant.[27])

known as the Utsonomiya reservoir, is constructed by bringing the distal ileum down to the pelvis and then looping it back on itself to form a J; the antimesenteric limbs of the ileum are opened and anastomosed to form a reservoir (Figure 9-8), and the spout is anastomosed to the anal canal. The S-reservoir is also known as the Parks pouch; it is constructed by opening three loops of ileum along their antimesenteric borders and then suturing the opened loops into a pouch configuration (Figure 9-9). The advantages and disadvantages of each approach are listed in Table 9-1, p. 334.

Another variation is the management of the mucosal layer in the retained rectal segment. Originally it was thought that this tissue layer *must* be removed to prevent recurrence of the disease; however, some surgeons prefer to leave the mucosa intact and to monitor the patient for any recurrence through periodic proctoscopy. Surgeons who favor this approach feel that retention of the transitional zone improves continence during the immediate postoperative period; in addition, they point out that there is very little mucosa retained (especially when the ileal-anal anastomosis is completed by means of a gastrointestinal stapling device, which fires a double row of staples and excises the excess tissue). Proponents of this approach recommend periodic

anoscopy to assess for recurrence at the anastomotic line, with cauterization of the mucosa as needed. (Some surgeons routinely cauterize the remaining mucosa a few months after surgery.)

INDICATIONS

Chronic ulcerative colitis requiring colectomy (because of intractability or development of dysplasia)
Familial adenomatous polyposis

CONTRAINDICATIONS

Crohn's disease
Obesity
Anal sphincter dysfunction

COMPLICATIONS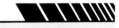

Anastomotic breakdown
Cuff abscess (abscess at junction of reservoir and anal canal)
Anastomotic stricture
Intractable diarrhea
Pouchitis (inflammation of reservoir thought to be caused by bacterial overgrowth)

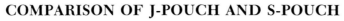

Table 9-1

COMPARISON OF J-POUCH AND S-POUCH

	Advantages	Disadvantages
J-pouch	Reservoir spout located at anorectal junction, so patient can empty reservoir effectively with Valsalva maneuver; does not require intubation or irrigation	Requires very mobile mesentery for tension-free anastomosis, because anastomosis is located deep in pelvis (may not be technically feasible in some patients); more prone to leakage than S-pouch (leakage more likely to be a problem during early postoperative period)
S-pouch	Can be performed on patients with less mobile mesentery (due to pouch configuration and point of anastomosis); less prone to leakage during early postoperative period than J-pouch	More difficult to empty spontaneously; may require intubation and irrigation

TWO-STAGE PROCEDURE: STAGE 1
(COLECTOMY, RECTAL MUCOSECTOMY, CONSTRUCTION OF RESERVOIR AND ANASTOMOSIS TO ANAL CANAL; TEMPORARY DIVERTING ILEOSTOMY)

PREPROCEDURAL NURSING CARE

NURSING DIAGNOSIS	NURSING INTERVENTIONS	RATIONALE
Anxiety related to creation of temporary ileostomy	Acknowledge negative feelings as normal, and emphasize the importance of honestly confronting one's feelings.	Recognizing that negative feelings are normal reduces feelings of guilt and improves the ability to cope.
	Explain the availability of ostomy visitors (trained volunteers from the United Ostomy Association who have had ileal reservoir–anal anastomosis), and arrange a visitor if desired.	Sharing concerns with others who have had similar experiences reduces patient's sense of isolation and provides additional support.
High risk for impaired skin integrity (postoperative) related to suboptimal stoma placement with resultant difficulty in maintaining pouch seal	Collaborate with ostomy care nurse and physician to select and mark optimum site for stoma placement (within rectus muscle; within patient's visual field; and on flat pouching surface); evaluate patient in lying, sitting, and standing positions.	An appropriately sited stoma facilitates self-care by improving pouch seal security and preventing frequent and unplanned pouch changes.

NURSING DIAGNOSIS	NURSING INTERVENTIONS	RATIONALE
High risk for infection related to opening of large bowel	Complete bowel preparation as ordered (e.g., laxatives, enemas, oral antibiotics); monitor results and notify physician if preparation does not produce clear returns.	Cleansing the colon of stool and bacteria reduces the risk of intraabdominal contamination and sepsis.

POSTPROCEDURAL NURSING CARE

NURSING DIAGNOSIS	NURSING INTERVENTIONS	RATIONALE
Altered renal, cerebral, cardiopulmonary, gastrointestinal, and peripheral tissue perfusion related to intraabdominal infection and septic shock	Monitor patient for signs and symptoms of anastomotic breakdown and peritoneal inflammation (increasing abdominal tenderness and distention, tachycardia, tachypnea, fever, hypotension, and drainage of small bowel contents through drains).	Prompt detection of complications permits early intervention.
	Monitor patient for increasing abdominal distention; irrigate N/G tube as needed to maintain patency.	Decompression of the stomach and proximal small bowel reduces distention and prevents tension on suture lines.
	Administer antibiotics as ordered.	Antibiotics reduce bacterial proliferation and help prevent or control infection.
	Administer IV fluids as ordered.	Fluid balance must be maintained to provide adequate tissue perfusion.
	Monitor patient's hemodynamic status (Swan-Ganz or CVP readings, urine output, BP, and pulse).	Continual monitoring provides data that guide treatment modifications.
	If patient fails to respond to above measures, prepare him for surgery.	Immediate surgical intervention may be required for anastomotic repair.
High risk for impaired skin integrity related to mucoid drainage from ileal reservoir	Monitor perianal skin for erythema or denudation.	Mucoid drainage from the newly constructed reservoir may contain proteolytic enzymes.
	Protect perianal skin with skin sealants or moisture barrier ointments (if skin is denuded, apply pectin-based powder such as Stomahesive before applying sealant or ointment).	Skin sealants provide a copolymer film that protects the skin from moisture; ointments repel moisture and reduce contact between mucus and skin; pectin-based powders absorb moisture and form a protective coating over the denuded skin.

See also Preprocedural Nursing Care and Postprocedural Nursing Care under Abdominal Surgery, pp. 303-306.

PATIENT TEACHING

1. Explain the rationale for the ileal-anal procedure (i.e., to remove the diseased colon and rectum while preserving the ability to store and voluntarily eliminate stool) and for the temporary diverting ileostomy (to protect the newly constructed reservoir and anastomosis). Explain that a second procedure will be needed for ileostomy takedown and that this procedure is performed when the reservoir and anastomosis are well healed.
2. Teach the patient ileostomy management. (See patient teaching guide for Ileostomy.)
3. Explain to the patient that leakage of irritating mucus may occur until the sphincter tone improves (the sphincter is stretched during transanal mucosectomy); teach the patient how to protect perianal skin (e.g., using skin sealants and moisture barrier ointments, using absorptive pads tucked between the buttocks).
4. If applicable (collaborate with physician to determine appropriateness and guidelines for initiation), teach the patient to perform sphincter exercises (pelvic muscle exercises, Kegel exercises) to strengthen sphincter tone. Instruct the patient to squeeze the pelvic muscles as if trying to prevent a bowel movement, to hold the contraction for 10 seconds, and then to relax. Provide written guidelines for the number of repetitions (usually about 50 per day). Emphasize the importance of keeping the abdominal, gluteal, and quadriceps muscles relaxed.
5. Instruct the patient to note the correlation between ingestion of various foods and the volume and consistency of output. (This information will guide dietary modifications for controlling diarrhea after ileostomy takedown.)
6. Teach the patient the signs and symptoms to report to the ostomy nurse specialist. Arrange follow-up with the ostomy nurse specialist.

TWO-STAGE PROCEDURE: STAGE 2 (TAKEDOWN OF ILEOSTOMY)

PREPROCEDURAL NURSING CARE

NURSING DIAGNOSIS	NURSING INTERVENTIONS	RATIONALE
High risk for infection related to opening into small bowel	Complete bowel preparation as ordered (e.g., liquid diet, oral antibiotics).	The small intestine has low bacterial counts, so effective cleansing usually can be achieved with liquid diets; laxatives usually are contraindicated for patients with ileostomies because of the risk of fluid and electrolyte imbalance.

See also Preprocedural Nursing Care under Abdominal Surgery, p. 303.

POSTPROCEDURAL NURSING CARE

NURSING DIAGNOSIS	NURSING INTERVENTIONS	RATIONALE
Diarrhea related to loss of colon's absorptive capacity	Monitor frequency, volume, and consistency of stools.	Continual assessment of stool volume and consistency provides data needed for treatment modifications.
	Administer antidiarrheal agents (e.g., diphenoxylate, loperamide, and codeine) as ordered and needed.	Antidiarrheal agents reduce peristaltic activity and thus reduce diarrhea.
	Administer bulking agents (e.g., psyllium products) as ordered and needed.	Bulking agents absorb fluid in the bowel and help thicken stool.

NURSING DIAGNOSIS	NURSING INTERVENTIONS	RATIONALE
	Monitor patient for signs and symptoms of fluid-electrolyte imbalance (e.g., output exceeding intake, oliguria, diminished skin turgor, dry mucous membranes, tachycardia, hypotension).	Prompt recognition of fluid-electrolyte deficits permits prompt intervention for restoration of fluid and electrolyte balance.
	Provide fluid replacement (oral or IV) as ordered and tolerated; encourage fluids containing Na^+ and K^+ (e.g., broth, fruit and vegetable juices, tea, sports drinks).	Fluid balance must be maintained to provide tissue perfusion and maintain neuromuscular function. Small bowel drainage contains large amounts of Na^+ and K^+; replacement must include these essential electrolytes.
	Collaborate with dietitian and patient to provide diet that reduces stool volume and thickens stool consistency (e.g., low-fiber, bland diet with constipating foods such as cheese, dairy products, and starches).	Constipating foods help thicken stool; high-fiber foods stimulate peristalsis and should be avoided; spicy foods can also stimulate peristalsis and may need to be avoided.
	Teach patient to monitor response to various foods and to modify diet according to tolerance.	Individual response to foods varies; each patient must assume responsibility for modifying his diet according to tolerance.
High risk for skin integrity (perianal) related to diarrhea	Monitor perianal skin for erythema and denudation.	Perianal skin is subject to breakdown caused by exposure to proteolytic enzymes.
	Cleanse skin after each bowel movement, using water or commercial cleanser and gentle technique (no scrubbing).	Skin must be kept free of stool containing enzymes; gentle cleansing technique must be used to prevent trauma.
	Protect perianal skin with skin sealants or moisture barrier ointments; if skin is denuded, apply pectin-based powder before applying sealants or ointments.	Skin sealants coat the skin with a copolymer film; moisture barrier ointments repel stool; pectin powders absorb moisture and form a protective coating.
	Apply a soft, absorptive dressing between the buttocks.	This absorbs moisture and helps prevent friction.
	Instruct patient to use unscented, white toilet paper and white cotton underwear.	Dyes and fragrances may irritate fragile or damaged skin; cotton underwear absorbs moisture.

See also Postprocedural Nursing Care under Abdominal Surgery, p. 304.

PATIENT TEACHING

1. Explain that takedown of the ileostomy may result in temporary diarrhea and that occasional daytime or nighttime leakage may occur during the adaptation phase.
2. Explain that the number of bowel movements will gradually decrease and that the degree of control over bowel movements will gradually increase; explain the factors that cause this (stretching of the reservoir, with resulting increase in storage capacity; strengthening of the sphincter muscles, which improves voluntary control and the ability to delay defecation; antidiarrheal medications, which slow intes-

tinal activity and help bulk up the stools; and dietary modifications, which help thicken the stool and reduce intestinal peristalsis).

3. Emphasize the things the patient can do to improve sphincter control and reduce diarrhea (sphincter exercises, dietary adjustments based on individual tolerance, and adherence to prescribed medication plan).

4. Explain that the stool contains proteolytic enzymes that can be very destructive to the skin, and emphasize the essential nature of scrupulous skin care (gentle cleansing after each bowel movement; using skin sealants or moisture barrier ointments to protect the skin; using unscented white toilet paper and white cotton underwear to prevent skin irritation; using absorptive pads between the buttocks to absorb moisture and prevent friction; using pectin-based powder for areas of breakdown).

5. Instruct the patient to continue doing sphincter exercises, and check to be sure that he is performing them correctly. Tell the patient to squeeze the pelvic muscles as if trying to prevent a bowel movement and to keep the abdominal and gluteal and quadriceps muscles relaxed; the muscle contraction should be held for about 10 seconds. Tell the patient to do about 45 to 80 of these each day.

6. If the patient has an S-reservoir and requires intubation, instruct him in the correct intubation technique: Insert a lubricated catheter (usually a no. 28 French catheter) through the anus into the reservoir about 3 to 4 inches, and angle the catheter slightly toward the back; allow reservoir contents to drain. (If irrigation is required, instruct the patient to gently instill about 2 ounces of lukewarm tap water through the catheter into the reservoir and then to allow the reservoir contents to drain into the toilet. Irrigation may be repeated to facilitate drainage of thick stool.)

7. Instruct the patient to maintain a daily fluid intake of at least 10 glasses per day and to increase fluid intake during episodes of increased loss (e.g., diarrhea or sweating). Teach the patient the signs and symptoms of fluid and electrolyte imbalance (e.g., dry mouth, thirst, reduced urine output, fatigue and weakness, dizziness when standing), and teach him to report such symptoms to his physician promptly.

8. Explain to the patient that certain medications are contraindicated—time-released medications, enteric coated tablets, and large tablets, because they may be incompletely and unpredictably absorbed; laxatives should be avoided because they may cause severe fluid and electrolyte imbalance. Teach the patient to routinely consult his pharmacist about the best form of medication to take and to notify all prescribing physicians and dentists of the ileal reservoir and removal of the colon. Tell the patient pills should *never* be crushed without the pharmacist's approval.

9. Provide the patient with a MedicAlert application, and stress the importance of MedicAlert identification.

Cholecystectomy/Common Bile Duct Exploration

Cholecystectomy is the surgical removal of the gallbladder; it is most commonly performed for gallstone disease (cholelithiasis), although it may also be indicated for a gallbladder that is infected or nonfunctioning.

Cholecystectomy may be preferred over drug therapy or lithotripsy for treating gallstone disease, because cholecystectomy removes the source of the disease and prevents recurrence. Since the liver continues to produce bile and to deliver the bile to the small intestine,

cholecystectomy has minimal impact on the individual's ability to digest and absorb fats and usually is well tolerated.

Until recently cholecystectomy always required an open abdominal procedure. With this approach the abdomen is opened through a midline or right subcostal incision; the gallbladder, cystic duct, common bile duct, and associated vascular structures are identified and examined. The common bile duct is carefully palpated to determine the presence of stones; in addition, a cholangiogram usually is obtained during surgery to determine the patency of the common duct and whether stones are present. If stones are found, an attempt is made to manipulate them back into the gallbladder. If this cannot be done, the common bile duct is opened and the stones are removed. The common duct is then closed over a T tube that is brought through a stab wound on the abdominal wall; the T tube provides drainage and also stents the common duct to prevent stricture. The gallbladder and the cystic duct are then ligated and removed, a surgical drain is placed through a stab wound into the gallbladder bed, and the abdominal incision is closed. If no stones are found in the common duct or if manipulation is successful in returning them to the gallbladder, the common duct is not explored and no T tube is required.

Endoscopic cholecystectomy recently has been introduced as an alternative to the open abdominal procedure. With this approach four small incisions (about 1 cm in diameter) are made into the abdominal wall; specialized instruments are inserted through these incisions to permit resection and removal of the gallbladder. An ultrasound study is done before surgery to determine whether stones are present in the common bile duct, and a cholangiogram may be obtained during surgery as well. If stones are present, they usually are extracted by the endoscopic approach (either before, in conjunction with, or after the endoscopic cholecystectomy). The initial incision is made just above the umbilicus, and the abdominal cavity is filled with 3 to 4 L of carbon dioxide to improve visibility. The endoscope is then inserted through the supraumbilical incision; the endoscope has a light source that permits visualization of the surgical site, and a microscopic camera that is connected to closed-circuit monitors for magnified visualization. Additional incisions are made for insertion of the surgical instruments; grasping forceps are inserted through incisions along the right anterior axillary line and the right midclavicular line, and a dissection laser (or electrocautery) is inserted through an incision into the midabdominal wall. The grasping forceps are used to stabilize and then remove the gallbladder, and the laser (or electrocautery) is used to free the gallbladder and cystic duct from their attachments. The gallbladder must be completely deflated so that it can be removed through one of the small incisions; intraluminal contents are aspirated as needed before removal.

The endoscopic approach provides many advantages; patients have only minor postoperative pain, require very limited hospitalization (usually 24 hours or less), and can resume moderate activities within 2 to 3 days. However, the endoscopic approach is not always feasible; patients with extensive adhesions, atypical biliary or vascular anatomy, bleeding disorders, peritonitis, or undiagnosed disorders require the open abdominal procedure. Pregnancy is also an absolute contraindication to the endoscopic approach, although the procedure can be safely performed within 3 weeks of a normal delivery. Because adhesions, an unexpected disorder, or excessive bleeding may be encountered during the operation, patients scheduled for the endoscopic approach must also consent to an open procedure if intraoperative findings indicate the need.

INDICATIONS

Acute and chronic cholecystitis
Asymptomatic cholelithiasis in a patient with diabetes or sickle cell disease
Asymptomatic cholelithiasis when stones are larger than 2 cm
Nonfunctioning gallbladder
Calcified gallbladder
Trauma to gallbladder
Cancer of gallbladder
Typhoid carrier with positive bile cultures

CONTRAINDICATIONS

Critically ill patient
Endoscopic procedure contraindicated for:
  Pregnancy
  Acute cholangitis
  Septic peritonitis
  Bleeding disorders
  Extensive adhesions
  Atypical biliary or vascular anatomy
  Undiagnosed abdominal disorder

COMPLICATIONS

Common bile duct injury
Common bile duct stricture
Injury to vascular structures supplying biliary tree
Retained common duct stones
Bile peritonitis (anastomotic breakdown or dislodgment of T tube)
Biliary fistula
Pancreatitis

PREPROCEDURAL NURSING CARE

See Preprocedural Nursing Care under Abdominal Surgery, p. 303.

POSTPROCEDURAL NURSING CARE

NURSING DIAGNOSIS	NURSING INTERVENTIONS	RATIONALE
Altered renal, cerebral, cardiopulmonary, gastrointestinal, and peripheral tissue perfusion related to intraabdominal infection, pancreatitis, or septic shock	Monitor patient for signs and symptoms of peritonitis and sepsis: increasing abdominal tenderness and distention, tachycardia, tachypnea, fever, hypotension, oliguria, or drainage of bile through incision (drainage of bile through surgical drains is expected).	Prompt detection of complications permits early intervention; peritonitis may result from bile leakage into the peritoneal cavity, bacterial contamination of the peritoneal cavity, or pancreatitis.
	Monitor output through surgical drains; for closed-suction catheters, monitor function of suction apparatus to optimize drainage. Collaborate with physician to remove drains as soon as the drainage ceases or becomes scant.	Drains are placed in the gallbladder bed to drain any biliary seepage, which could cause bile peritonitis; the drains are removed when drainage becomes minimal, because the drain can provide an entry port for bacteria.
	If applicable, stabilize T tube on abdominal wall; keep tubing dependent and patent to promote drainage.	Accidental dislodgment of the T tube can lead to biliary leakage and peritonitis; failure to maintain T tube drainage can lead to biliary leakage.
	Use strict aseptic technique when dressing and stabilizing drains and tubes. Administer antibiotics as ordered.	Drains and tubes provide a potential entry port for bacteria. Antibiotics reduce bacterial proliferation and help control infection.
	Administer IV fluids as ordered.	Fluid balance must be maintained to provide adequate tissue perfusion.
	For patient with signs of septic shock; monitor hemodynamic status (e.g., Swan-Ganz or CVP readings, urine output, pulse, BP).	Continual monitoring provides data for treatment modifications.
	If patient fails to respond to above measures, prepare her for surgery.	Emergency surgery may be required for repair of biliary leaks or drainage of intraabdominal abscess.

See also Postprocedural Nursing Care under Abdominal Surgery, p. 304.

PATIENT TEACHING

1. Explain the surgical procedure and its rationale (to remove a diseased or nonfunctioning gallbladder). If the patient is scheduled for the endoscopic procedure, explain that the open abdominal procedure might be required if the initial examination reveals atypical anatomic features or other conditions that make the endoscopic approach inadvisable. Explain that a biliary drainage tube (T tube) may be left in place and connected to a drainage bag for 1 to 2 weeks if the common bile duct requires exploration.

2. Explain that cholecystectomy has minimal impact on digestion and absorption of fats, because the liver will continue to make bile and to deliver it to the small intestine. Explain that a low-fat diet may be better tolerated during the initial postoperative period but that a regular diet may then be resumed.

3. If the patient is to be sent home with a T tube, explain that the T tube is in place to keep the bile duct open during the healing process and to maintain biliary drainage during the healing process. Explain that the T tube will be removed once the bile duct has healed and the swelling has resolved; explain that an x-ray will be done to check for any stones or obstruction in the duct before the tube is removed.

(Tell the patient that the x-ray is done by injecting dye through the tube, and explain that if any stones are found they usually can be removed through an endoscopic approach.) Teach the patient how to stabilize the tube, how to change the dressing around the tube with aseptic technique (if indicated), and how to maintain dependent drainage.

4. Instruct the patient in incisional care (keep incision dry until sutures have been removed) and in recognizing the signs of infection (redness, swelling, tenderness, purulent drainage). Teach the patient to report signs of infection to the physician promptly.

5. Instruct the patient in allowed and restricted activities during the early postoperative period (e.g., if the patient had an open abdominal procedure, lifting and strenuous activity are restricted but walking and general activity are encouraged). Teach the patient to begin abdominal strengthening exercises when the abdominal muscles have healed.

6. Teach the patient what signs and symptoms to report to her physician (fever, increasing abdominal tenderness and swelling, nausea and vomiting, calf and leg pain and swelling, dislodgment of the T tube, and signs of incisional infection).

Partial and Total Pancreatectomy (Pancreaticoduodenectomy; Pancreatectomy)

The pancreas is a complex organ with important endocrine and exocrine functions, and its anatomic location precludes simple removal of the gland itself; for many years it was considered unresectable. Today it is recognized that the pancreas and its contiguous organs can be removed; however, this is a complicated procedure that produces lifelong derangements in endocrine and exocrine function and can result in significant postoperative complications. **Partial and total pancreatectomy** therefore are limited to life-threatening conditions such as malignancies or severe trauma. Occasionally pancreatic resection may be performed for severe chronic pancreatitis; in this condition pancreatic function has already been seriously compromised, and the diseased gland is causing additional problems by obstructing the biliary ducts.

The goals in performing partial or total pancreatectomy include effective removal of the disease process (e.g., en bloc removal of a malignancy), optimum reconstruction of the gastrointestinal tract, and establishment of secure, leak-proof anastomoses. Specific procedures vary with the disease process and its location within the pancreas.

Proximal pancreatectomy (pancreaticoduodenectomy, or the Whipple procedure) may be indicated for cancer or for chronic pancreatitis resulting in obstruction of the common bile duct. Proximal pancreatectomy for removal of malignant lesions should always be preceded by a thorough workup to rule out metastatic disease; metastatic disease contraindicates pancreatic resection.

Proximal pancreaticoduodenectomy involves resection of the distal stomach, duodenum, gallbladder, distal common bile duct, and proximal pancreas. In resecting the proximal pancreas, care is taken to preserve the patency of the pancreatic duct, which facilitates subsequent anastomosis of the duct to the jejunum. Some patients are candidates for a pylorus-saving procedure, in which the duodenum is divided about 2 cm distal to the pylorus; this procedure may be feasible for benign disease or for tumors of the pancreatic head or ampulla that can be effectively resected while preserving the pylorus.

In reconstructing the gastrointestinal tract, the goals are to optimize nutrient digestion and absorption and minimize complications, such as anastomotic breakdown or ulceration of the anastomotic margins (from acidic chyme). Continuity must be reestablished between the bile duct, pancreatic duct, stomach, and jejunum. The proximal jejunal stump is closed, and the pancreas is anastomosed to the jejunum in an end-to-side manner just distal to this closure; a small opening is made between the jejunum and the pancreatic duct to permit drainage of pancreatic secretions into the jejunum. The common bile duct is then anastomosed to the jejunal loop about 10 to 15 cm distal to the pancreaticojejunostomy, and the gastric remnant (or duodenal stump) is anastomosed to the jejunal loop at a point about 40 to 50 cm from the choledochojejunostomy. This anastomotic sequence helps prevent ulceration of the anastomotic margins, because the alkaline pancreatic and biliary secretions drain into the jejunum proximal to the stomach, helping to neutralize the acidic chyme.

A major complication of this approach is leakage at the anastomosis between the pancreatic duct and the jejunum; therefore some surgeons prefer to anastomose the pancreas and pancreatic duct directly to the stomach (or gastric remnant). This anastomosis has a very low leakage rate.

Total pancreatectomy may be required for curative resection of cancers involving the head of the pancreas, and some surgeons recommend total pancreatectomy for all malignancies involving the head of the pancreas.

Total pancreatectomy involves resection of all structures involved in partial pancreatectomy. The difference is that the entire pancreas and the spleen are removed along with regional lymph nodes. Reconstruction involves closure of the jejunal stump with a proximal choledochojejunostomy and a distal gastrojejunostomy (or duodenojejunostomy). Thus continuity between the biliary tree and the proximal and distal gastrointestinal tract is restored, but pancreatic function is lost.

A number of postoperative complications are associated with partial and total pancreatectomy. Common complications during the early postoperative period include anastomotic breakdown with peritonitis, pulmonary complications, fluid shifts resulting in intravascular depletion, thrombophlebitis, and pulmonary emboli. Several drains are placed during surgery to provide proximal decompression of the reconstructed gastrointestinal tract, to prevent stricture of the common bile duct and pancreaticojejunostomy (if applicable), and to minimize leakage of biliary and pancreatic secretions into the abdominal cavity; closed-suction drains are placed near anastomotic lines, a T tube is placed into the common duct, and some type of stent is placed through the pancreaticojejunostomy (with partial pancreatectomy). In addition to the postoperative complications associated with pancreatic resection, long-term morbidity may be associated with partial or total loss of insulin and pancreatic enzyme production.

Liver Transplantation

Liver transplantation is a treatment option for patients with advanced liver disease. The average 1-year survival rate currently is around 75%, and most patients who survive the first year enjoy long-term survival.

Liver transplantation is indicated for treatment of progressive, irreversible liver disease that does not respond to alternative therapy. The most common indication for transplantation in adults is cirrhosis, which is the end result of most progressive liver diseases. The role of transplantation in the treatment of hepatic and biliary cancers remains unclear; recurrence is a common complication in many cases, although some tumors are associated with long-term survival.

A successful transplantation requires extensive coordination among many different professionals in diverse settings; this coordination is facilitated by a national computer system maintained by the United Network of Organ Sharing (UNOS). Patients thought to be candidates for liver transplantation are referred to a transplant center, where a thorough diagnostic evaluation is done. This evaluation is performed to determine the patient's candidacy for transplantation, the acuity of the liver condition, and the urgency for transplantation. Once the patient's acuity and need for transplantation have been determined, the patient's name, ABO type, geographic location, and urgency status are entered into the computer.

Patient and family education and support are major priorities throughout the evaluation and pretransplant periods.

Most donors are trauma victims who are declared brain dead and whose families have consented to organ donation. Successful transplantation requires screening of the donor to ensure viability and functioning of the donated liver and to prevent transmission of potentially fatal diseases. Factors generally considered contraindications to donation include prolonged episodes of hypotension or hypoxia; systemic or intraabdominal infection; cancer (except skin cancer or primary brain cancer); history of chronic liver disease or substance abuse; laboratory evidence of HIV infection, hepatitis B or C, or syphilis; and compromised cardiac, renal, or pulmonary function (while on ventilator support). Another contraindication is administration of large doses of vasopressors to maintain blood pressure (vasopressors may cause liver injury).

When a decision has been made to donate organs and the donor has been determined to be an appropriate candidate for liver donation, information about the donor is entered into the computer; the computer then matches the donor liver to the compatible recipient who has the highest acuity and urgency rating in that region.

Donor hepatectomy begins with a rapid but thorough evaluation of the abdominal cavity to rule out any tumors or other intraabdominal conditions that would preclude donation. The donor liver is mobilized, along with its vascular and biliary attachments; immediately before ligation of the major vessels, the liver is flushed with a cold preservative solution that maintains liver viability for up to 24 hours. The liver is then removed, packed in the preservative solution, and transported on ice to the recipient.

The recipient is readied for transplantation by another surgical team. The recipient's liver is mobilized in preparation for removal. Before ligation of the major vessels and the biliary duct, the patient is placed on venovenous bypass; this preserves cardiac output, prevents mesenteric congestion, and reduces bleeding during removal of the liver and anastomosis of the donor liver. When venous bypass has been established, the recipient's liver is removed, and the donor liver is placed into the abdominal cavity. Anastomoses are then established between all major vessels and between the bile ducts (or between the bile duct and the jejunum). The venovenous bypass is removed when the vascular anastomoses are complete, and the liver is flushed with warm blood. All bleeders are ligated, and clotting is returned to normal by administration of fresh frozen plasma, platelets, and cryoprecipitate. Drains may be placed, and the abdomen is closed; the patient is rewarmed and transferred to intensive care.

Common postoperative complications include hypothermia, bleeding, pulmonary complications, primary nonfunction of the donor liver (usually as a result of preservation injury), hepatic artery or portal vein thrombosis, biliary obstruction or biliary leaks, rejection of the donor liver, and infection. Renal failure may be seen in patients who had compromised renal function before transplantation; this is a serious concern, since the anti-rejection drug cyclosporine can further compromise renal function.

Treatment of complications depends on the causative factors. The two major long-term complications associated with liver transplantation are rejection and infection. To prevent rejection, immunosuppressive drugs are begun immediately following operation and continued on a lifelong basis. The most commonly used drugs are cyclosporine (CyA), azathioprine, and Minnesota antilymphocyte globulin (MALG); specific immunosuppressive regimens vary.

Postoperative infection is prevented by scrupulous technique in managing lines and drains and by prophylactic administration of antibiotics and antifungal agents. If infection occurs, it must be promptly recognized and vigorously treated; immunosuppression may be temporarily reduced until the infection is controlled. Lifelong prevention requires lifestyle modifications by the patient (e.g., avoidance of sick individuals, frequent dental and medical examinations, and monitoring for signs and symptoms of infection). Thus patient and family education is an essential component of posttransplant care.

CHAPTER 10

Patient Teaching Guides

Patient teaching has always been an important part of the nursing process. Nurses caring for patients with gastrointestinal disorders are responsible for teaching these patients how to prevent gastrointestinal problems by choosing healthy foods and adopting habits that promote general good health. These nurses also teach patients how to detect early signs of a gastrointestinal problem and show them ways to manage diet and lifestyle when the gastrointestinal system is impaired. Gastrointestinal nurses instruct patients who have undergone bowel surgery, such as ileostomy or colostomy, to manage their bowel functions on a day-to-day basis. Patients learn how to change their stoma pouches and how to care for their stoma and skin. Because these functions usually are taken care of in private, the nurse's responsibilities are not only to educate these patients on how to manage their disorders, but also to protect patients' privacy and to provide them with the tools to maintain their dignity. Teaching patients to cope with life after bowel surgery is an important part of the gastrointestinal nurse's responsibilities.

Written teaching guides can help reinforce patient teaching and encourage compliance. This chapter provides written handouts that can be photocopied and given to patients or their caregivers to take home and use for self-care. The handouts list step-by-step instructions for certain procedures. More than one guide may be needed for a particular patient.

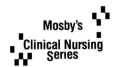

Constipation

Constipation is a term for difficulty in eliminating stool; it usually is associated with hard, dry stools.

Should everyone have a bowel movement daily?

The frequency of bowel movements varies greatly. It is not necessary to have a bowel movement every day; some healthy people have bowel movements every 2 or 3 days, whereas others may move their bowels twice or more a day. Bowel movements are considered normal as long as the stool is soft and easily eliminated.

What causes constipation?

Constipation may result from a number of conditions, but the most common causes are constipating diets, constipating medications, poor bowel habits, and inactivity. Constipating diets are low in fiber, or roughage; lack of fiber contributes to hard, dry stools that are difficult to pass. Inactivity and pain medications contribute to constipation, because they slow the bowel down and result in delayed passage of hard stools.

Poor bowel habits involve failure to respond to the urge to have a bowel movement; delay causes increased absorption of water from the stool, which makes the stool harder to eliminate. Painful anorectal conditions such as hemorrhoids also result in constipation by causing the person to delay bowel movements.

What are the complications of constipation?

Prolonged constipation can result in impaction, or being unable to empty the rectum. This may be accompanied by paradoxical diarrhea, in which watery stool is passed *around* the mass of hard stool. Impaction requires medical treatment.

How is constipation treated?

Treatment of constipation depends on its cause. Any painful condition, such as hemorrhoids, must be relieved. A diet containing plenty of fiber should be followed, and breakfast should be a meal of adequate bulk. Fiber can be found in cereal bran, the skins of fruits and potatoes, whole grain breads, and vegetables such as beans, peas, celery, and broccoli. Fiber, or roughage, is important to your diet because it provides the bulk your large intestine needs to carry away body wastes.

If you are unable to eat enough high-fiber foods, you may need a bulk laxative or a bran mixture. Bulk laxatives are available in powder form, capsule form, and wafer form; the dose must be individualized according to your response (the goal is to create soft stools that are easily eliminated). A suitable bran mixture is made from 1 cup of miller's bran, 1 cup of applesauce, and ¼ cup of prune juice. You should take 1 to 2 tablespoons of this mixture daily; you may increase the dose if needed to create soft stools.

It is essential that you get adequate fluids when adding bulk to your diet; you should drink at least 8 to 10 8-oz. glasses of fluid a day. This prevents clumping of the bulk laxative and helps keep your stools soft.

You should also increase your activity as much as possible; a simple walking program is very effective in stimulating normal intestinal activity. Another very important step in preventing constipation is to establish regular bowel habits and to respond promptly to the urge to defecate.

A common approach to constipation is routine use of stimulant laxatives or enemas; this is not recommended, because chronic use of stimulants creates bowel dependency, a state of reduced intestinal activity.

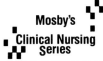
Peptic Ulcer

Peptic ulcer is a general term that refers to ulcers occurring in the lower esophagus, the stomach, or the duodenum (upper part of the small intestine).

What is the difference between a duodenal ulcer and a gastric ulcer?

A duodenal ulcer is a break in the lining of the upper part of the small intestine (the duodenum); a gastric ulcer is a break in the lining of the stomach.

What causes duodenal and gastric ulcers?

Duodenal ulcers are much more common than gastric ulcers. The primary cause of duodenal ulcers is increased production of acid by the stomach; factors that may contribute to this include cigarette smoking, excessive alcohol intake, chronic emotional stress, and certain drugs (aspirin, antiinflammatory drugs, and corticosteroids). Gastric ulcers, on the other hand, are thought to be caused by changes in the stomach lining that make it more susceptible to damage by the acid normally produced by the stomach. The stomach lining may be damaged by chronic gastritis, reflux of bile, and the same drugs that cause increased acid production.

What are the symptoms of ulcers?

Duodenal ulcers are characterized by pain that occurs when the stomach is empty and is relieved by eating; the pain usually is in the midabdominal area. Vomiting may occur but is uncommon. Some people have mild diarrhea with black stools (black stools indicate the presence of blood).

Symptoms of a gastric ulcer include pain, a feeling of fullness, nausea, and vomiting. The pain is not necessarily relieved by eating; in fact, it may become worse after eating. The pain is located in the upper abdomen, either in the middle or to the left.

If vomiting occurs, the vomit may be streaked with blood. Later symptoms include fatigue and weight loss.

Attacks of pain caused by an ulcer are subject to remission, and the pain may be absent for some weeks or months (this is particularly true of duodenal ulcers). Pain seems to depend on inflammation of the ulcer and not merely on its presence.

What are the possible complications?

Chronic slow bleeding can cause your stools to look dark ("tarry"); over time, slow bleeding can cause anemia and fatigue. Sudden major bleeding can cause you to vomit large amounts of blood or to pass bloody stools. Major bleeding requires prompt treatment. (Major bleeding is more likely to occur in a patient who has had ulcer symptoms for a long time.)

Other, uncommon complications that may occur include perforation and obstruction. Perforation means that the ulcer erodes through the wall of the stomach or the duodenum; this creates a hole that allows stomach or intestinal contents to leak into the abdominal cavity. Perforation causes severe abdominal pain and necessitates immediate treatment. Obstruction occurs when there is scarring or swelling that blocks passage of food and digestive juices from the stomach into the small intestine. This causes persistent vomiting, and medical treatment is required to relieve the obstruction.

How are ulcers treated and managed?

Many peptic ulcers heal spontaneously, but medical treatment usually is required, involving (1) learning ways to reduce stress or improve your ability to manage stressful situations; (2) eliminating foods and beverages that cause pain or delay healing (spicy foods may cause pain; alcohol and caffeine increase acid production and cause further tissue damage; small, frequent meals usually help neutralize acid and reduce pain); (3) avoiding aspirin, antiinflammatory medications, and corticosteroids; and (4) using antacids (to neutralize acid) and "antiulcer" drugs such as Tagamet or Zantac (to reduce the amount of acid produced and promote healing).

Because the symptoms sometimes disappear before the ulcer has completely healed, some ulcer patients give up before the course of treatment has been completed. It is essential to follow your doctor's instructions to the letter if medical treatment is to succeed.

Malignant changes sometimes occur in gastric ulcers, but these changes can only be diagnosed through specific tests. Thus it is foolish to try to cure ulcers by yourself or to ignore ulcer symptoms in the hope that the condition will get better by itself. It is important to obtain medical evaluation and advice in treating ulcer symptoms.

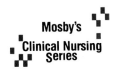
Irritable Bowel Syndrome

Irritable bowel syndrome is a condition encompassing a number of symptoms, rather than a specific disease. The symptoms include abdominal pain, increased gas, and altered patterns of bowel elimination (i.e., diarrhea, constipation, or both). Irritable bowel syndrome is not the same as inflammatory bowel disease or ulcerative colitis; the bowel is not inflamed or ulcerated, and there is no obvious disease process. In irritable bowel syndrome, the bowel seems to respond to certain stimuli (such as stress) with abnormal muscular contractions. It is important to realize that many people react to stress with some change in bowel habits; only when this becomes extreme is the individual considered to have irritable bowel syndrome.

What causes irritable bowel syndrome?

The anatomic cause of irritable bowel syndrome is unknown. However, a common theory is that patients with this condition respond to environmental stress and dietary irritants with abnormal muscle contractions in the large and small bowel. Another theory is that individuals with the disorder are more sensitive to intestinal "stretching" and more likely to feel this normal stretching as abdominal pain.

What are the symptoms?

Symptoms vary in pattern and intensity. The most common symptoms are abdominal pain, excessive gas, and altered bowel patterns (constipation, diarrhea, or both). Some individuals also have heartburn, nausea, and belching. Abdominal pain is more common during episodes of constipation; the diarrhea that occurs with irritable bowel syndrome usually is associated with fecal urgency but not pain. Diarrhea is most common after breakfast and does not occur during sleep. You may notice that certain foods such as fresh fruits and vegetables, coffee, and alcohol aggravate the diarrhea. The symptoms of irritable bowel syndrome may be worse when you are tense, anxious, or upset. Also, the disorder commonly is episodic, meaning that it comes and goes.

Irritable bowel syndrome sometimes appears after an episode of gastroenteritis (inflammation of the digestive tract), but usually its onset is gradual. Symptoms usually start before the age of 30, and teenagers may be affected. Although the discomfort can be severe, irritable bowel syndrome is not related to other chronic or life-threatening conditions and does not cause complications that reduce life expectancy.

How is irritable bowel syndrome managed?

Treatment is individualized according to the symptoms. A high-fiber diet commonly is prescribed for patients with constipation. Patients with diarrhea may be placed on a low-residue diet and given antidiarrheal medications. Patients with alternating constipation and diarrhea may benefit from bulking agents (such as a bulk laxative) to normalize stool consistency. Any foods found to trigger symptoms should be eliminated from the diet. Stress management techniques help most patients, and some patients benefit from psychiatric counseling. Antidepressants sometimes are prescribed and have proven beneficial in some cases. Cigarette smoking and alcohol intake generally should be reduced or discontinued.

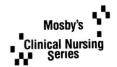
Mosby's
Clinical Nursing
Series

Living with Inflammatory Bowel Disease

Because the symptoms and complications of Crohn's disease and ulcerative colitis are similar, the two are often referred to as *inflammatory bowel disease*. Both diseases are characterized by inflammation of the wall of the intestine. The inflammation is a result of damage to tissues that causes them to become red, painful, and swollen. Inflamed tissue may leak fluid containing blood cells, and ulcers may form.

What causes inflammatory bowel disease?

The causes of inflammatory bowel disease are not known, but there are several theories. Crohn's disease and ulcerative colitis tend to be familial, with studies showing that 15% to 20% of patients may have a close relative with one of the diseases. However, researchers have not yet been able to find specific genes that carry these diseases. Therefore, inflammatory bowel disease is not considered genetic.

Inflammatory bowel disease involves inappropriate or prolonged activation of the body's normal defense system. While it is not clear exactly what causes inflammation, it is known that inflammatory bowel disease involves a persistent inflammation of the bowel wall.

It is true that stress can influence the course of Crohn's disease, ulcerative colitis, or any other illness. However, researchers do not believe that these diseases are caused by emotional stress. Acute emotional problems occasionally precede the onset or recurrence of inflammatory bowel disease; however, this sequence does not imply a cause-and-effect relationship.

What are the symptoms and complications?

Nausea, diarrhea, pain, weight loss, and cramping are common signs of inflammatory bowel disease. The earliest symptoms of Crohn's disease are usually abdominal pain and diarrhea; the pain is often felt in the area of the navel or on the right side and often occurs following a meal. In addition to the intestinal problems, the patient may experience joint pains, fever, and a variety of sores in the anal area; these sores include skin tags that mimic hemorrhoids, fissures (cracks in the skin), fistulas (abnormal openings from bowel to skin surface near the anus), and abscesses around the anus and rectum. The most common complication of Crohn's disease is partial bowel obstruction.

The first symptoms of ulcerative colitis are progressive diarrhea (which is usually bloody), cramping abdominal pain, and severe urgency to move the bowels. Symptoms may develop slowly or may begin suddenly. Joint pains and skin lesions may occur. In addition, a small percentage of patients suffer from iritis, which is a painful inflammation of the eye. Complications of ulcerative colitis include profuse bleeding and perforation of the colon, which is uncommon.

How is inflammatory bowel disease treated?

Treatment of inflammatory bowel disease might include medication, changes in diet, and, if necessary, feeding by intravenous fluids. Sometimes surgery may be necessary to remove diseased bowel or to treat complications. Once your disease has been diagnosed, you and your doctor will discuss treatment. You and your doctor will work as a team to decide what is needed for your particular disease.

What are the suggested management guidelines for inflammatory bowel disease?

With proper treatment and diet and stress management, you will be less likely to develop serious complications. Along with proper medical treatment, improved nutrition can reduce your symptoms and help an inflamed bowel to heal. While there is no single diet for inflammatory bowel disease, certain suggestions may help. A low-residue diet may help you feel better and have fewer symptoms during periods when the disease is active. Examples of high-residue foods are raw or dried fruits, raw vegetables, nuts and seeds, bran, and whole grains; these are foods you may need to avoid during periods of active disease.

You might also avoid foods that seem to cause problems in your own system. For example, some people cannot properly digest milk sugar (lactose) and either do not drink milk or drink only small amounts of it. Your doctor and a dietician may work with you to determine an appropriate diet for you during periods of active disease.

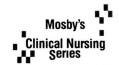

Ileostomy

An ileostomy is a surgical procedure in which an opening, or stoma, is created by bringing the ileum (the last part of the small intestine) through the abdominal wall. The stoma provides an opening for eliminating stool.

What will my stoma look like?

Your stoma should be bright red, the normal color of the inside of the bowel. Because your stoma will have no sensory nerve endings, it will not be sensitive to touch and it will not be painful. Immediately after surgery, your stoma will look swollen. This swelling probably will be gone after 8 weeks, but your stoma may continue to change size and shape during the first year, while further healing occurs.

How do I take care of my stoma?

You will not be able to control when your bowels move, so you will always wear an odor-proof, drainable pouch to collect the stool and protect your skin. Your ileostomy will drain at unpredictable intervals during the day, and the stool will be a thick liquid or mushy consistency. (Right after surgery it is normal to have a lot of very watery stool.)

How do I empty the pouch?

You should empty your pouch when it is about one-third to one-half full of gas and stool. (If the pouch gets too full, the weight may cause it to pull away from your skin.) To empty the pouch:

- Sit on the commode. Remove the clip or rubber band from the bottom of the pouch, and turn the bottom of the pouch back on itself to form a cuff. (This helps keep the end of the pouch clean.)
- Drain the stool into the commode. You may rinse the pouch with cool water (use a small squirt bottle) *if you wish.*
- Clean the bottom of the pouch with toilet paper, a damp paper towel, or a baby wipe. It is *very important* to clean the bottom of the pouch to prevent odor.
- Uncuff the pouch, attach the clip or rubber band.

How do I change the pouch and care for my skin?

Pouches are designed to stick to the skin for about 5 to 7 days; your pouch may stay on a little longer or may have to be changed a little more often. The important thing is to change your pouch on a routine basis to prevent accidental leakage. Also, you should change your pouch *anytime* your skin begins to burn or you notice stool leaking onto your skin; this is *very important,* because the stool from your ileostomy contains digestive enzymes that can cause serious skin damage.

Follow these steps (or the directions of your ostomy nurse) in changing your pouch:

- Gently remove the old pouch by pushing down on your skin while pulling up on the pouch.
- Clean your skin with warm water. Check for any reddened or irritated areas. If you have skin irritation, you should notify your ostomy nurse or doctor. To treat the irritation, you may sprinkle on a little Stomahesive or Premium powder and then blot the powder with a wet finger to make it gummy. **Note:** If the skin around your stoma is hairy, it is best to remove it with a safety razor or an electric razor; always shave away from the stoma.
- Check the size of your stoma; make sure your pouch is sized to fit right around the base of your stoma.
- Apply a skin barrier paste or protective wipe to the skin around your stoma (if instructed to do this by your ostomy nurse).
- Center your pouch around the stoma, and press securely into place.

How will an ileostomy affect my diet?

You eventually will be able to return to *most* of your normal dietary habits. After you recover from surgery, you may be kept on a low-residue diet for 6 to 8 weeks to allow your small bowel to adjust and heal. You may then begin to resume your regular diet.

You will need to make some dietary adjustments to prevent food blockage and to minimize gas. Food blockage can occur if you eat large amounts of undigestible foods, especially if you do not chew these foods well. The undigestible fiber clumps together and becomes stuck at a narrow place in your small bowel. The blockage may be partial or complete.

A partial blockage causes cramping and watery diarrhea, and your stoma and abdomen may become swollen. If you have a *partial* blockage, you should (1) stop eating solids; continue to drink liquids as long as you are not vomiting; (2) try sitting in a warm tub to relax your muscles; (3) try massaging around your stoma to try to push the blockage out; (4) change your pouch if your stoma is swollen. If you do not get relief, or you start feeling dehydrated (weak, thirsty, dizzy), call your doctor or ostomy nurse.

A complete blockage causes the following symptoms: *No output* from your stoma; abdominal cramping and swelling; nausea and vomiting. If you have a *complete* blockage, you should (1) stop eating and drinking; (2) try sitting in a warm tub and relax your abdominal muscles; (3) try massaging around your stoma to push the blockage out; (4) change your pouch if your stoma is swollen.

If you do not get relief within 1 to 2 hours, call your doctor or ostomy nurse.

Obviously it is much better to prevent a food blockage than to manage one. Here are some guidelines:

- Avoid high-fiber foods until the swelling in your stoma has gone (about 6 weeks after surgery).
- Add high-fiber foods one at a time and in small amounts.
- *Chew all foods thoroughly* and drink plenty of fluids.

What can I do to reduce gas?

Controlling gas is a common concern for people with an ostomy. You will have less gas with an ileostomy than you did when your colon was intact. Gas from an ileostomy may be caused by swallowed air or by certain foods (because of bacterial action). You can reduce swallowed air by limiting the use of straws and limiting smoking and gum chewing.

Foods likely to cause gas include beans, the cabbage family, and beer. Notice which foods cause you to have more gas; you may wish to limit these foods or to eat them when you will not be out in public.

What about fluids and dehydration?

You lose more fluid every day from your ileostomy than you did when your colon was intact. You can make up this loss by increasing your fluid intake by 1 to 2 8-oz. glasses a day. However, the increased loss of fluid means you are more likely to get dehydrated if you sweat excessively or if you have diarrhea or vomiting. Symptoms of dehydration include weakness, dizziness, dry mouth, ex-

treme thirst, dark urine, reduced urine output, abdominal cramping, and shortness of breath; these symptoms must be reported to your physician immediately.

To help prevent dehydration, follow these rules:
- Drink extra fluids every day (10-12 glasses).
- During episodes of increased sweating or diarrhea:
  - Drink an extra glass of fluid each time you empty your pouch;
  - Be sure to drink fluids and eat foods that replace sodium and potassium as well as water (e.g., sports drinks, broth, vegetable and fruit juices, tea, crackers).
- Notify your doctor immediately if you have symptoms of dehydration or if you have vomiting that persists longer than 4 hours.
- During periods of diarrhea, follow a bland, constipating diet (e.g., bananas, applesauce, smooth peanut butter).

How will the ileostomy affect my medicines?

Notify your pharmacist and any other doctor you see (including your dentist) that you have an ileostomy. Because medicine may pass through your bowel in as little as 2 hours, you may need to alter the types of medicines you take. Remember, *never* take laxatives; they can cause severe diarrhea, cramping, and dehydration. Carry a Medic Alert card, stating that you have an ileostomy and listing the drugs you do not take. **Note:** *Always* check with your pharmacist before crushing any large or coated pills; this is almost always the *wrong* thing to do, because you could cause stomach damage or could make the drug inactive.

Will an ileostomy affect my daily activities?

The only limits imposed by your ileostomy involve contact sports, which could injure the stoma. Even though you will have to adjust your lifestyle, you can manage your recovery and minimize the effect this change will have on your life. One of the first steps is to resume your daily activities. Concerns or fears about your social and sexual relationships are normal, although most people can resume these activities and find their friends and loved ones very supportive. Remember that you are still the same person you were before the surgery. Concerns should be discussed with your doctor or nurse, and with your partner.

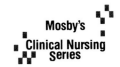
Colostomy

A colostomy is a surgical procedure that creates an opening, or stoma, between the colon (large intestine or bowel) and the abdominal wall to provide an alternative route for elimination of stool from the body. A colostomy is performed when a portion of the large bowel, including the colon, rectum, or anus, is diseased and must be bypassed or removed.

Colostomies are most commonly located in the transverse colon or in the descending or sigmoid colon. Since the stool is changed from liquid to solid during its passage through the colon, transverse colostomies drain mushy stool, whereas descending or sigmoid colostomies drain more solid stool.

There are three types of colostomies: end stoma, double-barrel stoma, or loop stoma.

In an end stoma, the bowel is divided into two sections; the distal (lower) section is removed or sewn shut, and the proximal (upper) section is brought out to the abdominal wall as a stoma.

In a double-barrel stoma, the bowel is divided, and both ends of the bowel are brought out to the abdominal wall as stomas; stool drains from the upper stoma and mucus drains from the lower stoma.

In a loop colostomy, the bowel is not divided; instead, an opening is made in the abdominal wall, and the loop of the bowel is brought to the abdominal surface and held in place with a support device until the bowel heals to the skin. An opening is made into the front wall of the bowel to allow stool to pass out of the body. A loop colostomy usually is intended to be temporary.

When is a colostomy needed?

Colostomy surgery is performed on thousands of people in the United States each year, most commonly for diverticulitis, tumors, injuries, or birth defects.

Your stoma is formed by turning the colon back on itself and suturing the edges of the colon to the skin. Your stoma should appear moist and bright red; the red, healthy color shows that its blood supply is adequate. Because the blood vessels in your stoma are superficial, you may sometimes find blood on the cloth when you clean the stoma. This slight bleeding is similar to that which occurs when

you brush your teeth, and clears up just as fast. Because there are no sensory nerve endings in your stoma, you will have no feeling in it. Stomas usually are round but can be irregularly shaped. Loop colostomy stomas tend to be oval and larger than end stomas. Because the stoma has no sphincter muscle, you will not be able to control the passage of stool.

How do I care for the stoma?

The drainage from your stoma can irritate your skin; to prevent this, you must always wear a properly fitting pouch, which collects the stool from your colostomy, and change the pouch as necessary. If irrigation is part of your regimen, you will change the pouch when you irrigate.

Many kinds of pouches are available; your ostomy nurse will help you select the best one for you. As you recover from surgery and progress in daily activities, changes in your abdomen and other factors may necessitate a change in the type of pouch you use.

How do I empty the pouch?

A drainable pouch should be emptied whenever it is about one-third full of stool, or when it is full of gas. Sit on the toilet, and empty the pouch between your legs. When convenient, you can rinse your pouch with cool water. (Most people find it helpful to "cuff" the end of the pouch [turning the end of the pouch back on itself] before draining the stool; this keeps the end of the pouch clean.)

How do I change the pouch?

When changing the pouch, you should first assemble all items: a new pouch and skin barrier, pouch closure (rubber band or clip), paste (if needed), and equipment for disposing of used pouches. The skin is best cleansed with plain water; soap leaves a residue that may irritate the skin.

Follow the steps below in changing your pouch and caring for the skin around the stoma:

- Gently remove the soiled pouch by pressing down on the skin while pulling up on the pouch. Discard the soiled pouch in a plastic bag (save the pouch closure).
- Gently clean the skin and stoma with warm water, using a soft washcloth or a paper towel.
- If the area is hairy, remove hair with an electric razor or safety razor. Always shave from

the stoma out to prevent injury. (If you use a safety razor, use shaving cream and rinse the skin thoroughly.)

- Check the size of the pouch opening to be sure it fits around your stoma without leaving skin exposed.
- Apply paste around your stoma if needed. Then center the pouch, press it into place, and attach the clip or rubber band.

If your skin becomes red or irritated, notify your ostomy nurse or doctor. You may try a light application of pectin-based powder (e.g., Stomahesive) to any raw areas to provide protection and improve pouch adhesion.

How do I perform irrigation?

If you have a descending or sigmoid colostomy, you may be taught the irrigation procedure. This procedure is like an enema; it stimulates the bowel to move. Irrigation is done every day at the same time, because this regulates the colon to move once a day at a time that is convenient for you. It often takes weeks or months for the bowel to become regulated, and medication or postsurgical treatment often affects the bowel's usual habits. Your ostomy nurse can help you work out an appropriate schedule and solve any problems you may have.

What dietary guidelines should I follow?

There is no special diet for a person who has a colostomy. Your ability to digest and absorb nutrients has not changed, and there are no forbidden foods. However, you may want to modify your diet somewhat to reduce gas, since you will not be able to control the passage of gas.

Food will affect you the same way it did before your surgery. However, you may notice that certain foods make your stool looser or thicker. For example, some foods have a laxative effect on stool. This may be a concern if you are trying to regulate your colostomy with irrigations. Other foods may cause constipation. By experimenting you will find out what foods you can eat with confidence and what foods you may need to limit or avoid. Your doctor, ostomy nurse, or hospital dietitian will give you guidelines for setting up your diet.

How long does it take to adjust to a colostomy?

A colostomy is a major adjustment, and it is normal to feel sad, angry, frustrated, or depressed. Be honest about your feelings, and share them with loved ones if you feel comfortable doing so. If you deal honestly with your feelings, the sadness and anger will lessen and you will be able to adjust to life with a colostomy. You may find support groups helpful, and your ostomy nurse will also be available to talk with you.

Even though you will have to adjust your lifestyle, you can manage your recovery and minimize the effect this change will have on your life. The first step to successful recovery is to resume your normal activities. It is important to get back into the mainstream. Exercising and returning to work will help facilitate this process.

How is sexuality affected?

Concerns about intimacy are legitimate and should be discussed openly with your partner. Remember that you are the same person you were before the surgery, and you have the same capabilities to feel, love, and respond to others as you did before. The effect of this type of surgery on sexual function varies with each individual. Discuss any problems you may have with your doctor or ostomy nurse.

References

1. American Cancer Society: *Proceedings from national conference on colorectal cancer*, Atlanta, 1991, The Society.
2. Anderson B: Tube feedings: Is diarrhea inevitable? *AJON* 86(6):704-706, 1986.
3. Beck D, Welling D, editors: *Patient care in colorectal surgery*, Boston, 1991, Little, Brown, & Co.
4. Becker J: Questions and answers about strictureplasty vs. resection in Crohn's disease, *Foundation Focus* July 1991, pp. 10-11, Crohn's and Colitis Foundation of America.
5. Belcher A: *Cancer nursing*, St. Louis, 1992, Mosby–Year Book.
6. Block G, Nolan J: *Health assessment for professional nursing: a developmental approach*, ed 2, East Norwalk, CN, 1986, Appleton-Century-Crofts.
7. Bockus S: Troubleshooting your tube feedings, *AJON* 91(5):24-31.
7a. Brundage DJ, *Renal disorders*, St. Louis, 1992, Mosby–Year Book.
8. Bryant R, editor: *Acute and chronic wounds: nursing management*, St. Louis, 1992, Mosby–Year Book.
9. Bryant R: Diverticular disease, *J Ent Ther* 13(3):114-117, 1986.
10. Coellen D: Understanding diverticular disease, *J Ent Ther* 16(4):176-180, 1989.
11. Curtas S, Chapman G, and Meguid M: Evaluation of nutritional status, *Nurs Clin North Am* 24(2):301-311, 1989.
12. Doughty D: A step-by-step approach to bowel training, *Prog* 4(2):12-23, 1992.
13. Doughty D, editor: *Urinary and fecal incontinence: nursing management*, St. Louis, 1991, Mosby–Year Book.
14. Dudrick S, Latifi R, and Fosnocht D: Management of the short-bowel syndrome, *Curr Strat Surg Nurt* 7(3):625-642, 1991.
15. *Enteral nutrition ready reference*, Columbus, OH, 1992, Ross Laboratories.
16. Fazio V, editor: *Current therapy in colon and rectal surgery*, Philadelphia, 1990, BC Decker.
17. Fifield M: Relieving constipation and pain in the terminally ill, *AJON* 91(7):18-19, 1991.
18. Finne C: Advances in colorectal cancer, *J ET Nurs* 18(3):82-89, 1991.
19. Ganong WF: *Review of medical physiology*, ed 11, Los Altos, CA, 1983, Lange Medical Publications.
20. Gauwitz D: Endoscopic cholecystectomy: the patient-friendly alternative, *Nursing90* 20(12):58-59, 1990.
21. Ginsberg A: Newer medical therapies for inflammatory bowel disease, *Contemp Intern Med* October 1990:27-40, 1990.
22. Given B, Simmons S: *Gastroenterology in clinical nursing*, ed 4, St. Louis, 1984, Mosby–Year Book.
23. Grau P: Are you at risk for hepatitis B? *Nursing91* 21(3):44-45, 1991.
24. Greenberger N: *Gastrointestinal disorders: a pathophysiologic approach*, ed 4, Chicago, 1989, Year Book Medical Publishers.
25. Grimes J, Burns E: *Health assessment in nursing practice*, ed 2, Boston, 1987, Jones and Bartlett.
26. Guyton AC: *Testbook of medical physiology*, ed 6, Philadelphia, 1981, WB Saunders.
27. Hampton B, Bryant R, editors: *Ostomies and continent diversions: nursing management*, St. Louis, 1992, Mosby–Year Book.
28. Holmes K, Notarangelo P: Pseudomembranous colitis, *J Ent Ther* 14(3):190-112, 1987.
29. Kaminski M, Pinchcofsky-Devin G, Williams S: Nutritional management of decubitus ulcers in the elderly, *Decubitus* 2(4):20-30, 1989.
30. Konigsberg A: Keeping up with viral hepatitis, *Phys Assis* 16(7):25-36, 1992.
31. Kyba F, Ogburn-Russell L, Rutledge J: Magnetic resonance imaging: the latest in diagnostic technology, *Nursing87* 17(1):44-47, 1987.
32. Lancaster-Smith M, Chapman C: *Gastroenterology*, Littleton, MA, 1985, PSG Publishing.
33. Malasanos L, Barkauskas V, Stoltenberg-Allen K: *Health assessment*, ed 4, St. Louis, 1990, Mosby–Year Book.
34. Mash N, et al: *Standards of care: patient with colostomy*, Irvine, CA, 1989, International Association for Enterostomal Therapy.
35. Mash N, et al: *Standards of care: patient with ileostomy*, Irvine, CA, 1990, International Association for Enterostomal Therapy.
36. McCance K, Huether S, editors: *Pathophysiology: the biologic basis for disease in adults and children*, St. Louis, 1990, Mosby–Year Book.
37. McConnell E, Lawler M: Preventing postop complications: parts 1 and 2, *Nursing91* 21(11):33-48.
38. McDonagh A: Getting your patient ready for a nuclear medicine scan, *Nursing91* 21(2):53-57, 1991.
39. Mehl B: Pharmacology focus: overview of 5-ASA medications, *Foundation Focus* July 1991: 9, Crohn's and Colitis Foundation of America.
40. Meize-Grochowski A: When the Dx is Crohn's disease, *RN*, February 1991: 52-55.
41. Mudge-Grout CL: *Immunologic disorders*, St. Louis, 1993, Mosby–Year Book.
42. Murray N, Vanderhoof J: Short bowel syndrome in children and adults, *J Ent Ther* 14(4):168-173, 1987.
43. Ogorek C, Fisher R: Current drug therapy for inflammatory bowel disease, *Compr Ther* 17(4):31-37, 1991.
44. Olson E, Johnson BJ, Thompson L: The hazards of immobility, *AJON* 90(3):43-48, 1990.
45. Plankey E, Knauf J: What patients need to know about magnetic resonance imaging, *AJON* 90(1):27-28, 1990.
46. Preece P, Cuschier A, Wellwood J: *Cancer of the stomach*, Orlando, 1986, Grune and Stratton.
47. Romano J, Jennings T: Challenges in IBD research: inflammatory mediators, *Foundation Focus* July 1991: 13, Crohn's and Colitis Foundation of America.
48. Rowland M: Myths and facts about postop discomfort, *AJON* 90(5):60-64, 1990.
49. Rubin M: The physiology of bed rest, *AJON* 88(1):50-58, 1988.
50. Rudy E and Gray V: *Handbook of health assessment*, East Norwalk, CN, 1991, Appleton and Lange.
51. Schwartz S, Ellis H, editors: *Maingot's Abdominal Operations*, vols 1&2, ed 9, East Norwalk, CN, 1989, Appleton and Lange.
52. Seidel H, et al: *Mosby's guide to physical examination*, ed 2, St. Louis, 1991, Mosby–Year Book.
53. Seeley R, Stephens T, Tate P: *Anatomy and physiology*, St. Louis, 1989, Mosby–Year Book.
54. Sheets L: Liver transplantation, *Nurs Clin North Am* 24(4):881-889, 1989.
55. Smith A: When the pancreas self-destructs, *AJON* 91(9):38-48, 1991.
56. Thelan L, Davie J, Urden L: *Textbook of critical care nursing*, St. Louis, 1990, Mosby–Year Book.
57. Thompson J, et al, editors: *Mosby's manual of clinical nursing*, ed 2, St. Louis, 1989, Mosby–Year Book.
58. Thomson A, DaCosta L, Watson W, editors: *Modern concepts in gastroenterology*, vol 1, New York, 1986, Plenum Medical Book Co.
59. Walsh S, Banks L: How to insert a small-bore feeding tube safely, *Nursing90* 20(3):55-59, 1990.
60. Wardell T: Assessing and managing a gastric ulcer, *Nursing91* 21(3):34-42, 1991.
61. Whiteman K, et al: Liver transplantation, *AJON* 90(6):68-72, 1990.
62. Zuidema G, Condon R, editors: *Shackelford's surgery of the alimentary tract*, vols 1-5, ed 3, Philadelphia, 1991, WB Saunders.

Index

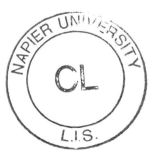

STAGING SYSTEMS FOR COLORECTAL CANCER

American Joint Committee on Cancer				Dukes' Classification
Stage 0	T_{is}	N_0	M_0	
Stage I	T_1	N_0	M_0	Dukes' A
	T_2	N_0	M_0	
Stage II	T_3	N_0	M_0	Dukes' B
	T_4	N_0	M_0	
Stage III	Any T	N_1	M_0	Dukes' C
	Any T	N_2, N_3	M_0	
Stage IV	Any T	AnyN	M_1	Dukes' D

T_{is}, Carcinoma in situ; T_1, tumor invading submucosal layer of bowel; T_2, tumor invading muscularis layer of bowel; T_3, tumor invading subserosal layer of colon or extending into nonperitonealized pericolic or perirectal tissues; T_4, tumor extending through visceral peritoneum or directly invading other organs or structures; N_0, no lymph node metastasis; N_1, metastasis involving one to three pericolic or perirectal lymph nodes; N_2, metastasis involving four or more pericolic or perirectal lymph nodes; N_3, metastasis to any lymph node along a named vascular trunk; M_0, no distant metastasis, M_1, distant metastasis.